Men's Fitness magazine

TOTAL TRAINING GUIDE

by Joe Warner

Art Editor Fanni Williams
Additional design Jo Gurney, Marc Southey
Chief Sub Editor Jo Williams
Sub Editor Chris Miller
Art Director Donovan Walker
Photography Tom Miles, Shutterstock
Model Sean Lerwill@WAthletic
Illustrations Sudden Impact
With thanks to Ultimate Performance (upfitness.co.uk)

MAGBOOK

Group Publisher **Russell Blackman**
Group Managing Director **Ian Westwood**
International Business Development Director **Dharmesh Mistry**
Digital Production Manager **Nicky Baker**
Operations Director **Robin Ryan**
Managing Director of Advertising **Julian Lloyd-Evans**
Newstrade Director **David Barker**
Commercial & Retail Director **Martin Belson**
Chief Operating Officer/ Chief Financial Officer **Brett Reynolds**
Group Finance Director **Ian Leggett**
Chief Executive Officer **James Tye**
Chairman **Felix Dennis**

TOTAL TRAINING GUIDE ISBN **1-78106-132-7**
To license this product please contact Nicole Adams on +44 (0) 20 7907 6134 or nicole_adams@dennis.co.uk

Advertising
Katie Wood katie_wood@dennis.co.uk
Emma D'Arcy emma_darcy@dennis.co.uk

The health and fitness information presented in this book is an educational resource and is not intended as a substitute for medical advice. Consult your doctor or healthcare professional before performing any of the exercises described in this book or any other exercise programme, particularly if you are pregnant, or if you are elderly or have chronic or recurring medical conditions. Do not attempt any of the exercises while under the influence of alcohol or drugs. Discontinue any exercise that causes you pain or severe discomfort and consult a medical expert. Neither the author of the information nor the producer nor distributors of such information make any warranty of any kind in regard to the content of the information presented in this book.

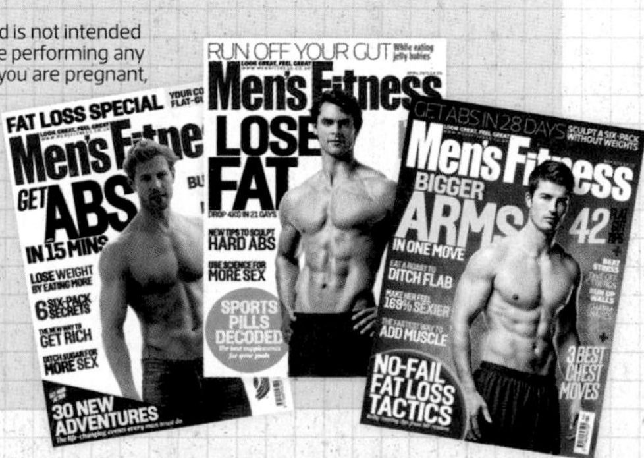

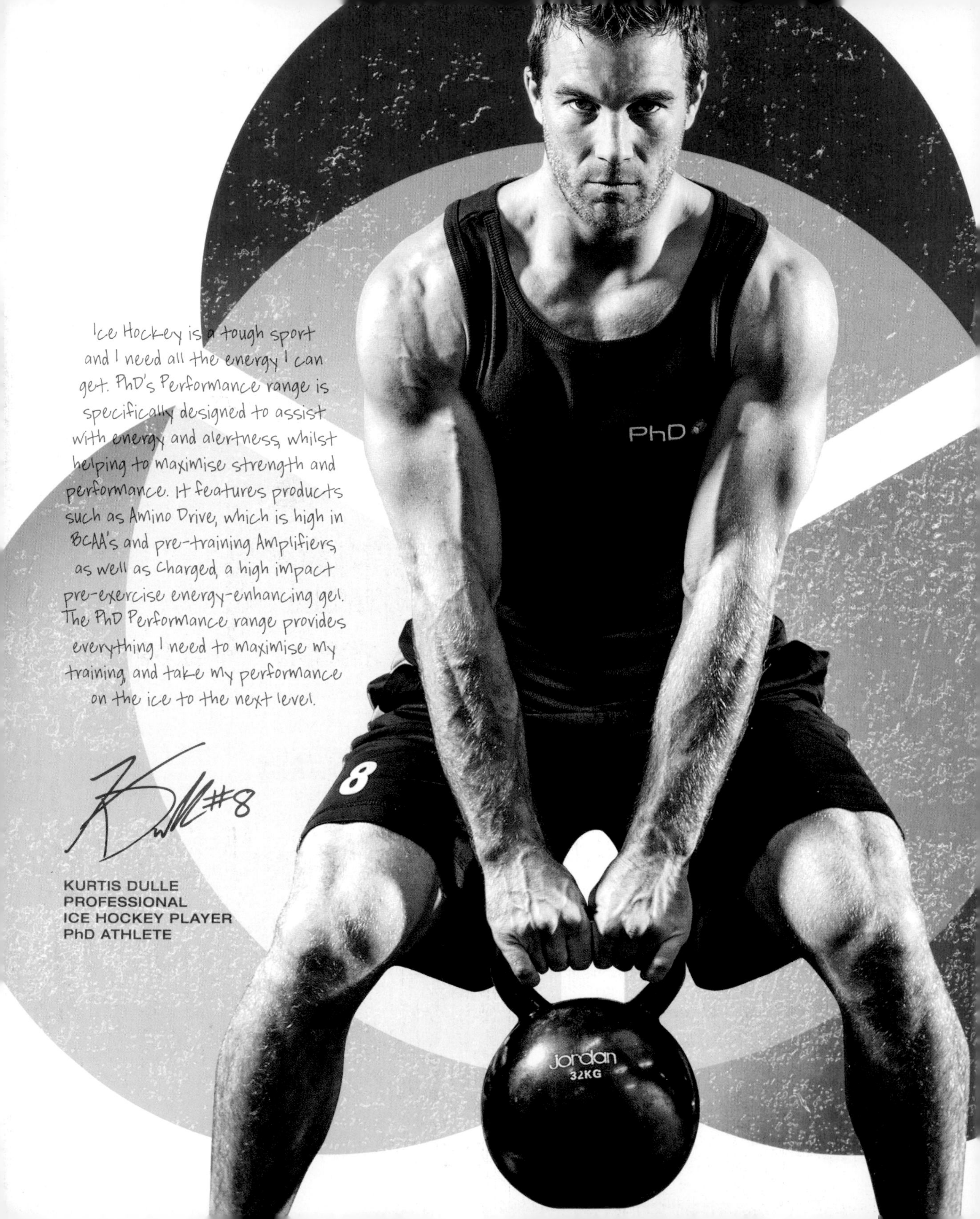
Ice Hockey is a tough sport and I need all the energy I can get. PhD's Performance range is specifically designed to assist with energy and alertness, whilst helping to maximise strength and performance. It features products such as Amino Drive, which is high in BCAA's and pre-training Amplifiers, as well as Charged, a high impact pre-exercise energy-enhancing gel. The PhD Performance range provides everything I need to maximise my training, and take my performance on the ice to the next level.
#8
KURTIS DULLE
PROFESSIONAL
ICE HOCKEY PLAYER
PhD ATHLETE
PhD
8
Jordan
32KG

Contents

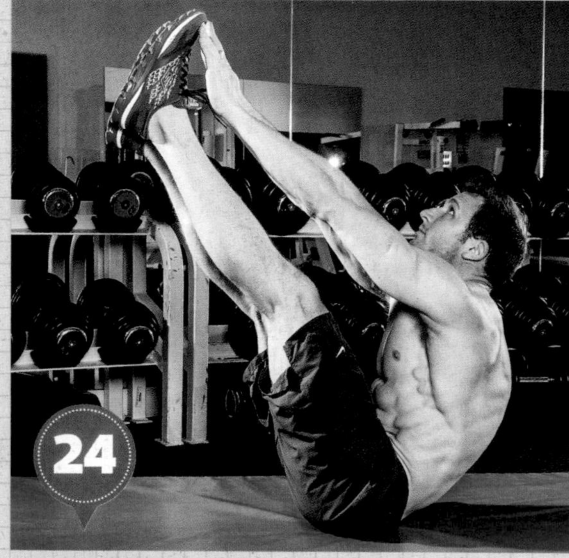

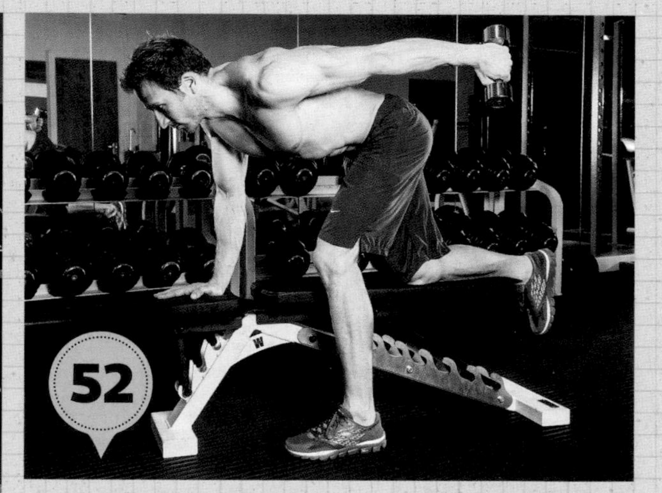

ABOUT THE BOOK 12
How to use this book to get the most out of your training sessions and build the body you want

BEFORE YOU BEGIN 18
Here's what you need to know about your major muscle groups, plus the truth behind common fitness myths

ABS 24
Essential moves that will strengthen your core and put you on course for an impressive six-pack

ARMS 52
Bulge out of your T-shirt sleeves with the exercises that will give you rippling biceps and triceps

BACK 76
The best moves to build a strong, muscular back for a well-balanced and injury-proof physique

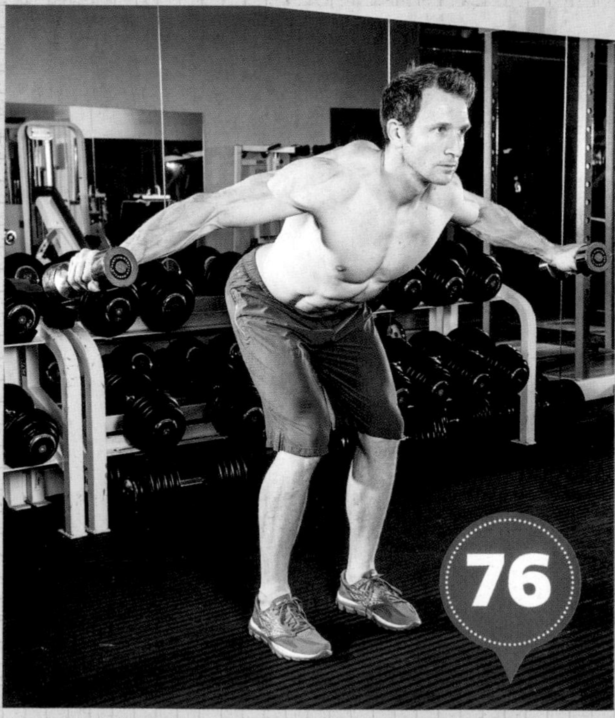

Contents

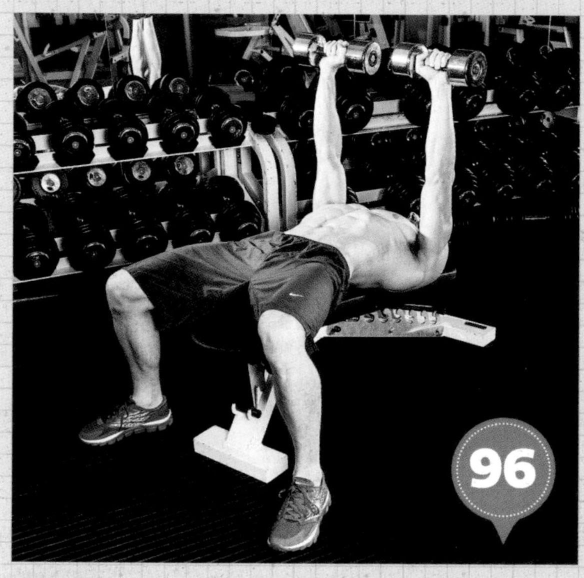

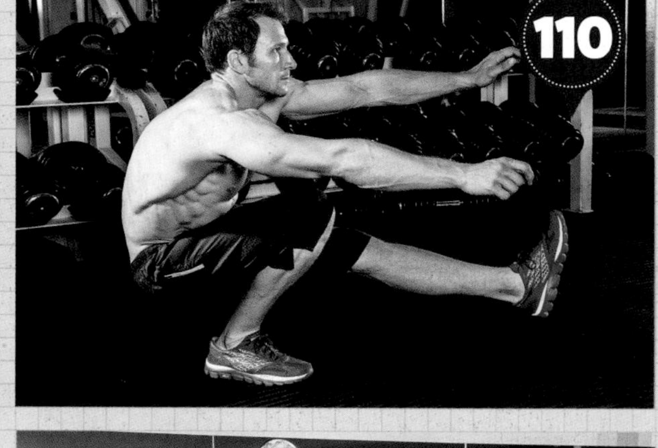

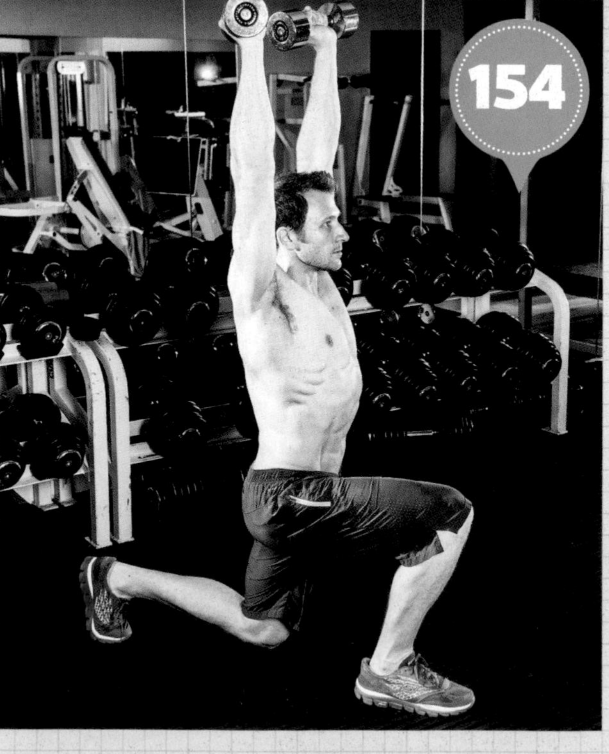

CHEST 96
Our guide to the classic bench press and 23 other ways to get powerful pecs

LEGS 110
Work the biggest muscle groups in your body and you'll pack on size everywhere

SHOULDERS 136
The exercises that will help you get the type of V-shaped torso that attracts admiring glances

TOTAL BODY 154
These super-effective compound moves recruit lots of muscle fibres for incredible gains

WORKOUT THEORY 174
Guidelines to help you design workouts for the best results in the shortest possible time

About this book

Get the most of this essential guide by learning the exercises then discovering how to put them together into an effective training plan

The most important part of any training programme – whether you want to build muscle, burn fat or improve sports performance – isn't which exercises you do for how many sets or reps, or even how often you train.

So what is the most important part? The ability to perform a move, whatever muscle it works, correctly and safely. If you don't know the right form, or movement pattern, for an exercise, at best you'll simply waste your time and not see results. At worst, you'll injure yourself. And the longer you have to spend away from the gym recuperating, the longer it will take for you to get the body you want.

That's why the *Total Training Guide* is your essential handbook for mastering all the exercises you'll ever need to build a bigger, stronger and leaner body.

Fitter, faster

The best way to improve your physique and get fitter and faster on the sports field is through weight training. Why? Lifting weights causes tiny tears in your muscle fibres. These are then repaired while you rest away from the gym and as a result your muscles grow back bigger and stronger. Resistance training is also one of the best ways to burn body fat.

However, many men stick to the same few exercises every time they go to the gym. That isn't the right way to keep improving because your muscles quickly adapt to the same stimuli and so no longer need to keep growing.

That's why this book contains more than 250 moves, so you can continuously change the exercises you perform. This will ensure your muscles are never allowed to stay in their comfort zone, forcing them to continue getting larger and stronger.

> **"Weight training is one of the most effective ways to burn fat and build muscle"**

Main moves

All the exercises in this book are divided into sections based on the primary muscle group they target. The sections appear in alphabetical order – abs, arms, back, chest, legs and shoulders – with the final section containing those exercises that target multiple muscle groups across the body.

The main moves in each section are featured on every left-hand page, with a description of why that move is so effective at building muscle and a detailed guide to performing it perfectly.

On the right-hand page opposite each main move are variations of the exercise, so you can understand how making key tweaks will keep your muscles guessing so they have no option but to pack on size and strength.

Workout theory

The final section of this book is a comprehensive guide to workout theory, including explanations of the key components of every workout, and how different workouts can be put together to form an effective training programme. This allows you to transform your newfound knowledge of how to perform all the exercises into an effective plan based on your ultimate fitness goal.

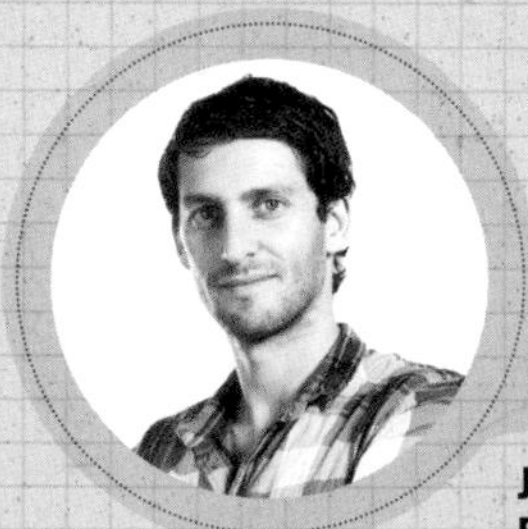

Joe Warner
Editor

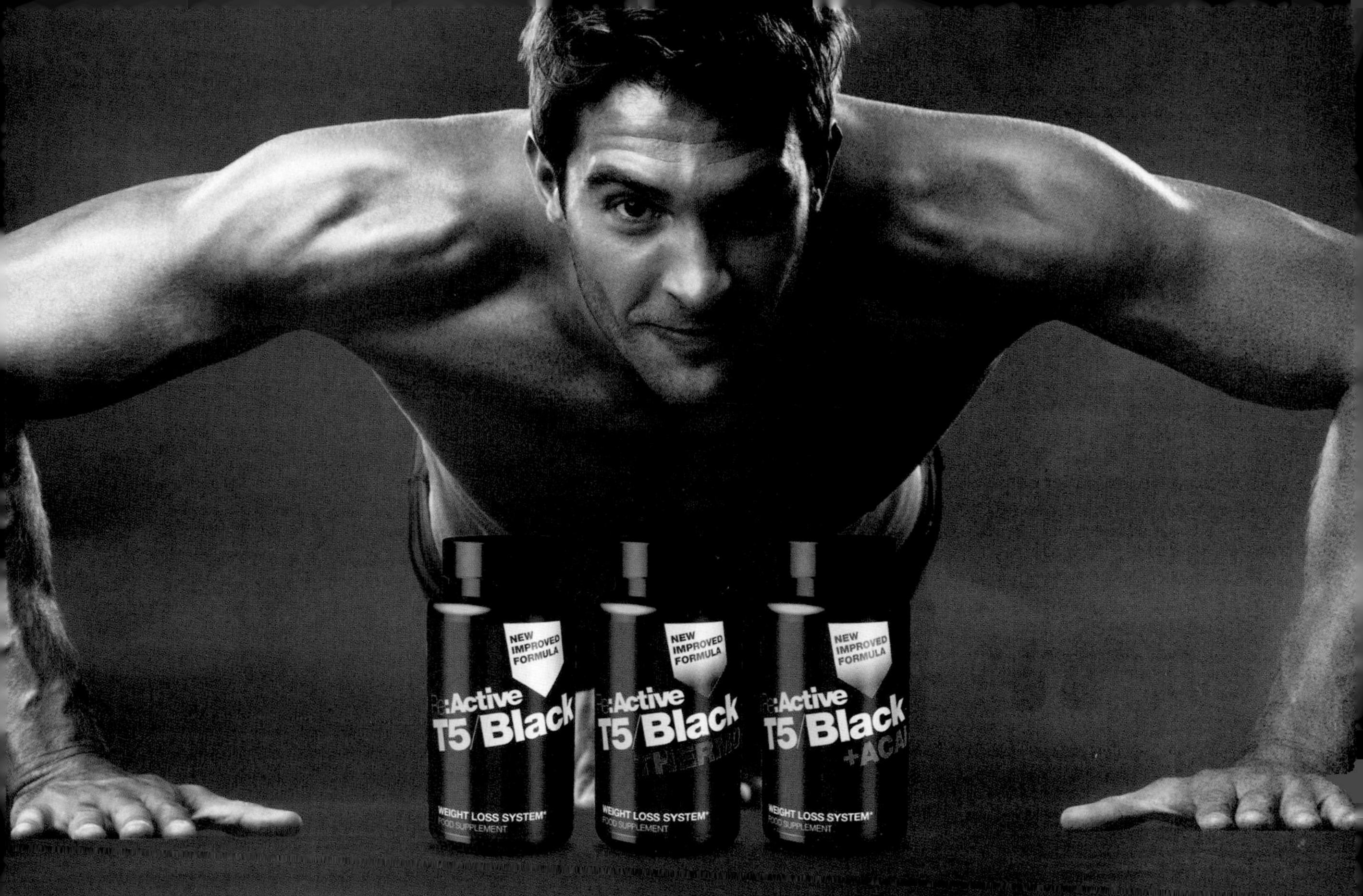
NEW IMPROVED FORMULA
Re:Active T5/Black
WEIGHT LOSS SYSTEM*
NEW IMPROVED FORMULA
Re:Active T5/Black
WEIGHT LOSS SYSTEM*
NEW IMPROVED FORMULA
Re:Active T5/Black
WEIGHT LOSS SYSTEM*

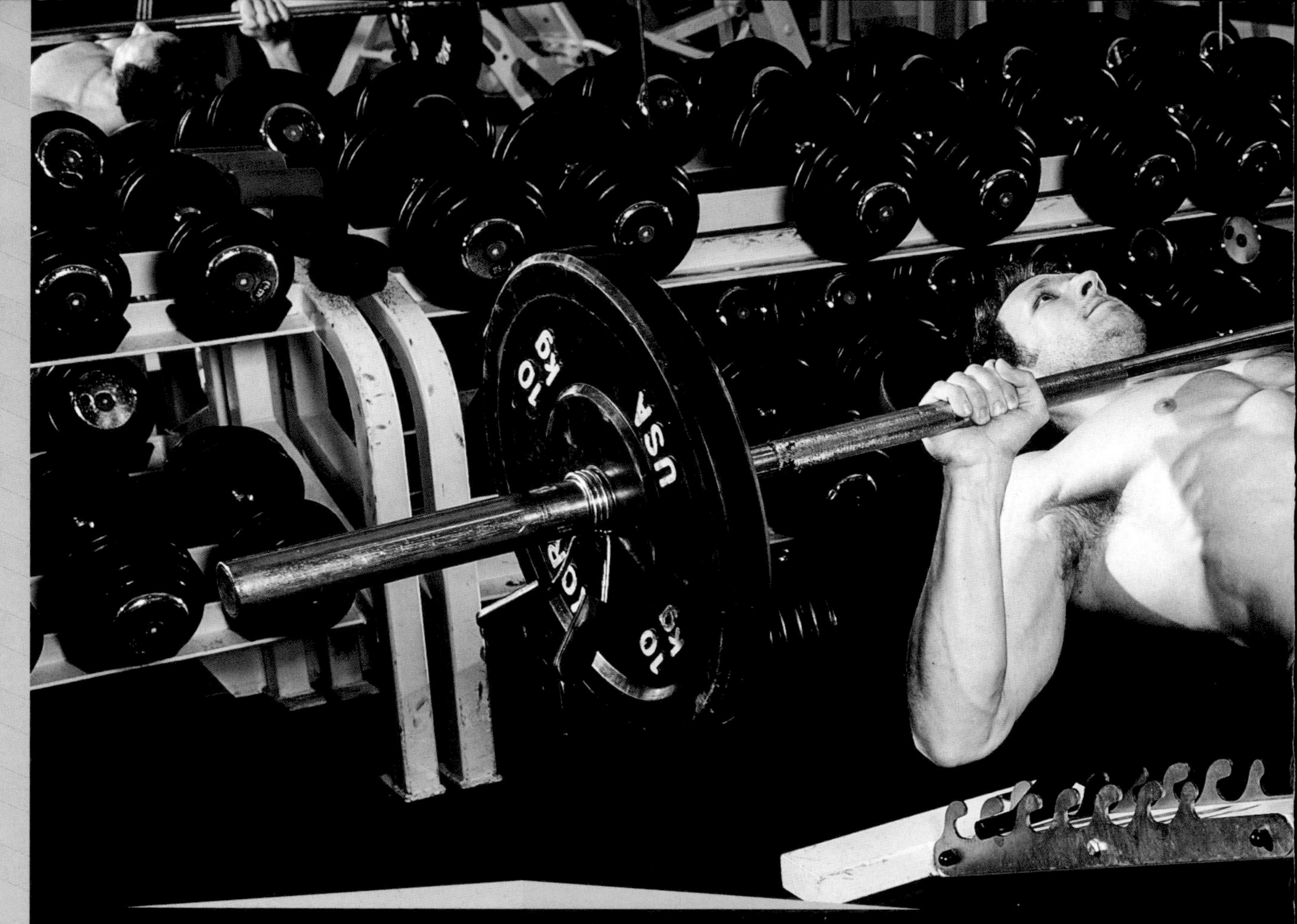

TOTAL TRAINING GUIDE

This is your comprehensive guide to working out for the best body you've ever had. Turn over to get started

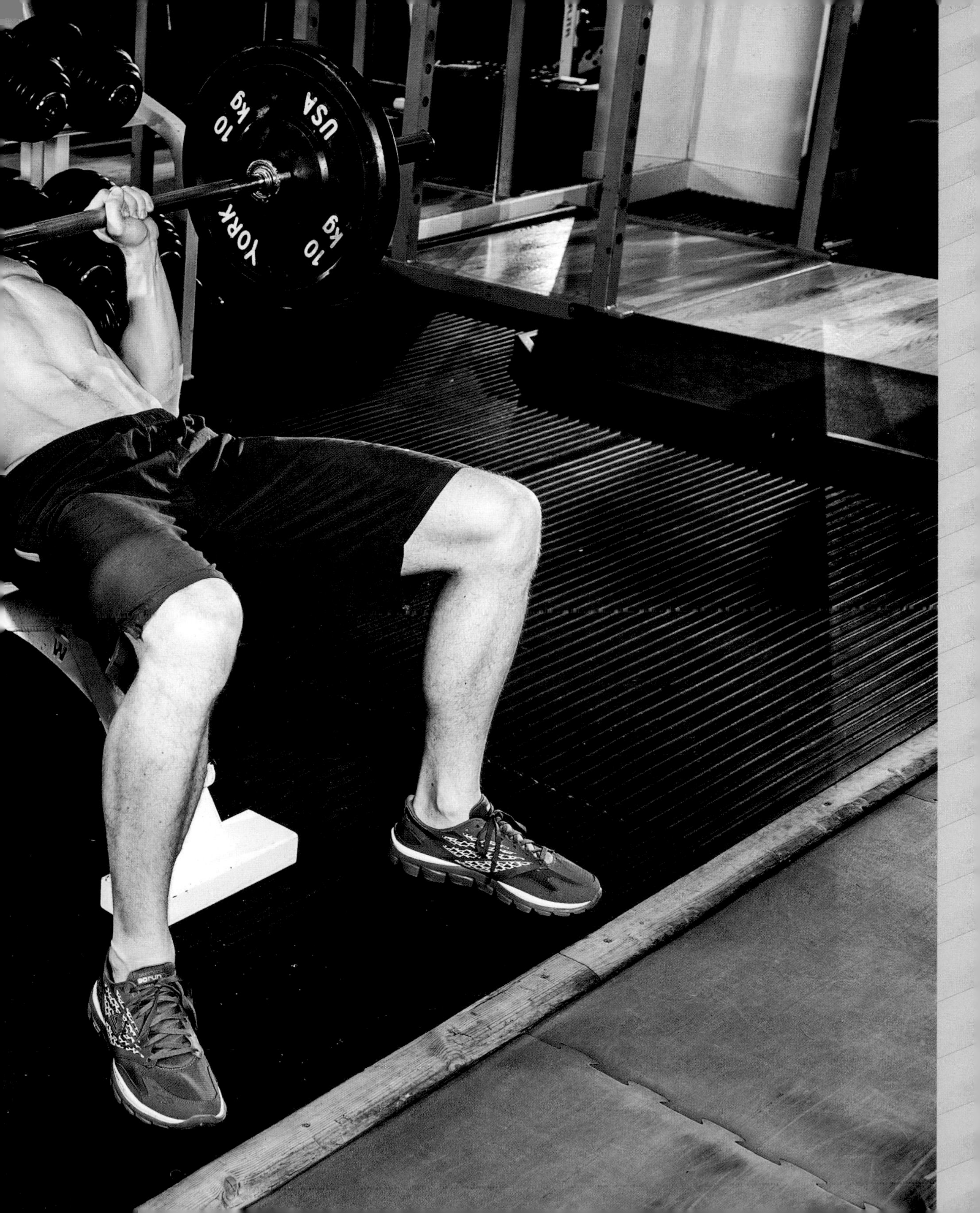
10 kg
USA
YORK
10 kg

How to use this book

Get more from your workouts whatever your training experience

This book, brought to you by the experts at *Men's Fitness* magazine, is your complete guide to the gym whatever your fitness level and includes everything you need to know about lifting weights safely and effectively.

If you've never stepped foot in a gym before but have always wanted to make a positive move towards building a better body, you can use this book to learn and master all the key exercises, and discover how to put them together to build the right workout for you.

If, on the other hand, you're an experienced gym-goer, you can use this book as a reference guide to the best exercises for each muscle group and the variations of these key moves you should introduce to your workouts to keep your muscles growing bigger and stronger.

Section guide

In this introductory section, you'll find a glossary of key workout terminology and an illustration of all the major muscles groups so you know what you should be targeting. We'll also bust some of the more common fitness and exercise myths.

Then come all the exercises you'll ever need to build the body you want. For simplicity, we've divided the exercises by body part, starting with abs before moving on alphabetically to the arms, back, chest, legs, shoulders and total body.

Of course, many exercises work different muscles groups at the same time, but we've listed each move under the muscle group it works the hardest. So, for example, the bench press is in the 'chest' chapter (on p98), even though it also trains the triceps and shoulders.

On every two-page spread we've demonstrated one main move and up to three variations. The main moves are the classic lifts that should be in every man's repertoire, while the variations ensure you always have an alternative when you need to shake up your training to keep making gains. These will either hit the muscle group from a different angle or use a different bit of kit to work your muscles in a different way.

> **"We'll show you how to change your workout so you keep moving forwards"**

Putting it into practice

The final section in this book is a comprehensive guide to how to arrange the exercises into the right workouts for your training goal.

Most fitness books give you a specific workout plan to follow, but this means their usefulness comes to an end once you've completed that plan. This guide, however, will teach you the basic principles behind different workout protocols so you can create the right workout for your needs, and then show you how to keep changing elements of it so you can always keep moving forwards.

So whatever your fitness experience, the *Total Training Guide* provides all the information and motivation you need to build the body you've always wanted.

Getting started

Before starting any exercise regime you should check with your GP, especially if you have a history of heart trouble, or long-standing joint or muscle issues.

It's also important to always warm up properly before doing any serious exercise (see p180 for a detailed guide). This will ensure your mind and muscles are fully prepared and less likely to suffer injury.

In many of the form guides in this book, you'll see instructions telling you to 'brace your core muscles' or 'engage your core'. This means you should contract the muscles around your midriff – especially your abdominals – to stabilise your spine.

To do this, ensure you're standing or sitting up straight, with your hips in line with your torso. Now imagine someone is about to punch you in the stomach and you have to tense your abdominal muscles to take the blow. You need to maintain that tension throughout each set to keep your torso stable.

For more advice on training, plus detailed workouts, nutrition and supplement tips, see *Men's Fitness* magazine, published every month, or go to mensfitness.co.uk.

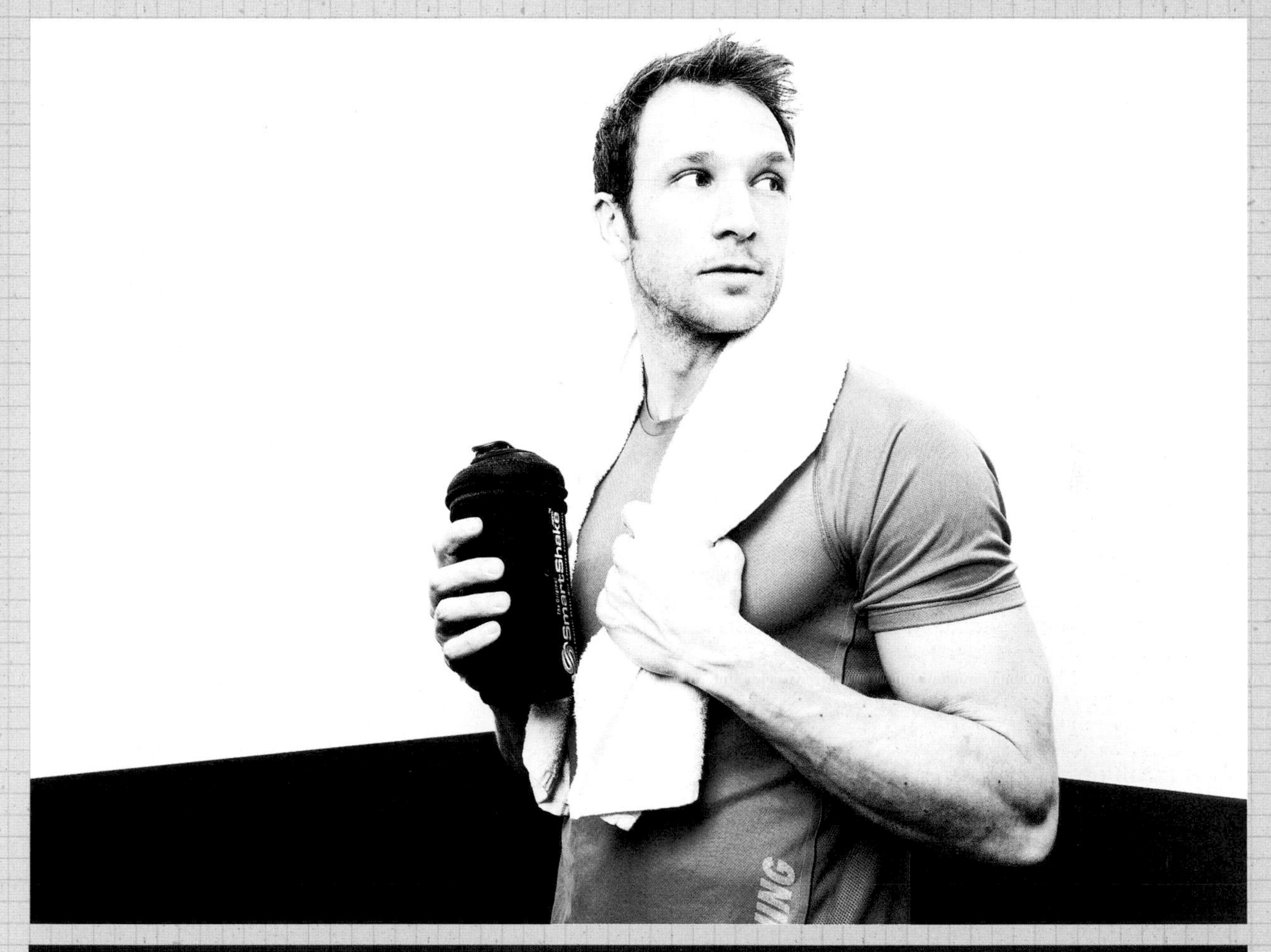

Advice for beginners

If you are new to exercise and the gym, here's what you need to know

▶ If you feel pain at any time during your workout, stop immediately. Don't be tempted to work through the pain or you could make a small problem significantly worse.

▶ Maintain perfect form for every repetition, or rep, of every exercise. Each exercise in this book comes with detailed notes on form and most gyms have fitness experts on hand who will be happy to help if you're still unsure about an exercise.

▶ Pick a weight you can manage easily the first time you do any lift. This allows can to concentrate on perfecting the form; the weight can be increased over time. Leave your ego at the door – choosing a weight that's too heavy is the fastest way to cut your training short through injury.

▶ It's worth remembering a few basic points of gym etiquette. Always return any equipment to its place after using it and don't hog equipment for too long. Wipe your sweat off machines, mats or benches after using them. If someone is using the equipment you want, ask to 'work in' with them, which means you take turns doing a set of exercises while the other person rests.

Glossary

Common workout terms explained

A

Anabolic
The metabolic phase during which nutrients from your diet, specifically protein, are synthesised by your body and turned into new muscle tissue.

Atrophy
Muscle atrophy is the wasting away of muscle tissue leading to a decrease in muscle mass, typically due to inactivity.

C

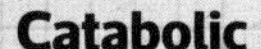

Catabolic
The metabolic phase when muscle tissue is broken down and used as energy – the opposite of anabolic.

Compound lift
An exercise that involves movement in two or more different joints. Good examples include the squat (movement at the hip and knee joints) and shoulder press (movement at the shoulder and elbow joints). These lifts should form the basis of all programmes where increased muscle size and strength are the objectives because they recruit more of the muscle fibres responsible for the development of these attributes.

D

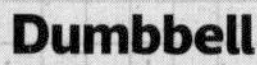

Dumbbell
One of the best known types of free weights, dumbbells can be used to added extra resistance to almost every exercise, typically by holding one in each hand.

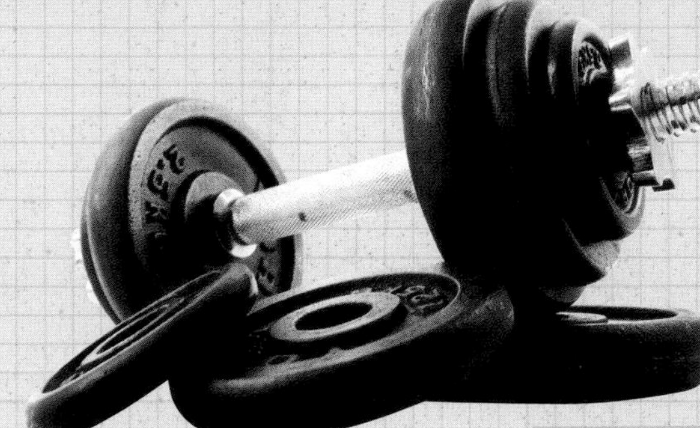

Dumbbells are the most common free weights

E

EZ-bar
A type of barbell with a series of kinks in the middle of the bar. It is designed to put less pressure on the wrists and elbows when lifting.

F

Form
The technique used when performing an exercise.

Free weights
Any weight-training equipment used to increase muscle size and strength that can be moved in any direction. The most common examples include barbells, dumbbells and kettlebells.

H

Hypertrophy
Greek for 'excess nourishment', hypertrophy is an increase in the volume of a muscle (or organ) caused by the enlargement of its cells. Hypertrophy occurs through sarcoplasmic hypertrophy, which focuses on increasing size; myofibrillar hypertrophy, which focuses on increasing strength; or a combination of the two.

I

Isolation lift
A move that involves movement in only one joint. Examples include the biceps curl (movement at the elbow joint only) and leg extension (movement at the knee joint only). These exercises are ideally placed at the end of a workout, when you can work the target muscle group to fatigue.

K

Kettlebell
Cast-iron balls of different weights, originating from Russia. They have a handle on the top so you can grip them with one or two hands while performing different exercises.

M

Muscle pump
When your muscles become engorged with blood after you have repeatedly shortened and lengthened a muscle. Typically this occurs after weight training

but sometimes it can be achieved simply by flexing your muscles repeatedly as hard as possible.

O

Olympic barbell
A key piece of weight training equipment used to perform all manner of lifts. It has thick 'sleeves' for the weight plates to slot on to, which means they can spin when you're doing lifts such as the clean or snatch. Full-length bars weigh 20kg before any weights are added.

R

Range of motion
The full extent or range of a muscle's movement. Performing lifts through a muscle's full range of motion is important in promoting muscle growth.

Reps
Abbreviation of repetition. One rep is the completion of a given exercise from start to finish through a full range of motion. The number of reps per set can vary from one to more than 20, depending on your training goals.

Resistance machine
A type of gym machine that allows you to target specific muscles in a predetermined controlled path of movement. Favoured by novices and bodybuilders, resistance machines reduce the risk of injury because of their set range of motion. However, as a consequence they don't work the smaller but vital stabilising muscles.

Rest interval
The time you take between exercises and/or sets, during which your muscles are given the chance to replenish their energy stores.

S

Sets
A given number of reps of a single exercise performed consecutively without rest. The number of sets performed of each exercise can vary, but three or four is most effective for building muscle mass.

Supercompensation
The period after a training session and subsequent recovery during which you're fitter and stronger than before. Training again during this window will result in further gains in strength, size and fitness. Training before this window, on the other hand, can result in overtraining and you becoming weaker, while training after the window has closed reduces your ability to make additional gains.

Supersets
Two different exercises done back to back without rest or with only a short rest period between them. Supersets are a great way to shake up your existing training regime because they shock your muscles into growth by increasing their workload. They also allow you to train with more volume in a much shorter period of time, improving your muscles' ability to work harder with less rest.

T

Tempo
The speed at which you lift and lower a weight during each rep. The slower the tempo, the longer your muscles are exposed to the stress of managing the weight. This is called 'time under tension' (see below for more detail). In exercise guides, the tempo is usually described using a four-digit code, such as 4010. The first number is the time in seconds the weight is lowered, the second is the time in seconds the move is held at the bottom position, the third is the time in seconds that the weight it lifted (if 'X' is shown this means lift explosively) and the final digit is the time in seconds the weight is held at the top of the move.

Time under tension
The duration in seconds that your muscles are exposed to controlling a weight through a range of motion, as in a squat or bench press, or in an isometric hold, such as a plank. Time under tension is dictated by the tempo of each rep and how many reps you perform in a given set.

Kettlebells add resistance to natural movements such as swings

KNOW YOUR MUSCLES

There are over 600 muscles in the human body. These are the major ones you'll be targeting during your workouts

DELTOIDS
1. Medial deltoid (middle)
2. Anterior deltoid (front)

PECTORALS
3. Pectoralis major
4. Pectoralis minor (beneath the pectoralis major)
5. Serratus anterior

BICEPS
6. Biceps brachii
7. Brachialis

FOREARMS
8. Brachioradialis
9. Flexor carpi radialis

ABDOMINALS
10. Rectus abdominis
11. External obliques
12. Internal obliques (beneath the external obliques)
13. Transverse abdominis (beneath the internal obliques)

QUADRICEPS
14. Vastus lateralis
15. Rectus femoris
16. Vastus intermedius (beneath the rectus femoris)
17. Vastus medialis

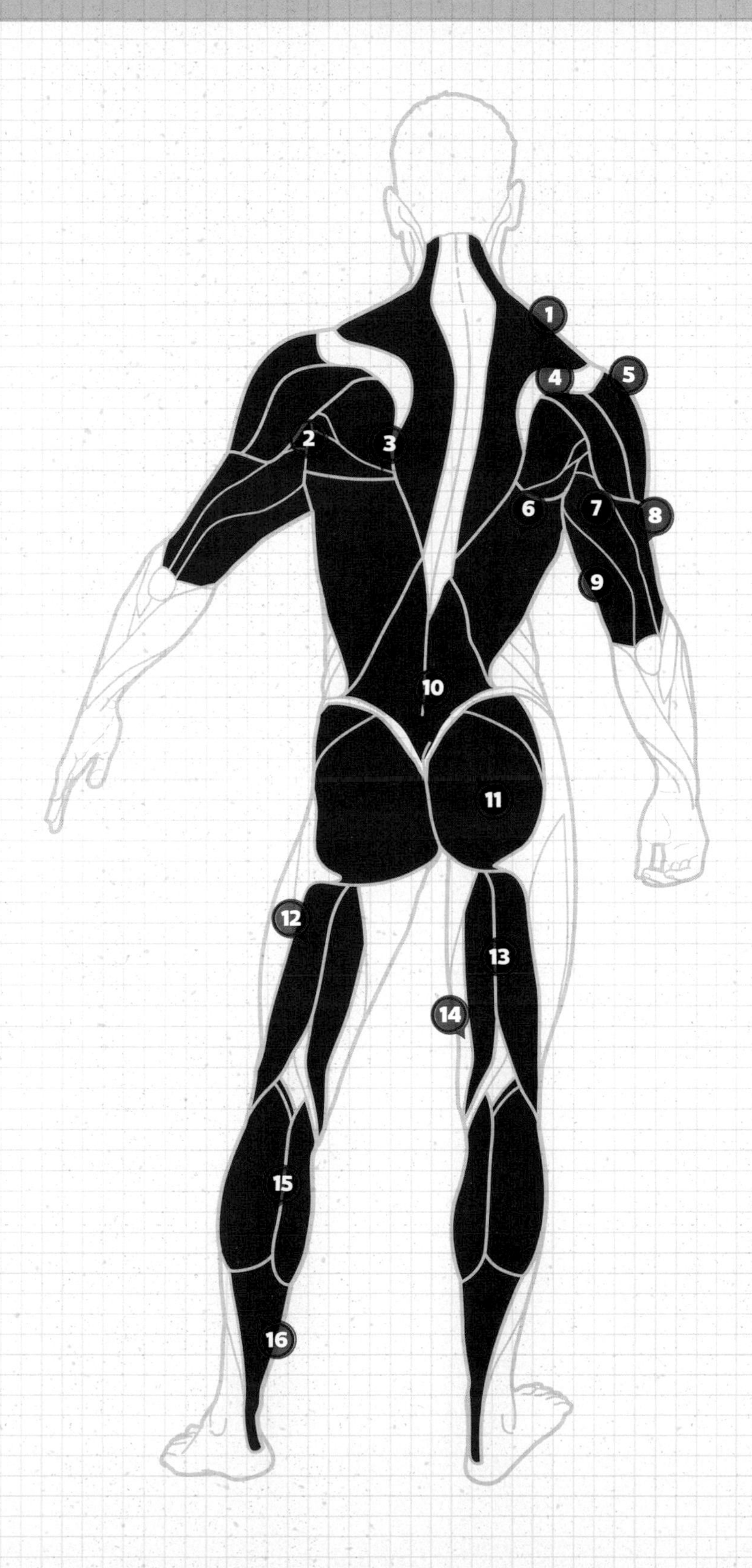

TRAPS

1. Trapezius

BACK

2. Teres major
3. Rhomboid (beneath the trapezius)

DELTOIDS

4. Rotator cuff (beneath the deltoids)
5. Posterior deltoid (back)

LATS

6. Latissimus dorsi

TRICEPS

7. Triceps brachii long head
8. Triceps brachii lateral head
9. Triceps brachii medial head

LOWER BACK

10. Erector spinae

GLUTES

11. Gluteus maximus

HAMSTRINGS

12. Biceps femoris
13. Semitendinosus
14. Semimembranosus

CALVES

15. Gastrocnemius
16. Soleus

Let's get this straight

The no-nonsense truth behind the most common fitness myths

1 The more often you train, the better the results

You need to train hard and regularly, but doing too much too often is counterproductive. If you're new to the gym, start with three sessions a week to give your muscles time to recover – and grow – before training them again. Too little rest between sessions can result in overtraining, when you feel tired, fatigued and demotivated. You are also more likely to suffer from injury.

2 Cardio training is the best for fat loss

High-intensity cardio training, such as sprints or hill runs, is great for fat loss. However, long and slow steady-state sessions, while good for heart and lung health, aren't that great at burning fat. This is because long sessions place your body in a state of stress, which encourages muscle mass to be broken down and instructs your body to store more of the energy you eat as fat. Weight training is one of the most effective ways to burn fat and build muscle, and should form the core of your training programme.

3 You can turn fat into muscle

Fat and muscle are two totally different types of tissue so it's impossible for one to turn into the other. Muscle is active tissue that burns calories, while fat tissues store excess energy. When you train hard it is possible to burn away fat and build muscle, giving the appearance that one has turned into the other, but that isn't actually the case.

4 Machines are better than free weights

Resistance machines have their place in a gym: they are a great way for beginners to learn movement patterns without the risk of danger, and allow experienced trainers to isolate specific muscles to lift heavier weights. But because the movement pattern is restricted, they're no good at working the stabilising muscles that are so important in staying injury free. Free weights require more skill to use, recruit these smaller stabilising muscles and allow you to move through a greater range of motion to work your muscles to their full extent, but both have merits.

> "Fat and muscle are different types of tissue. You can't turn one into the other"

5 Doing crunches will burn body fat

You can't lose fat from a specific part of your body, so no matter how many abs exercises you do they won't shift your belly. More often than not, the fat on your stomach is the last to go, so you need a well-structured training and nutrition plan to chip away constantly at your body-fat percentage.

6 Weight training makes you too bulky

Putting on serious amounts of lean muscle mass takes time, and only then if you have a progressive training plan and eat the right foods at the right time. No one has even woken up the day after a great chest and arms session to discover none of their T-shirts fit.

7 Light weights are best for muscle toning

There is no such thing as 'toning' a muscle. This made-up fitness phrase simply means building muscle and burning fat to give your muscles better definition. While light weights are great for training your small, stabilising muscles, especially those of the shoulders, the best way to build muscle and create a fat-burning response is to lift heavier weights to push your body out of its comfort zone.

FIT TIP
It's best to see your GP for a check-up before starting any new training programme

ABS

Sculpt a rock-solid six-pack with the must-do abs moves

Ask most men what body part they most wish to improve and their abs will feature high on the list. A rock-hard six-pack not only looks good, it also proves you take training seriously and know what you're doing when it comes to burning excess body fat and building hard, lean muscle mass.

Your abdominals are a collection of important postural muscles and are responsible for flexing your spine forwards, as when doing a crunch. The group also assists with breathing, stabilising the torso during exercise and protecting your internal organs from impact.

When people talk about the abs, they're often referring to the rectus abdominis, a paired muscle that runs vertically on either side of the front of the abdomen, separated down the middle by a band of connective tissue called the linea alba, or white line. It's this line, along with those that run horizontally across this muscle group, that creates the six distinct parts of a six-pack. There are actually four vertical sections, but the bottom pair are just above the pubic bone and not typically visible.

Heavy compound lifts, such as squats, deadlifts and overhead presses, are among the best moves for building your abs because they require your core to work hard to stabilise your upper body and to transfer power between your legs and your torso.

However, the abs are like every other muscle group in that they need to be targeted directly, from a variety of angles, to effectively elicit maximum muscle growth. This chapter reveals the best moves for sculpting a six-pack.

The role of the abs muscles

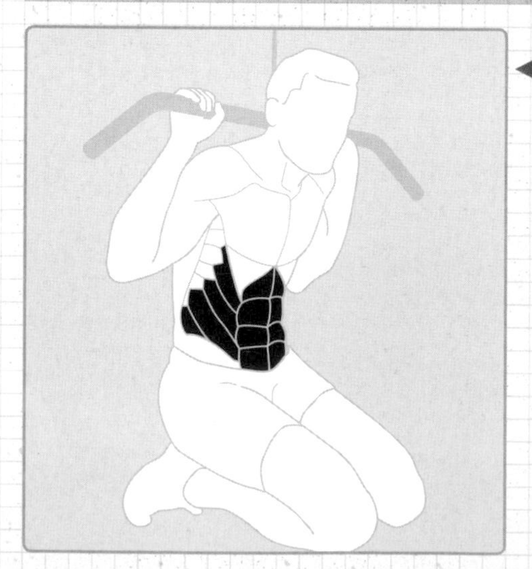

The abdominals are a collection of muscles in the front of your torso that play a variety of important roles. They are responsible for bending your spine forwards and rotating your torso left and right, and together with your lower back provide postural support and stability and allow the efficient transfer of power between you upper and lower body. They also assist in the respiration process and serve to protect the organs of your lower torso too.

Abs explained

Here are the major muscles of the core and what they do

- The rectus abdominis is a long, flat muscle that runs down the front of your stomach and is better known as your abs or six-pack. It's an important stabilising muscle and is responsible for flexing your spine, as when performing a crunch. It also assists with breathing and plays an important role when forcefully expelling air from the lungs. It creates intra-abdominal pressure that protects your internal organs. It's divided down the middle by the linea alba.

- The external obliques are the largest and most superficial of the obliques, which run either side of the rectus abdominis. Their function is to the pull the chest downwards. They also have limited actions in both the flexion and rotation of the spine.

- The internal obliques are deep-lying muscles that lie under the external obliques. They have two major functions: as antagonists to the diaphragm to inhale and expel air from the lungs, and to rotate and bend the torso. This is achieved when the right internal oblique and left external oblique contract together to flex and rotate the torso to bring the left shoulder towards the right hip.

- The transverse abdominis are the deepest muscles of the abdominals group, lying under the external and internal obliques, and stabilise your torso.

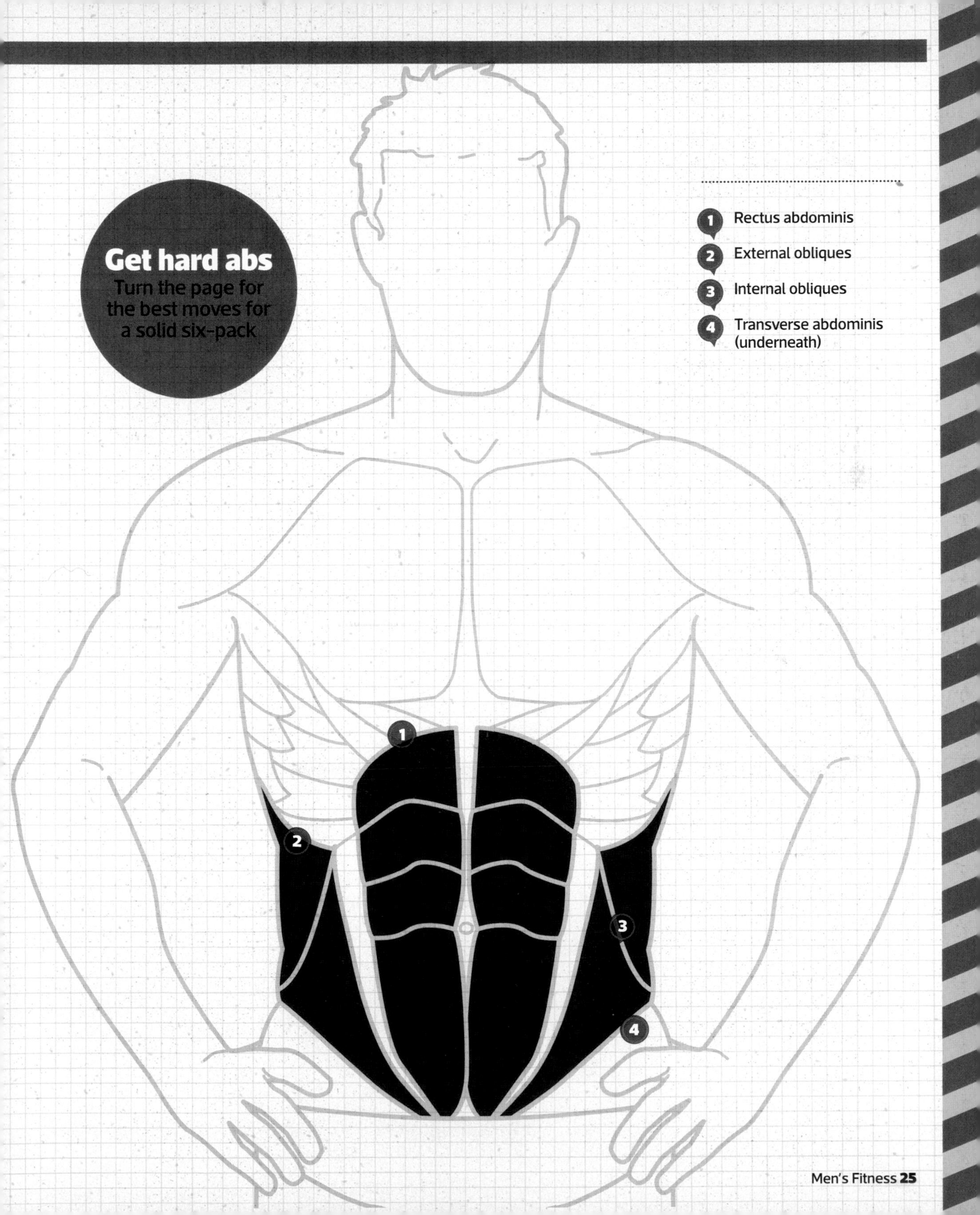
Get hard abs
Turn the page for the best moves for a solid six-pack
1 Rectus abdominis
2 External obliques
3 Internal obliques
4 Transverse abdominis (underneath)
1
2
3
4

CRUNCH

***Targets** Upper abs*

The classic move for working your upper abs

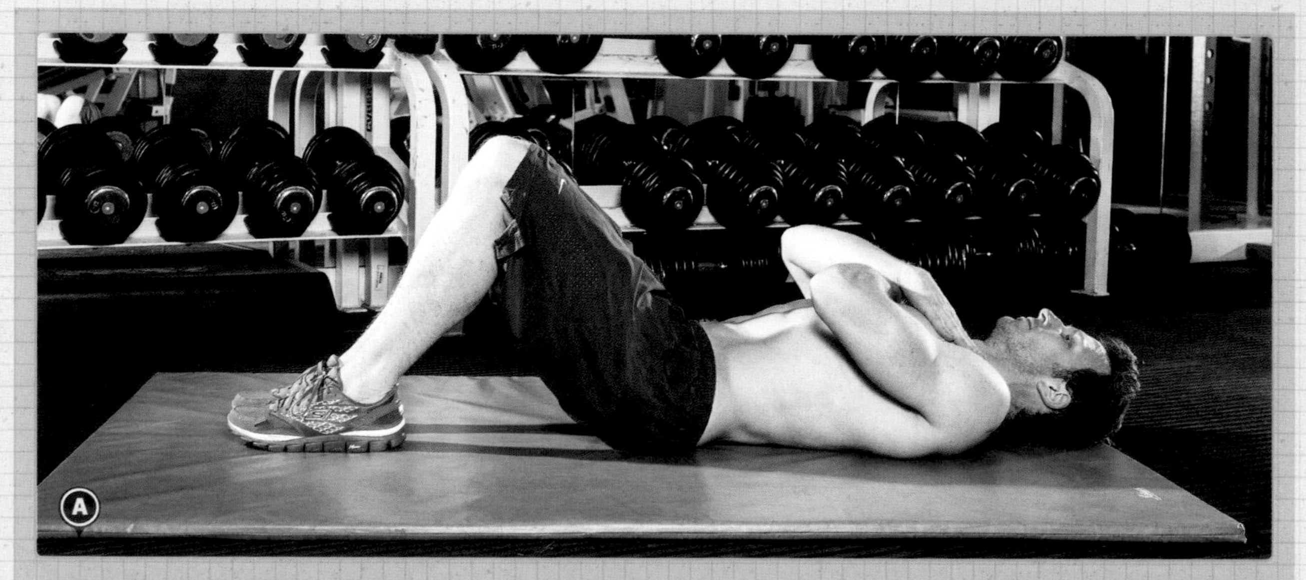

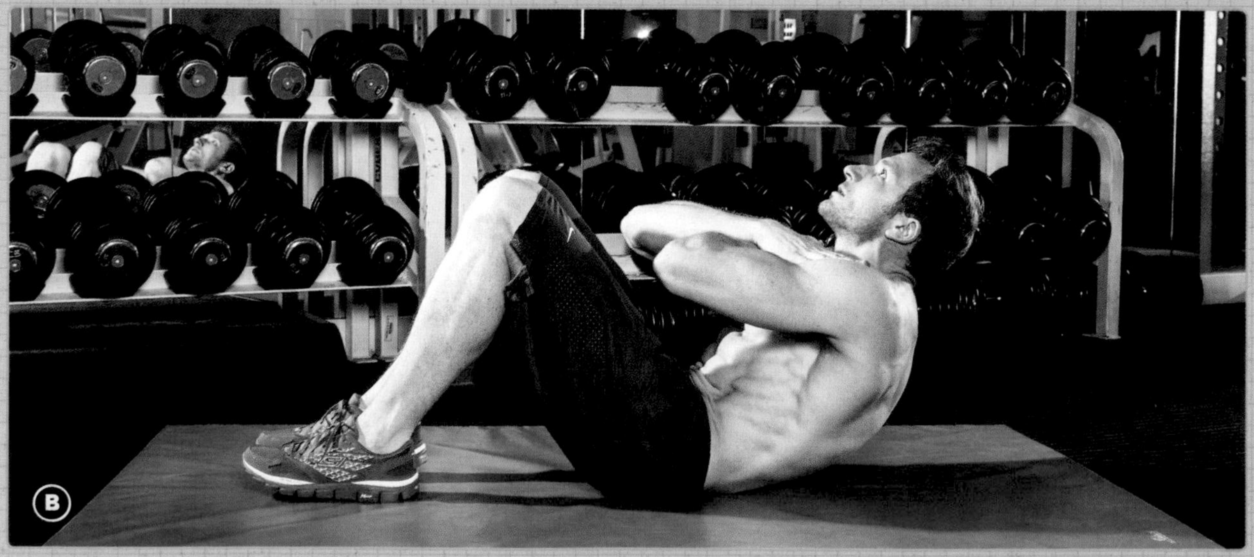

- Lie on a mat with your arms crossed and hands on the top of your chest, your feet on the floor and knees bent at 90°.
- Contract your abs to lift your upper back off the ground and curl your chest towards your knees.
- Pause at the top of the move, squeeze your abs, then slowly lower your torso back towards the floor.

Gym ball crunch

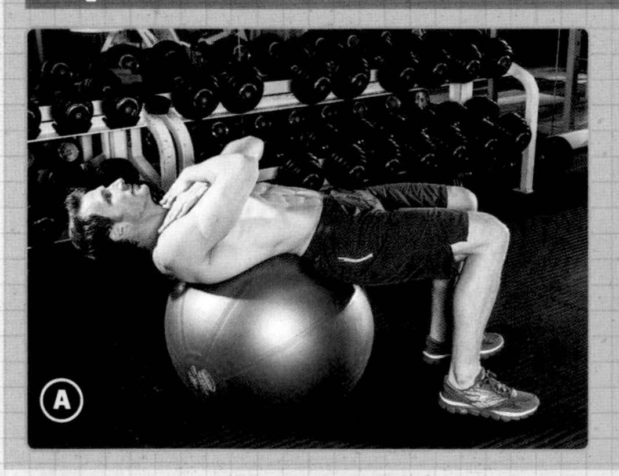

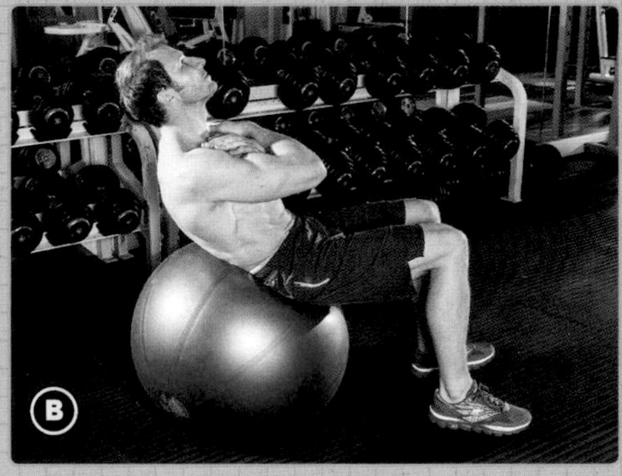

Lying over a gym ball works your core muscles because they must stabilise your body throughout the move. It also works your abs harder through a greater range of motion.

Dumbbell crunch

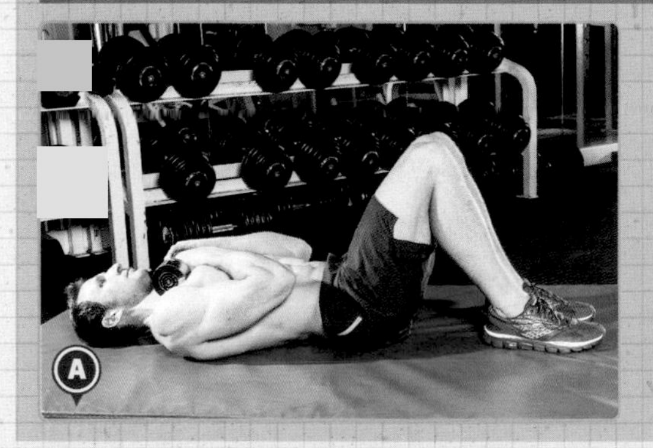

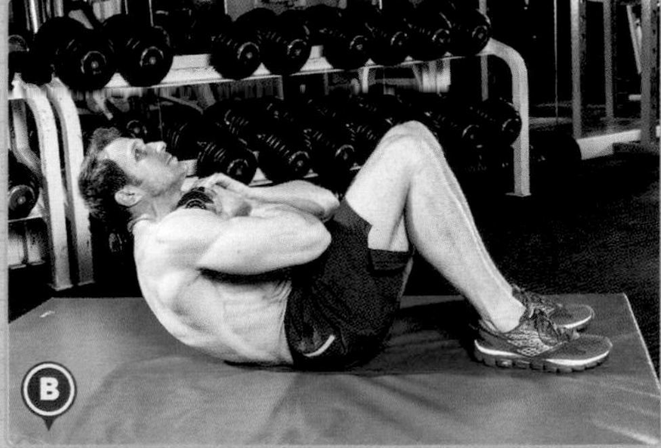

Holding a dumbbell with both hands over your chest increases the amount of weight your muscles must move and therefore works your abs even harder.

Cable crunch

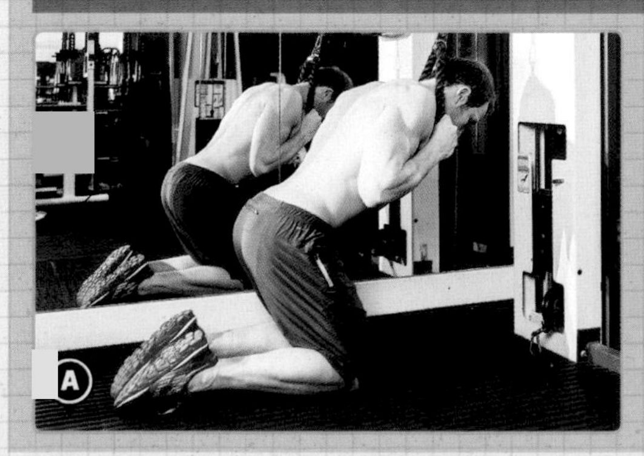

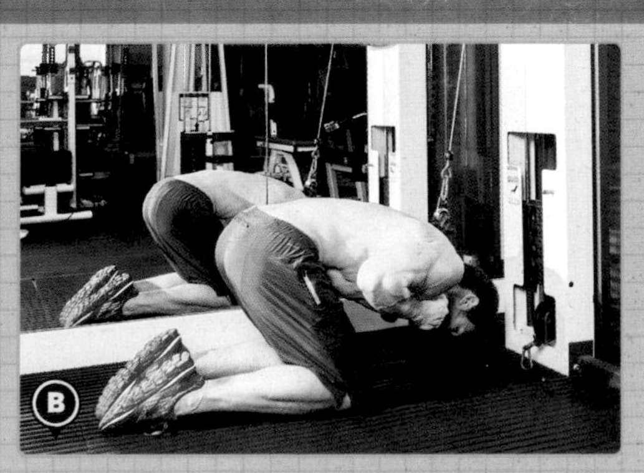

Using a cable as resistance forces your muscles to manage the weight throughout the entire rep and allows you to lift a lot of weight to work your abs harder.

REVERSE CRUNCH

***Targets** Lower abs*

One of the best moves to work the lower part of your six-pack

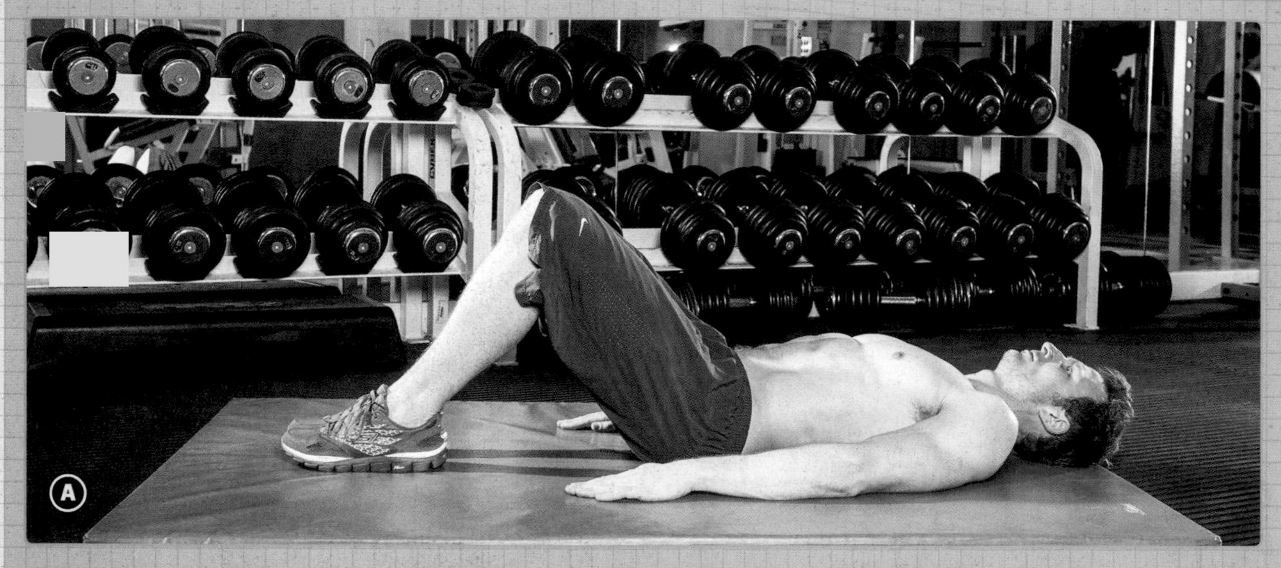

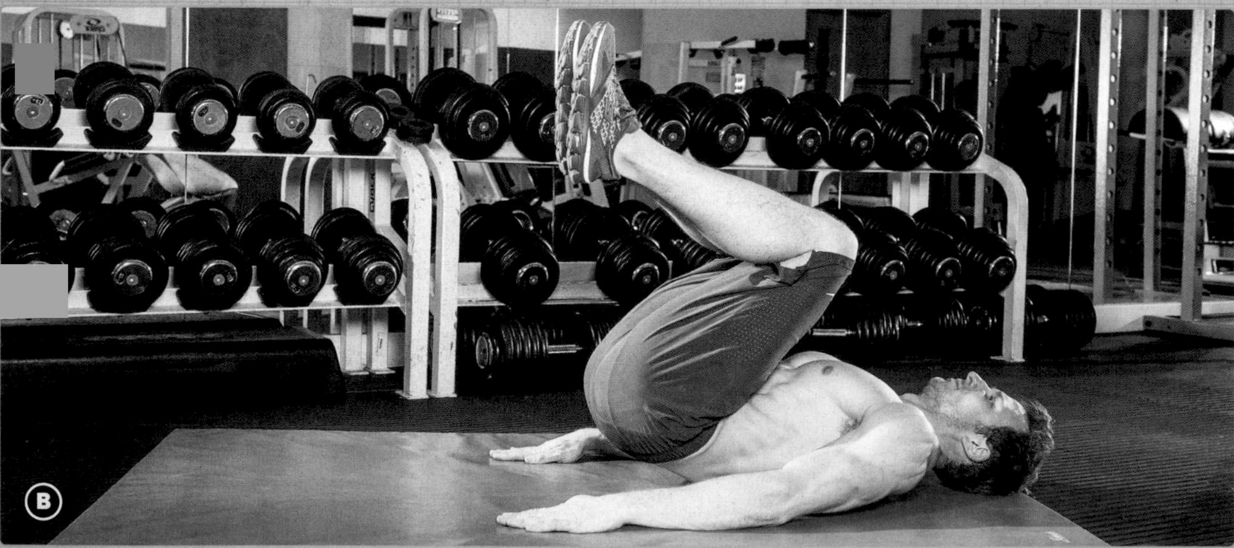

- Lie flat on a mat with your hands on the floor by your thighs, your knees bent at 90° and your feet on the floor.
- Contract your abs to raise your knees towards your chest.
- Pause at the top of the move, squeeze your abs, then slowly lower your feet back towards the floor.

Seated reverse crunch

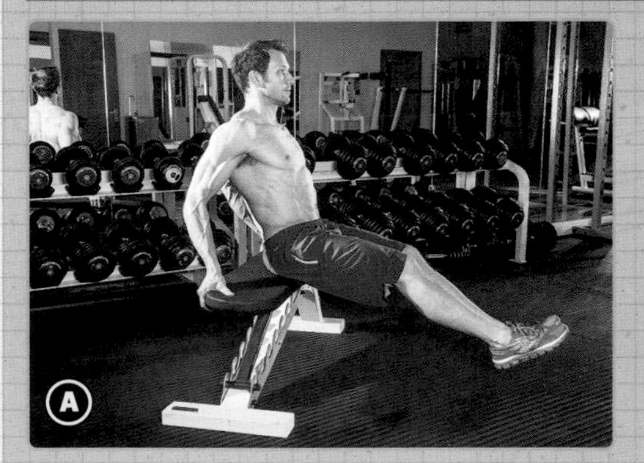

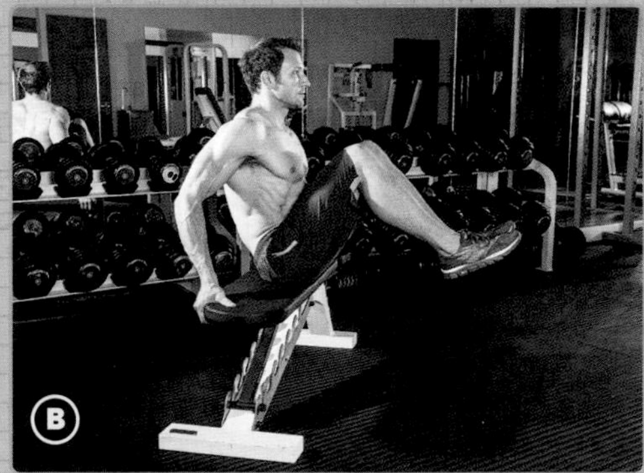

Sitting on the edge of a bench increases the workload on your lower abs and forces your deep-lying core muscles to stabilise your torso.

Medicine ball reverse crunch

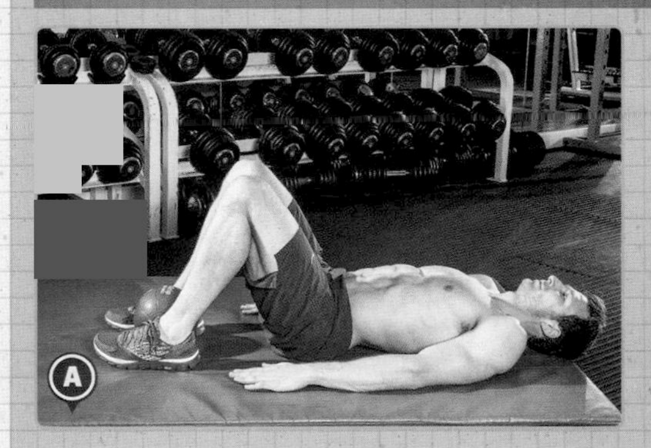

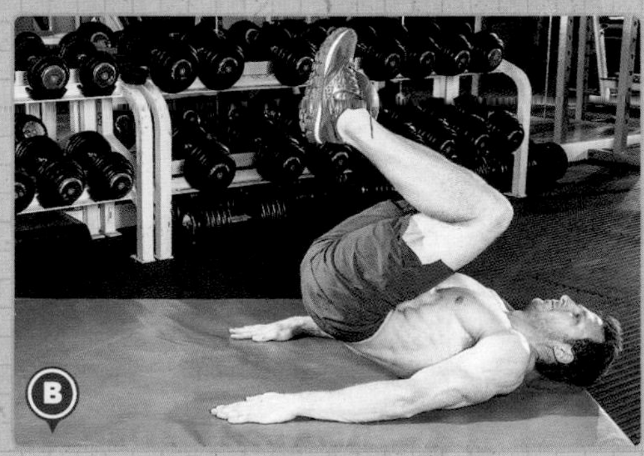

The additional weight of a medicine ball between your feet will stimulate greater muscle growth.

Tuck and crunch

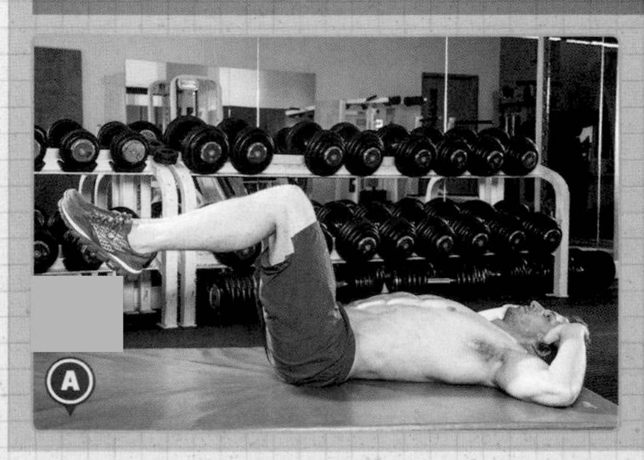

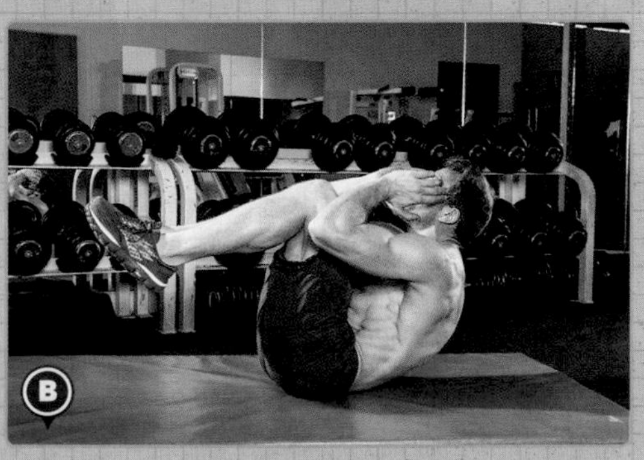

Raising your chest to meet your knees will target all your abs in just one move.

OBLIQUE CRUNCH

***Targets** Obliques*

Hit your side abs to complete your six-pack

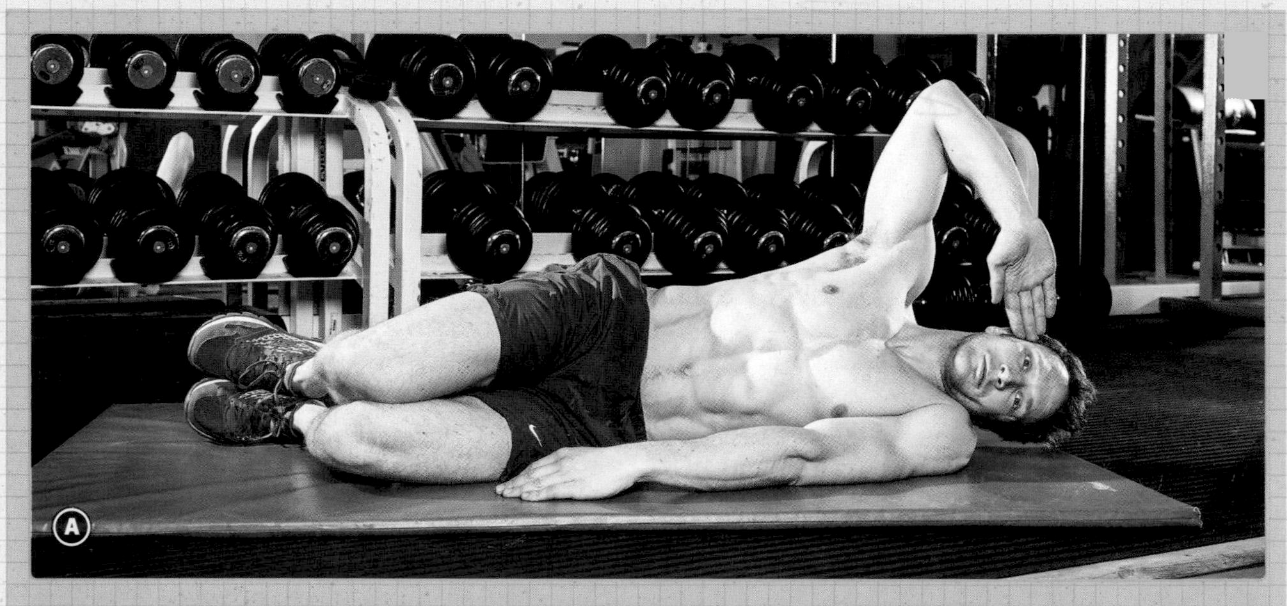

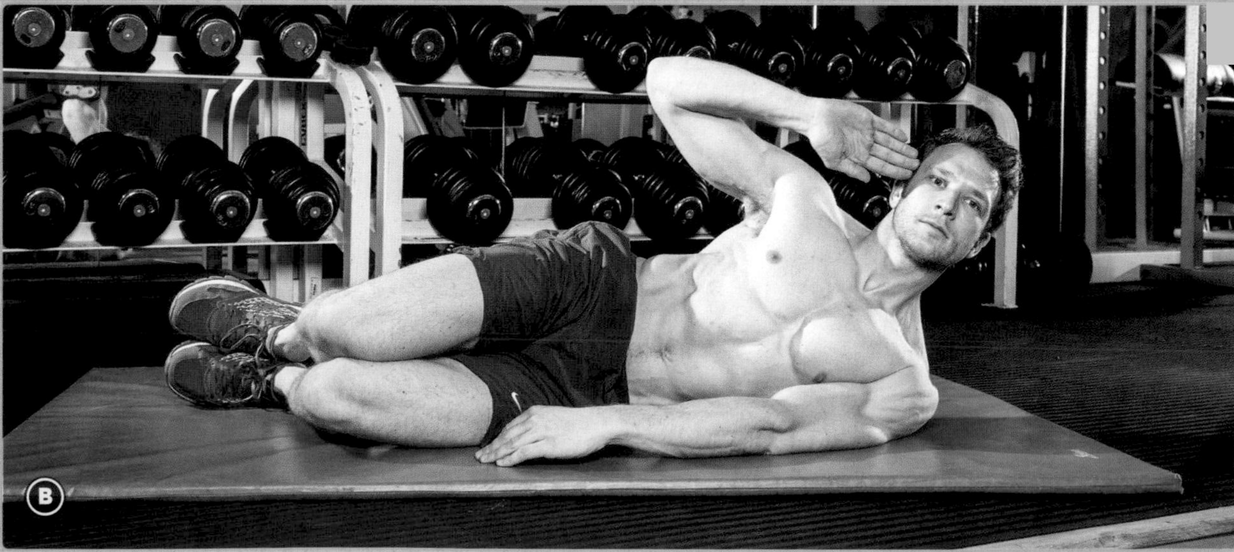

- Lie on your side on a mat with your knees bent.
- Crunch your torso up off the floor by squeezing your side abs.
- Pause at the top of the move, squeeze your abs, then slowly lower your torso back to the floor.

Dumbbell side bend

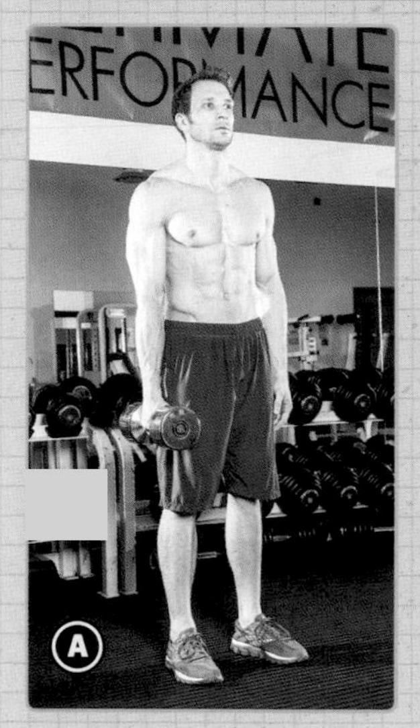

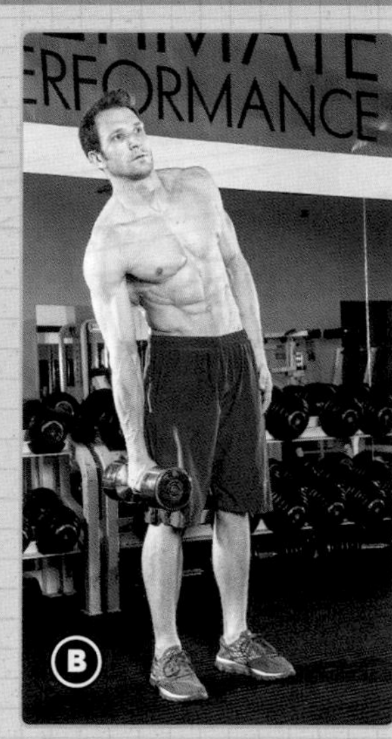

Increase the resistance you place on your obliques by holding a dumbbell in one hand and leaning towards the floor on the same side.

One-arm med ball slam

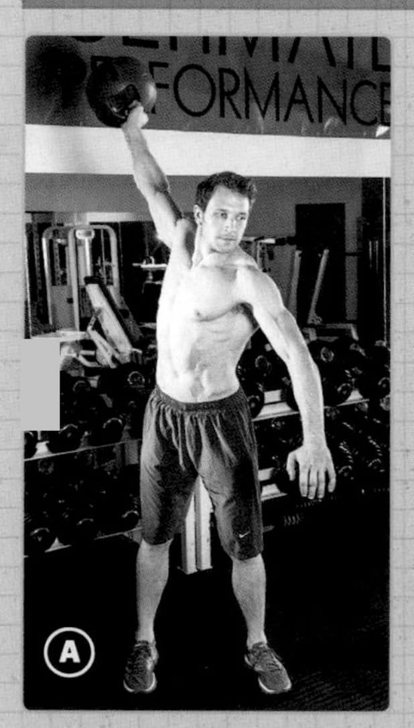

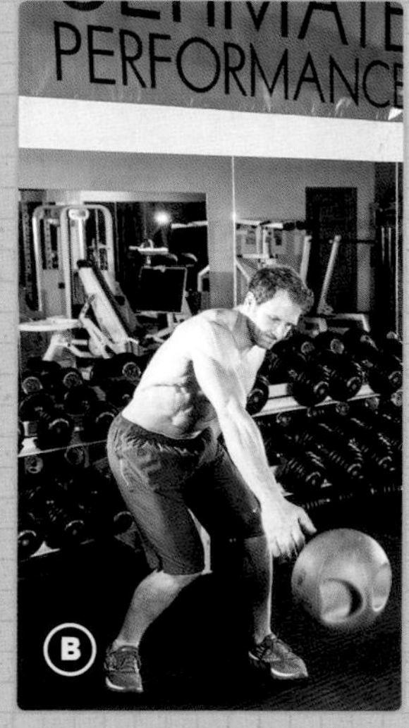

Holding a medicine ball in one hand above your head and explosively throwing it across your body and to floor fires up the fast-twitch muscle fibres of your obliques.

Gym ball oblique crunch

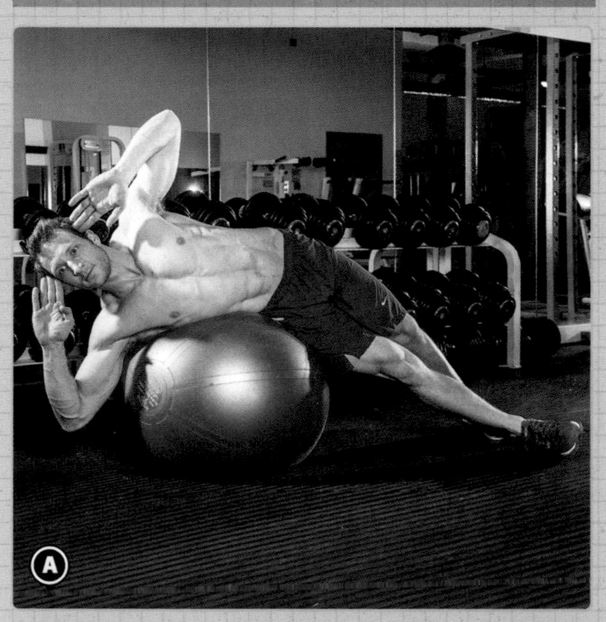

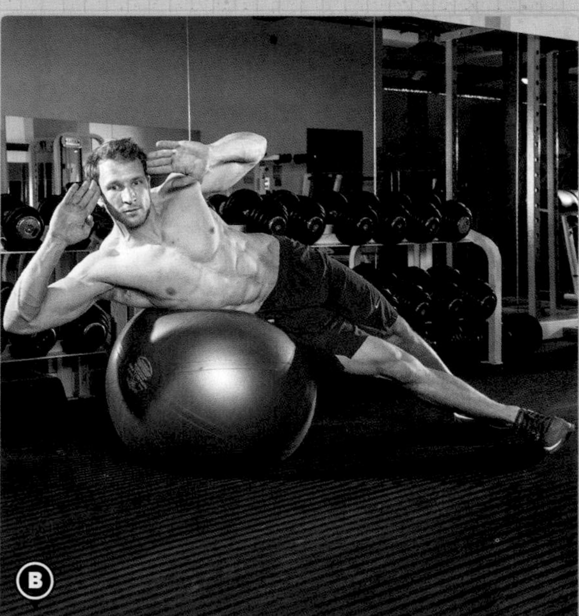

Using a gym ball allows for a greater range of motion to work your muscles, as well as activating your deep-lying core muscles to stabilise your body.

CROSSOVER CRUNCH

***Targets** Abs*

Adding a twist to the crunch works your abs and obliques in one simple move

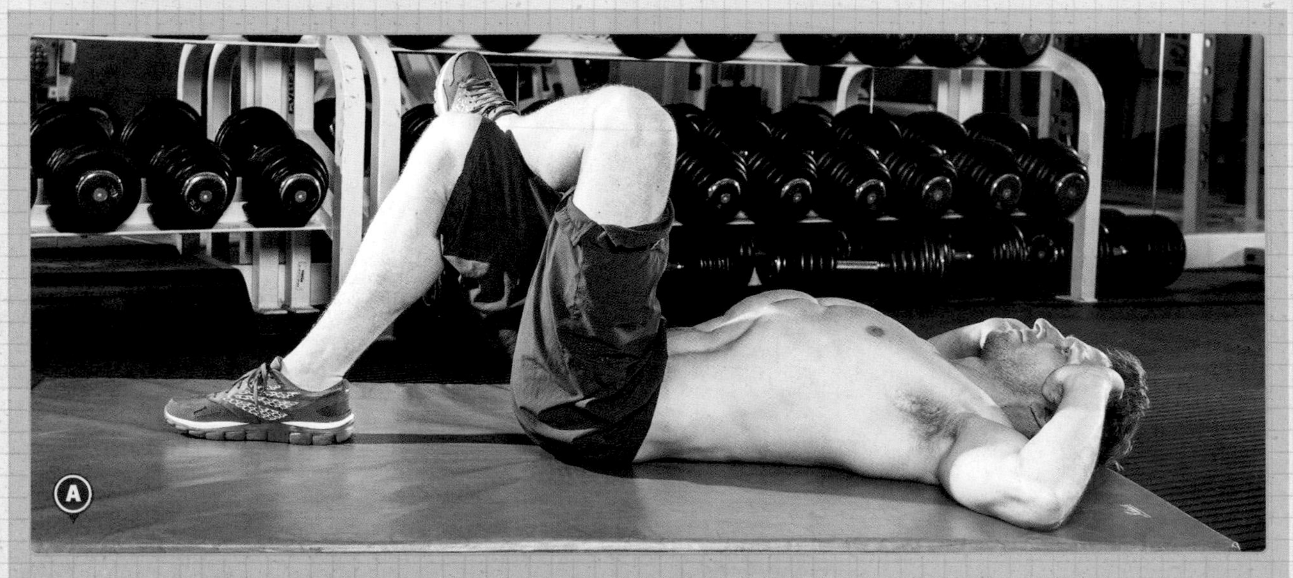

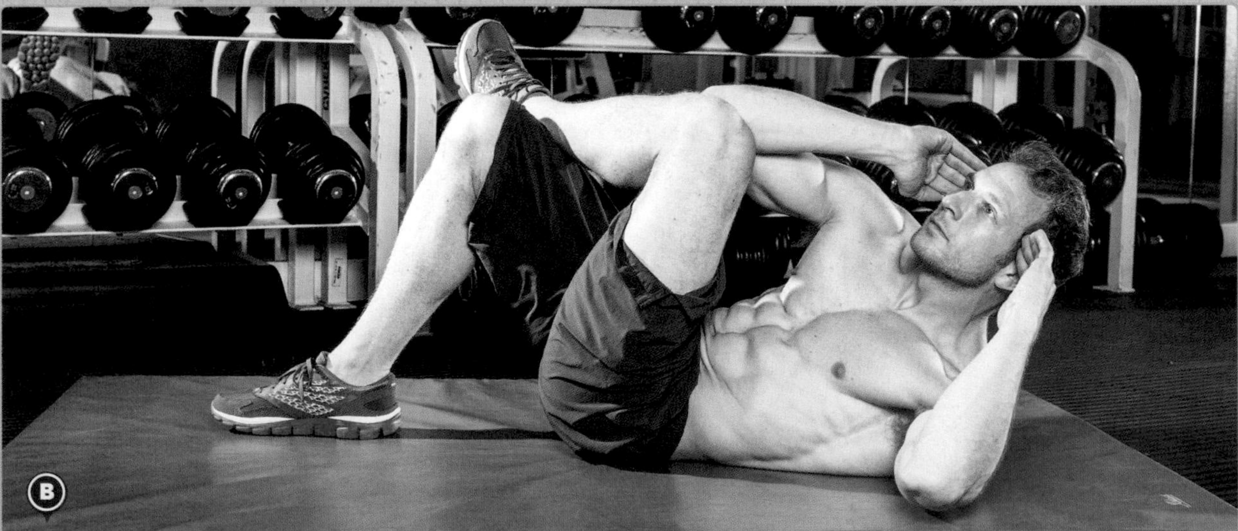

- Lie flat on a mat with your hands by your temples. Bend one leg and place that foot flat on the floor and bend your other leg and rest that foot on the opposite knee.
- Contract your abs to lift your upper back off the ground.
- As you crunch up, twist your torso so your elbow meets your knee.
- Pause at the top of the move, squeeze your abs, then slowly lower your torso back towards the floor.

Bicycle

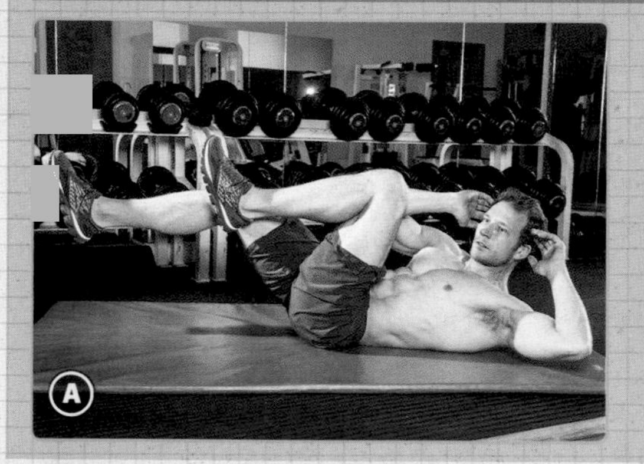
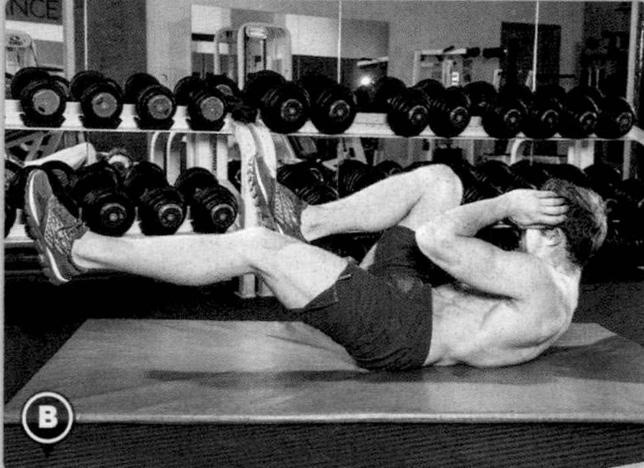

Crunching up to make opposite knees and elbows meet works your abs and obliques. Do them quickly and keep tension on your abs throughout.

Gym ball twist crunch

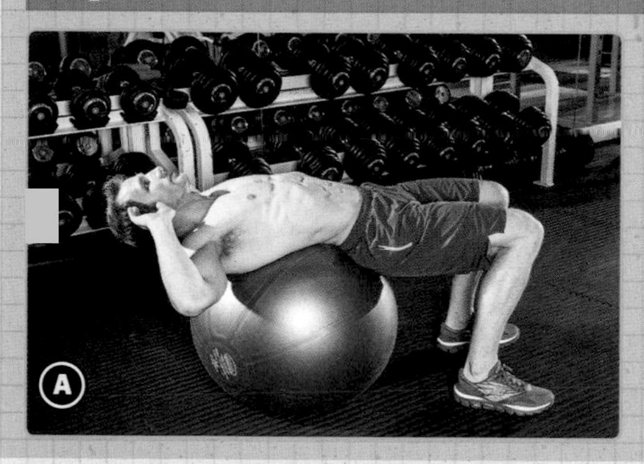
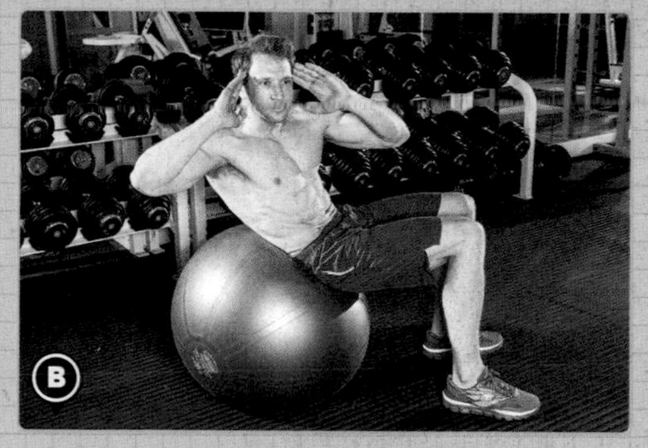

The instability of the gym ball recruits the entire core while also allowing for a greater range of motion.

One-arm cable cross crunch

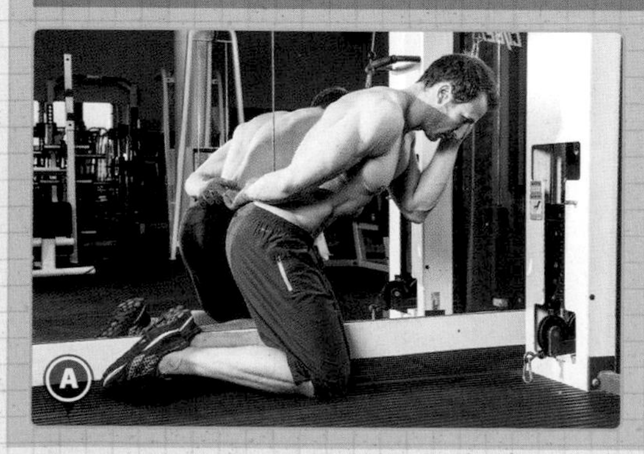
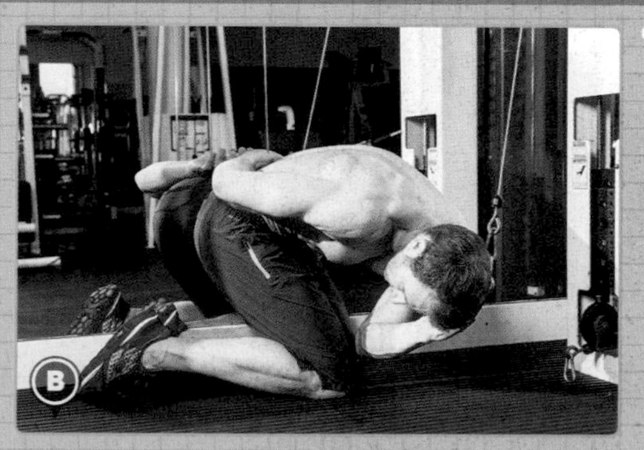

Crunch and twist against the constant resistance of a cable to work your entire midsection hard.

HANGING KNEE RAISE

***Targets* Lower abs**

A tough exercise that mainly works your lower abs but also activates the rest of your core to prevent your body swinging

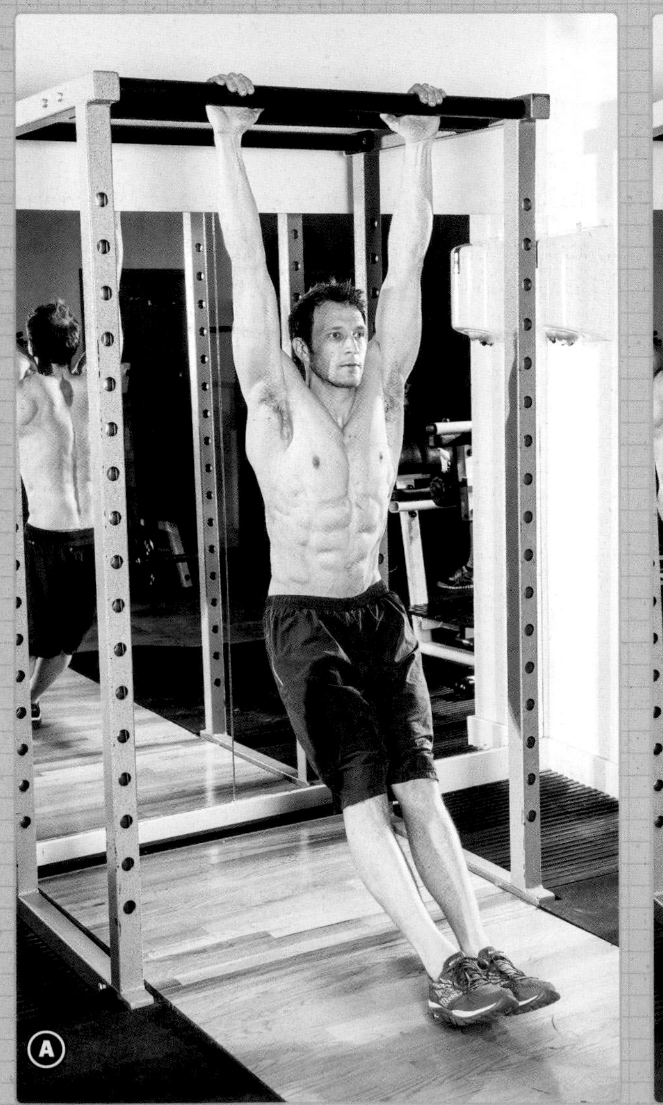

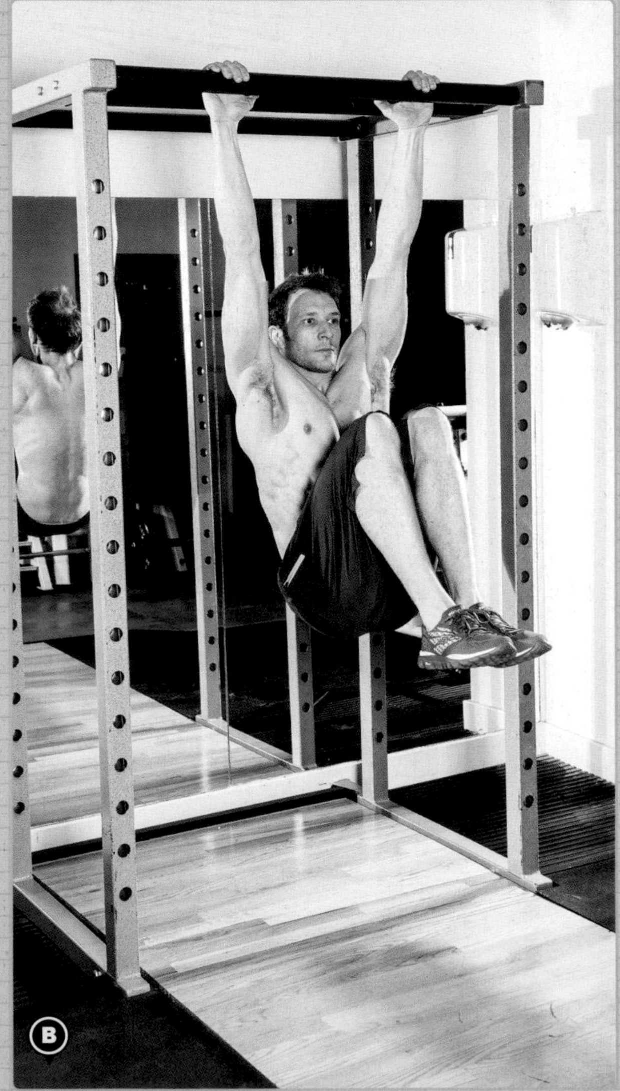

- Hang from a bar with your body straight.
- Bend your knees and draw them up by contracting your abs until your knees are almost touching your chest.
- Hold briefly then slowly lower back to the start.

Twisting knee raise

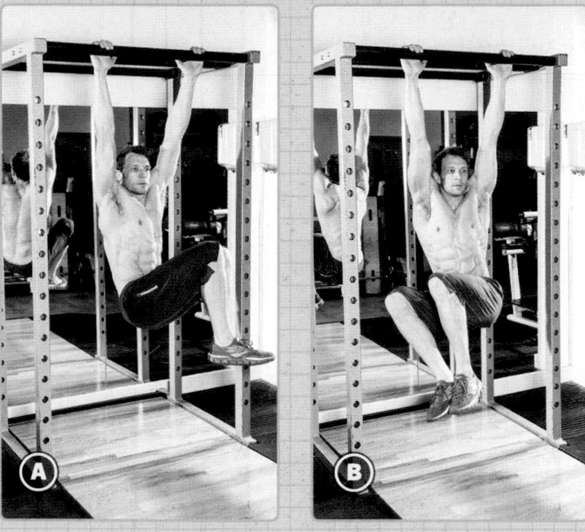

Bringing your knees up then twisting them to the sides brings your obliques into play.

Hanging leg raise

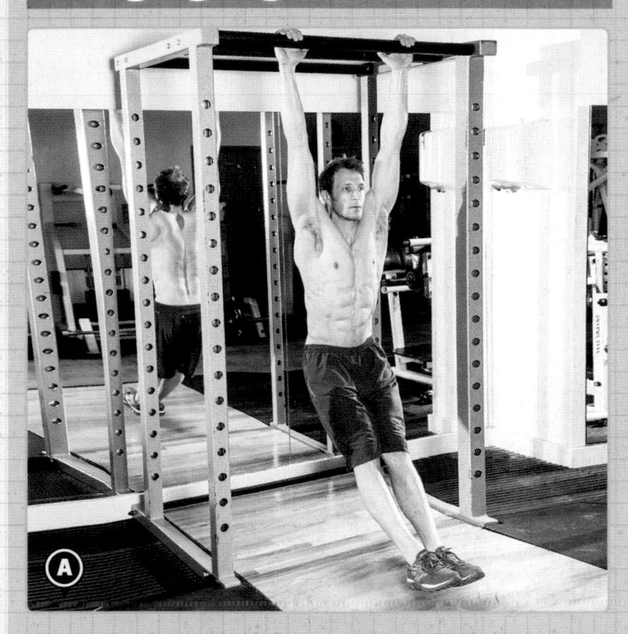

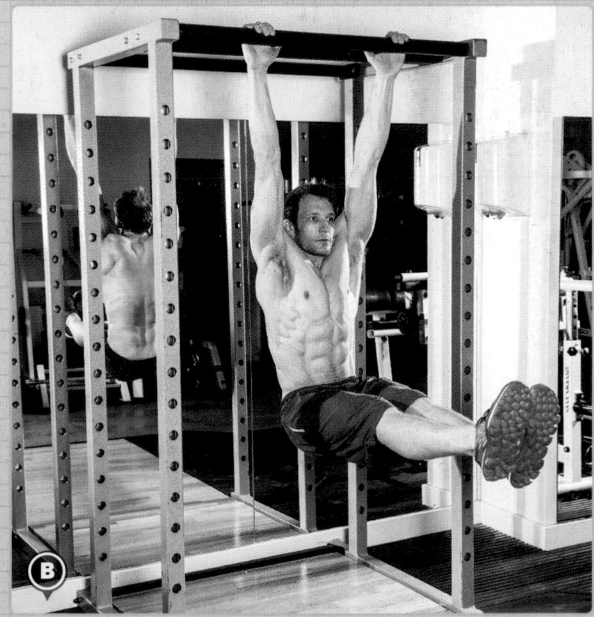

Keeping you legs straight throughout the move makes your lower abs and core work harder.

Medicine ball knee raise

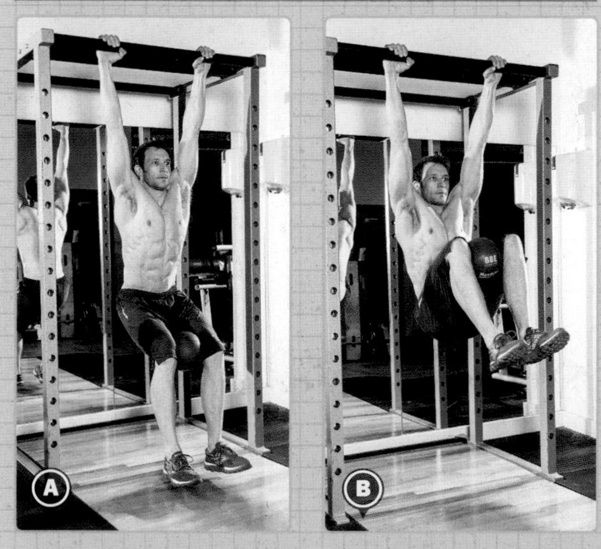

The additional weight of the medicine ball between your knees increases the workload your abs must manage.

TOES TO BAR

***Targets** Abs*

Raising your feet to meet your hands then lowering them slowly recruits all the major muscles of the abs, making this a very tough but rewarding move

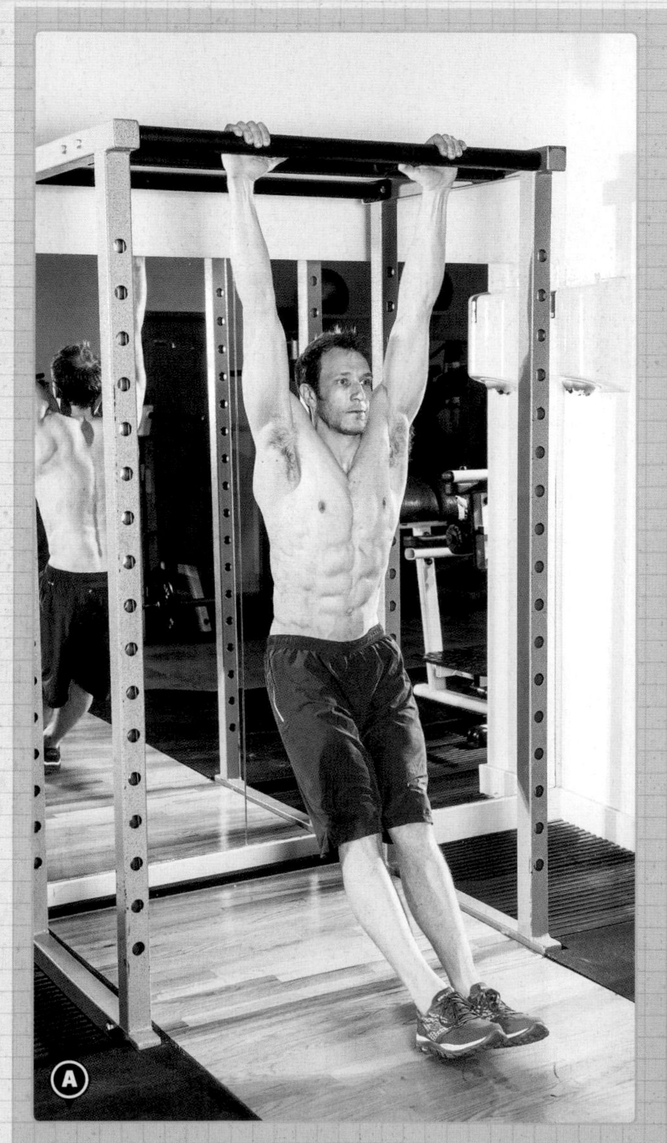

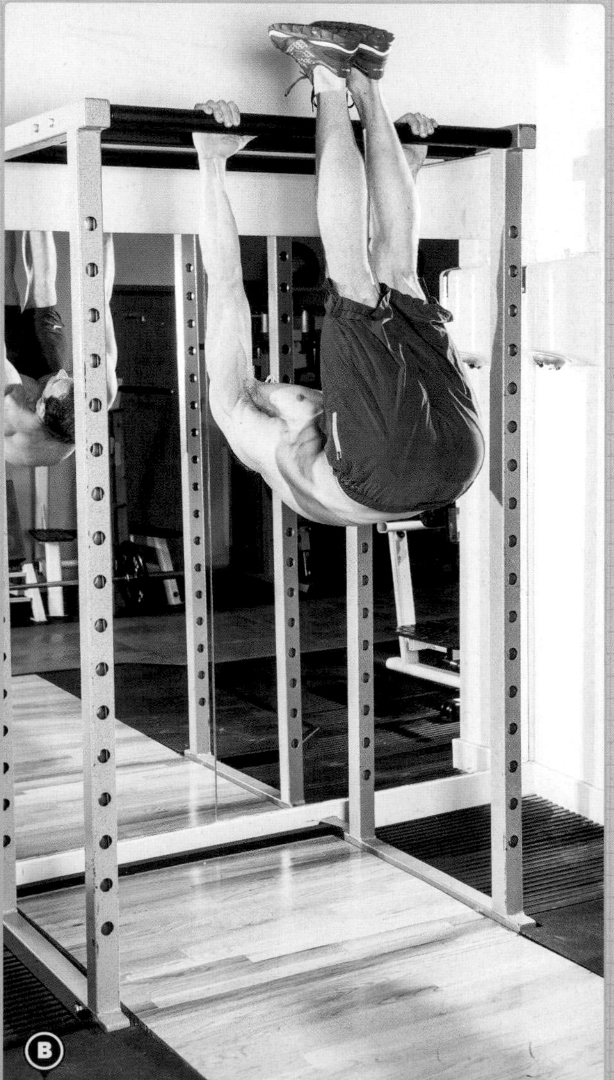

- Hang from a bar with your body straight.
- Keeping your legs straight, contract your abs to raise your feet above the bar.
- Hold briefly then slowly lower back to the start.

Windscreen wiper

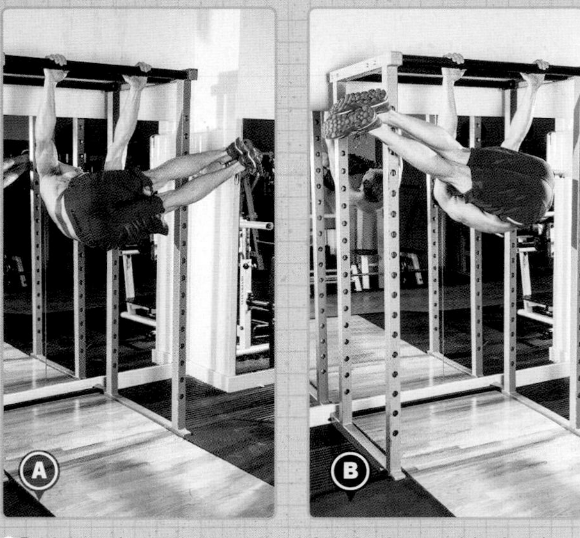

Raising your legs and rotating them left then right is tough but hugely effective at targeting your abs, obliques and other core muscles.

Garhammer raise

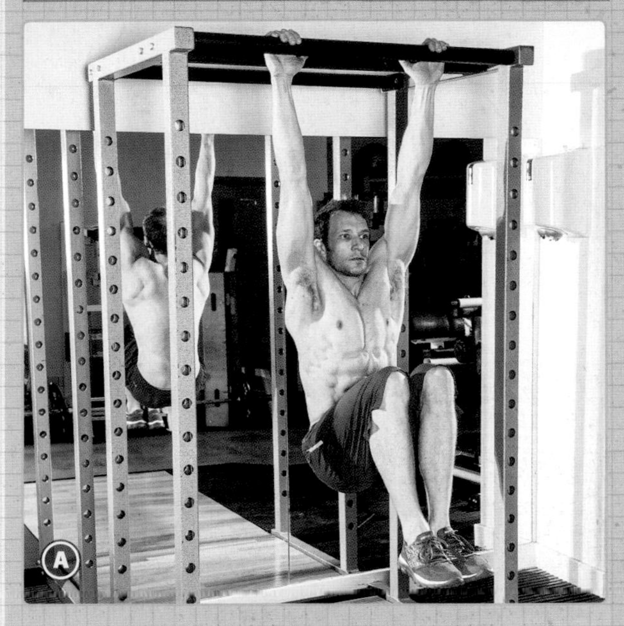

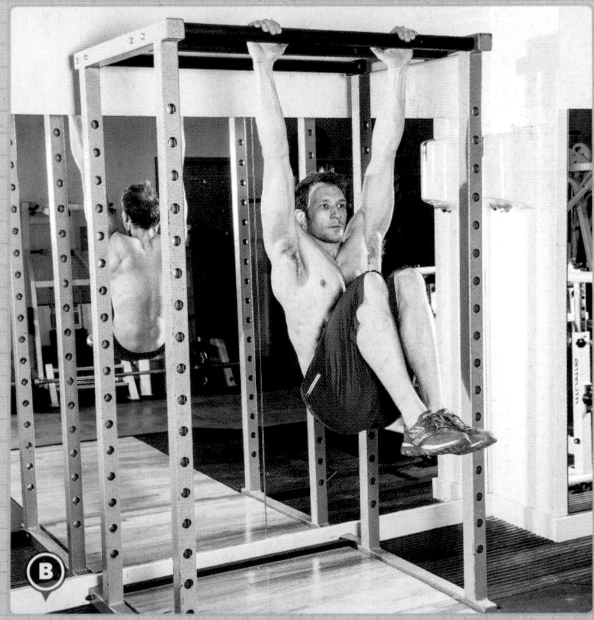

Quickly raising your bent legs towards your chest then back down again makes this a high-rep move that rapidly fatigues your abs.

Isometric leg raise

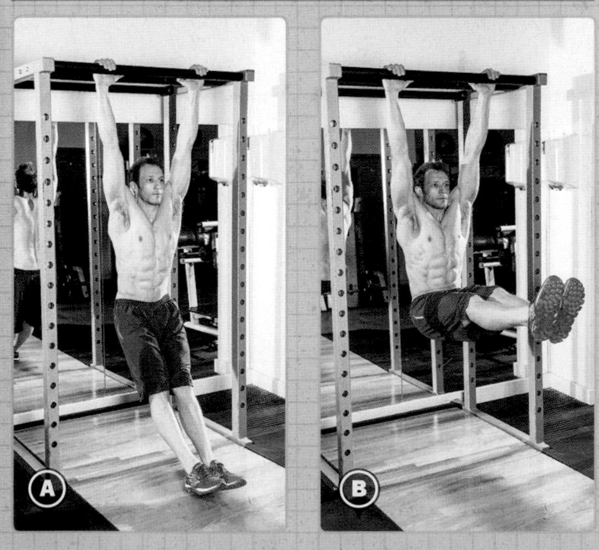

Holding your legs straight at a 90° angle to your body places your abs under a great deal of tension, which forces them to grow stronger.

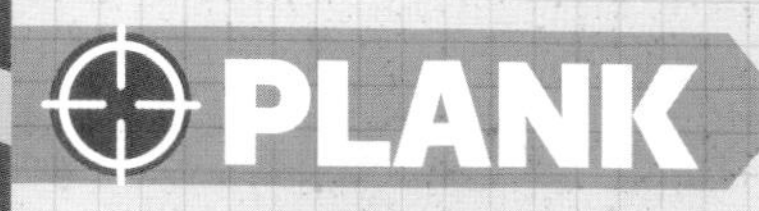

PLANK

***Targets* Core**

Maintaining your body in a straight line works your core and lower back to build better posture, increase muscle mass and improve power transfer between your upper and lower body

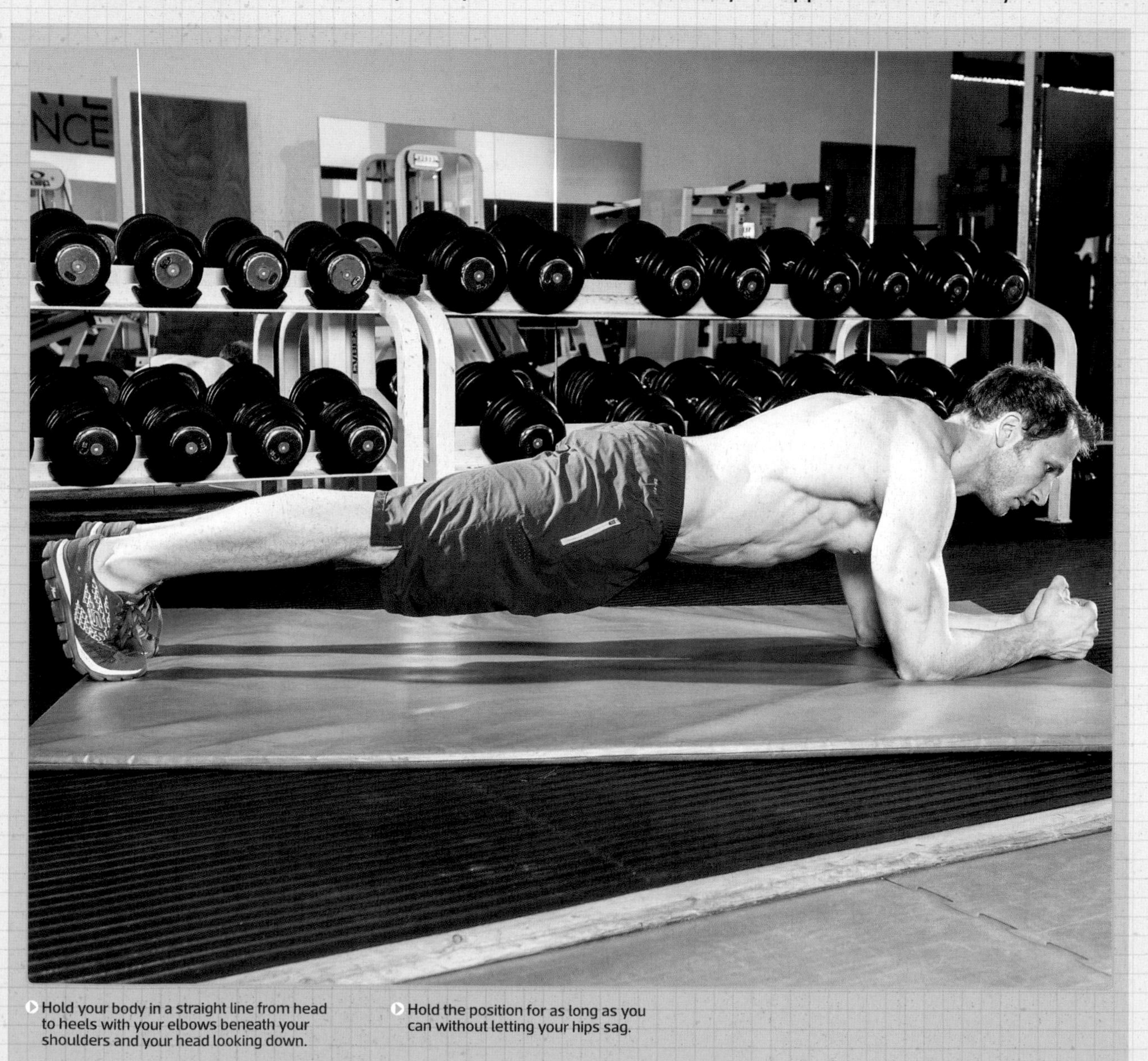

- Hold your body in a straight line from head to heels with your elbows beneath your shoulders and your head looking down.
- Hold the position for as long as you can without letting your hips sag.

Decline plank with alternate foot touch

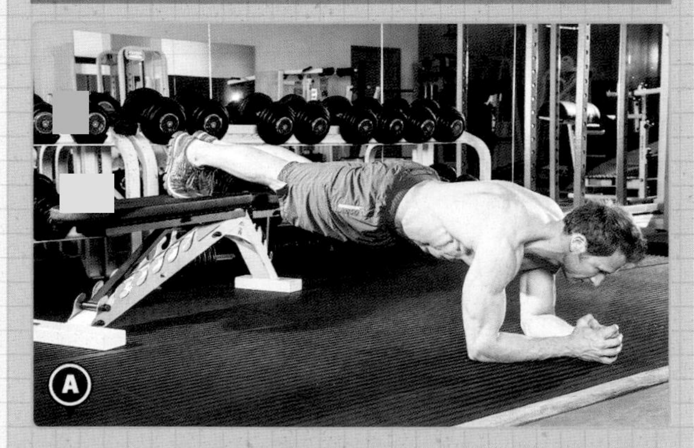

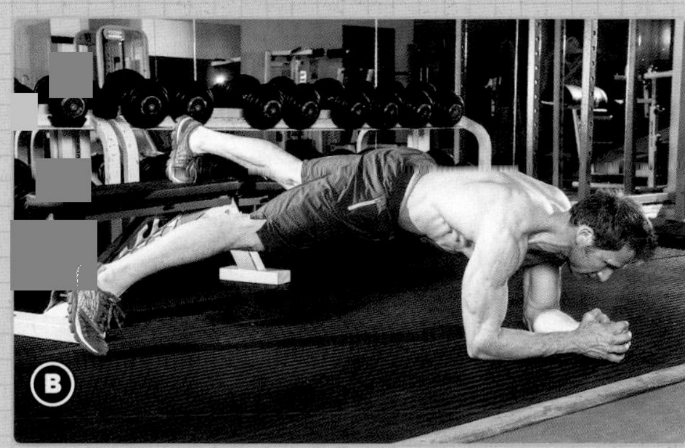

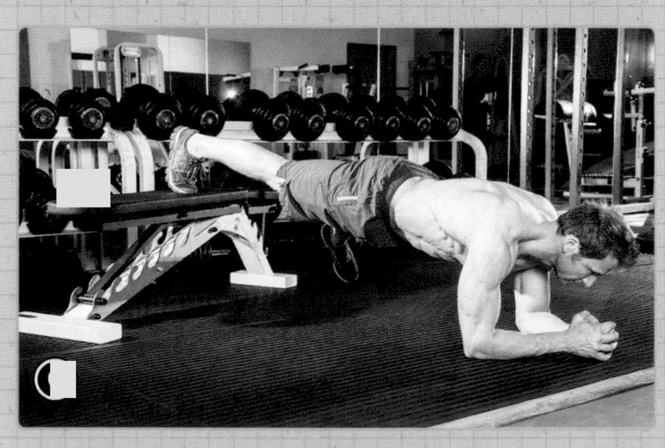

Starting with your feet in a raised position, then lifting one leg at a time and slowly lowering it to the floor, works the entire core region.

Decline plank

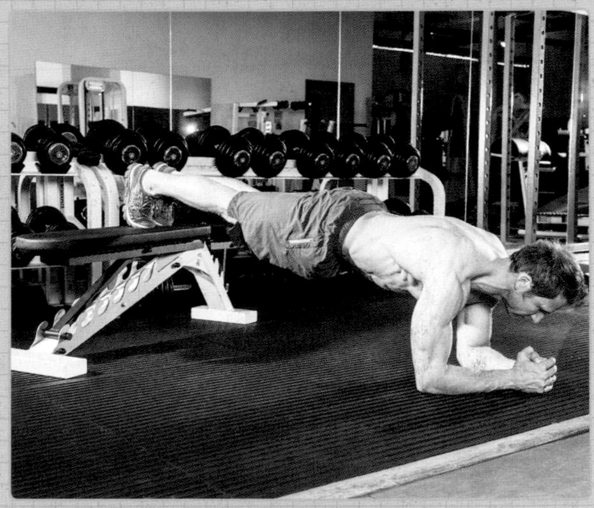

Elevating your feet increases the amount of bodyweight your abs must manage throughout the move, making this a more advanced version for building core strength.

Incline plank

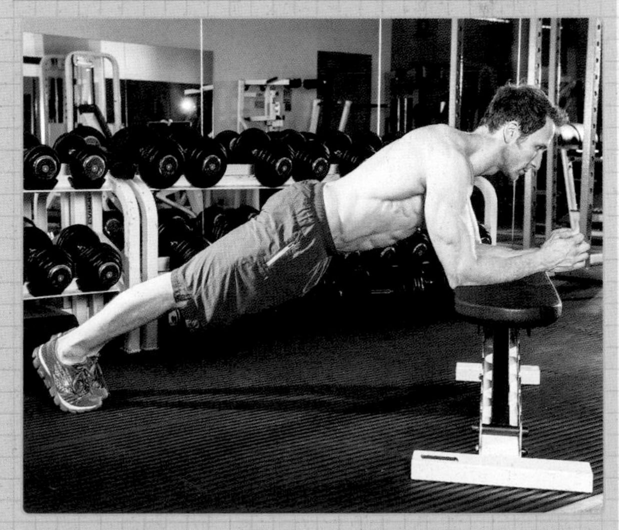

Resting your elbows above your feet reduces the amount of bodyweight your abs have to manage, making this a great foundation move for improving core strength.

SIDE PLANK

***Targets** Core*

Build a strong link between your upper and lower body and work your obliques with this twist on this classic stability move

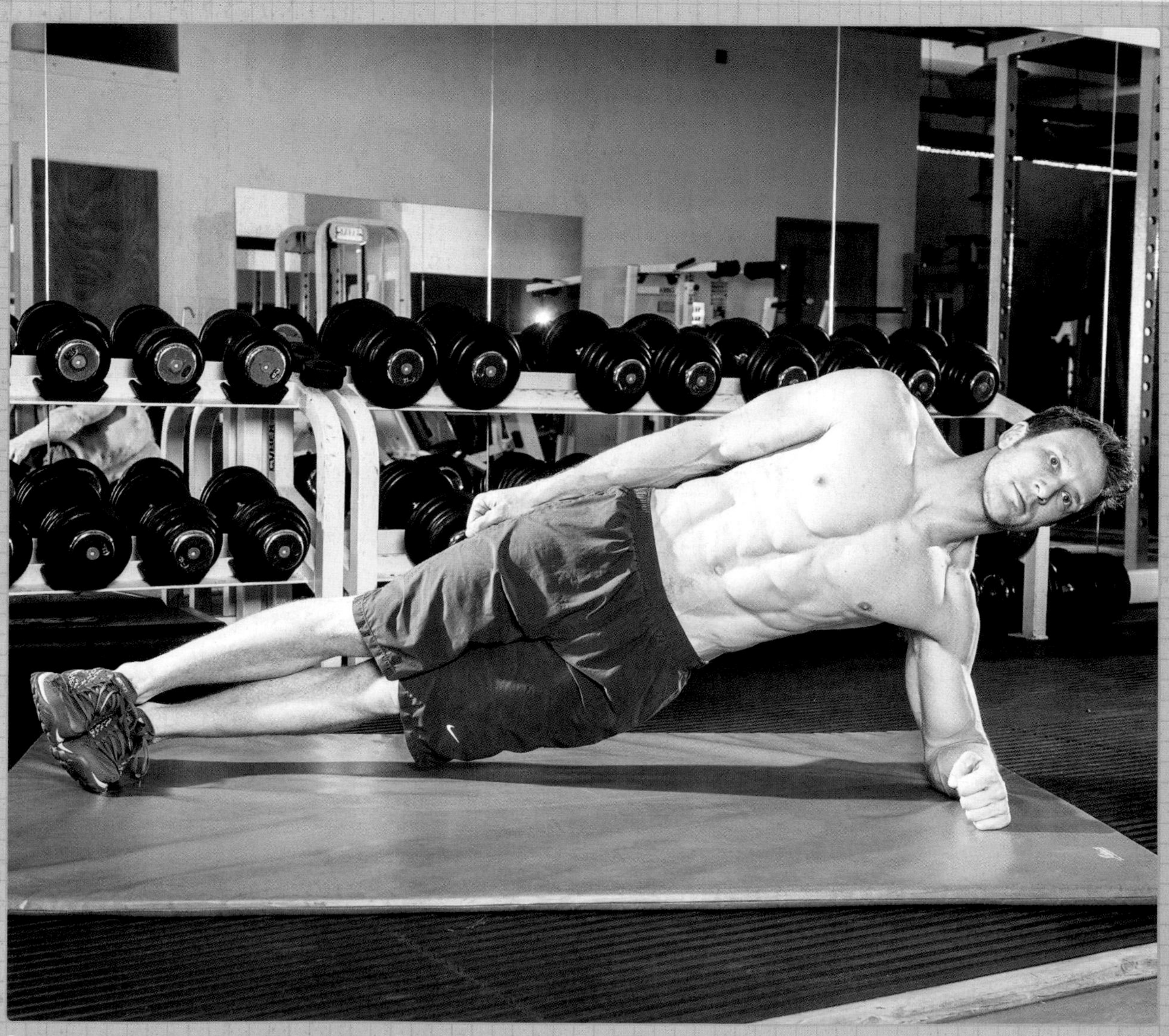

- Hold your body in a straight line from head to heels with one elbow directly beneath your shoulder and your legs together.
- Hold the position for as long as you can without letting your hips sag.

Side-plank star

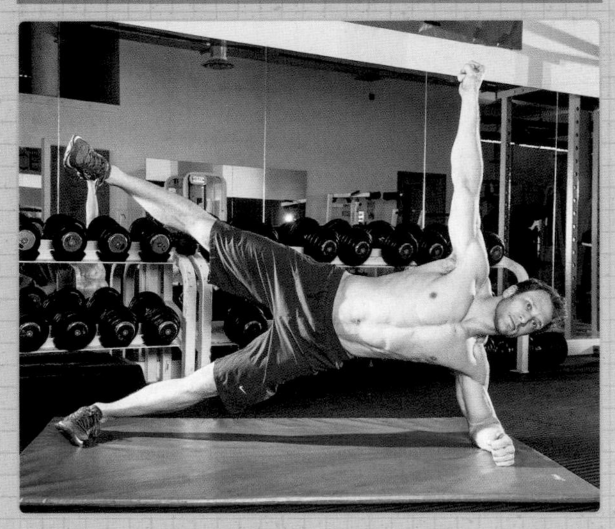

Lifting up one leg and arm at the same time increases the tension placed on your core to maintain balance.

Gym ball side plank

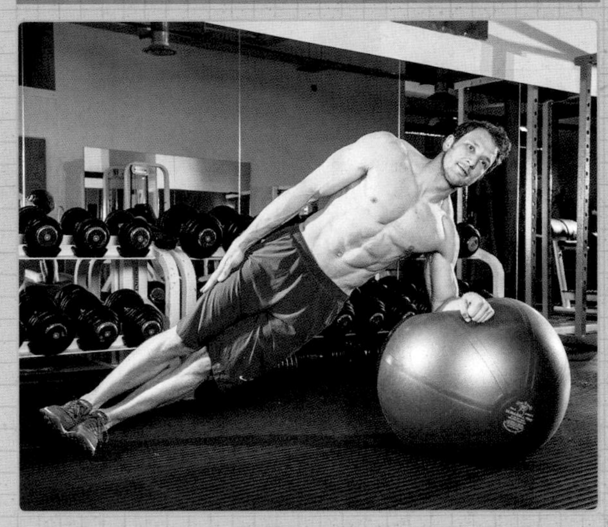

The instability of the gym ball makes every muscle of your core work together to keep your body balanced and stable.

Side plank with lateral raise

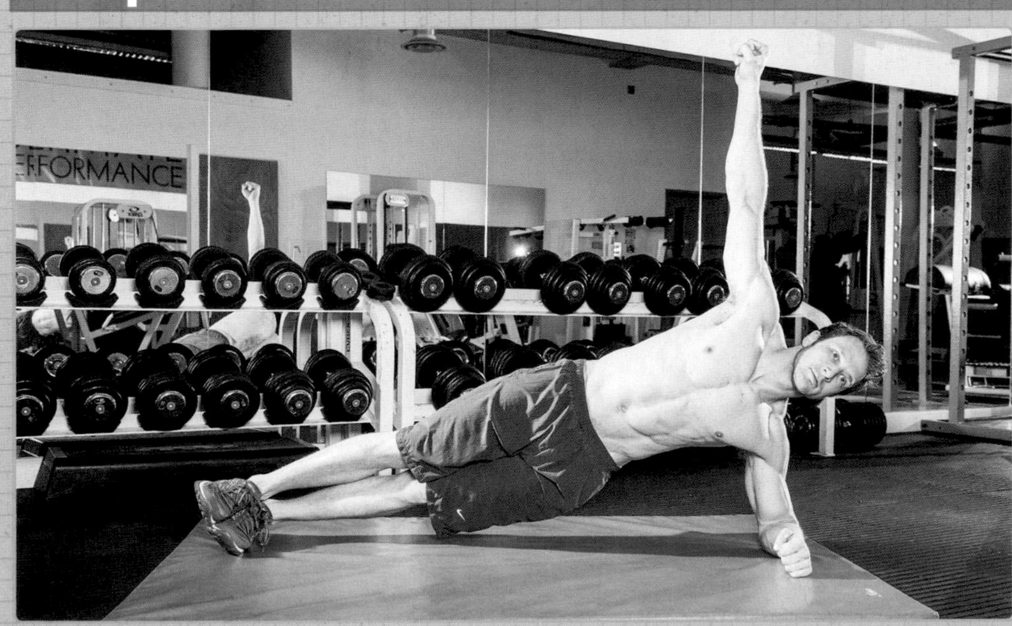

Raising one arm requires your core to work harder to keep your body stable.

BENCH LEG RAISE

***Targets** Abs, hip flexors*

This move works your abs and your hip flexors – the small but important stabilising muscles of your hips – which must work together to raise your legs effectively

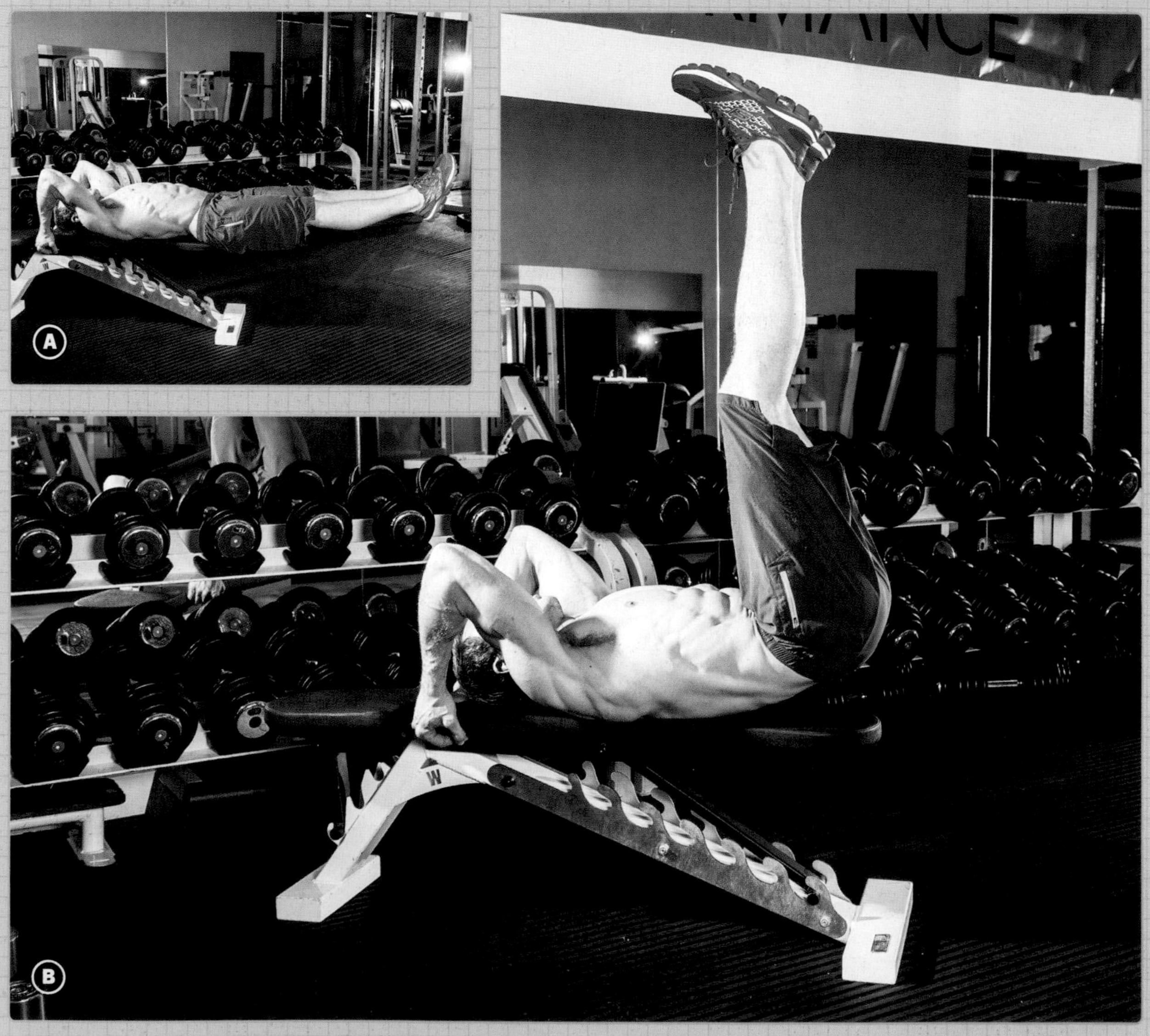

- Lie with your back and thighs on a bench so your lower legs and feet are suspended off the floor.
- Raise your legs until they are almost vertical.
- Contract your abs to raise your hips off the bench, then return slowly to the start position.

Hip raise

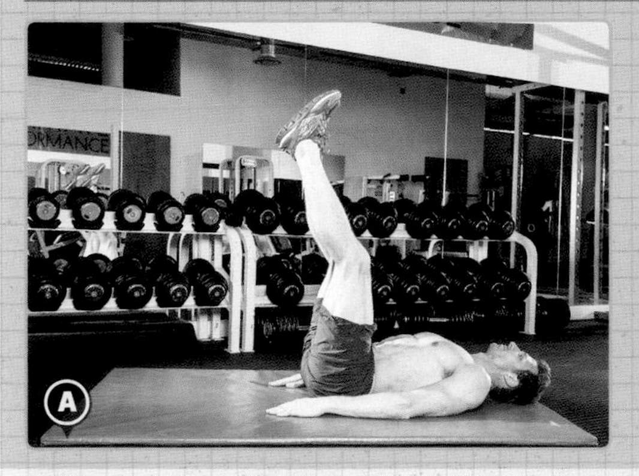

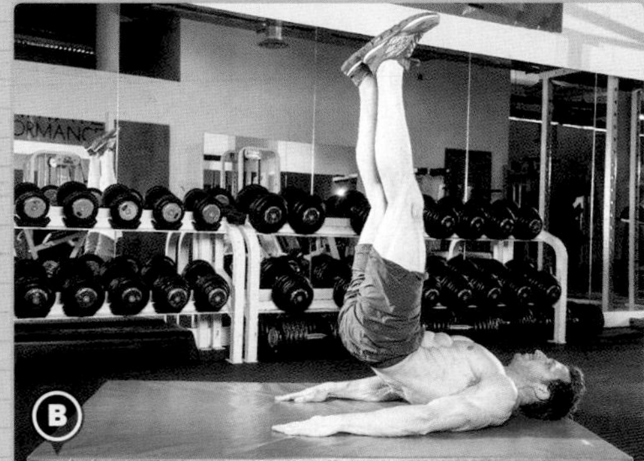

Performing this leg raise on a mat makes it slightly easier but you should still lift your hips off the floor to work the target muscles.

Medicine ball leg raise and hold

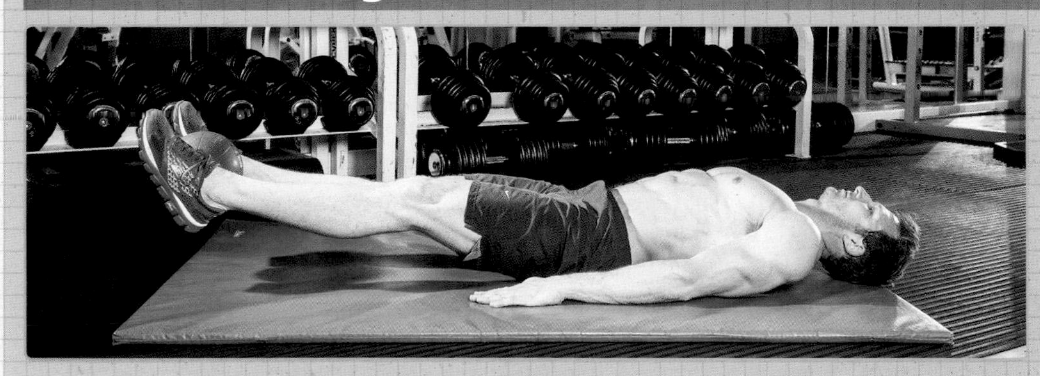

Holding your legs off the floor with a medicine ball between your feet places major tension on your abs.

Medicine ball leg raise

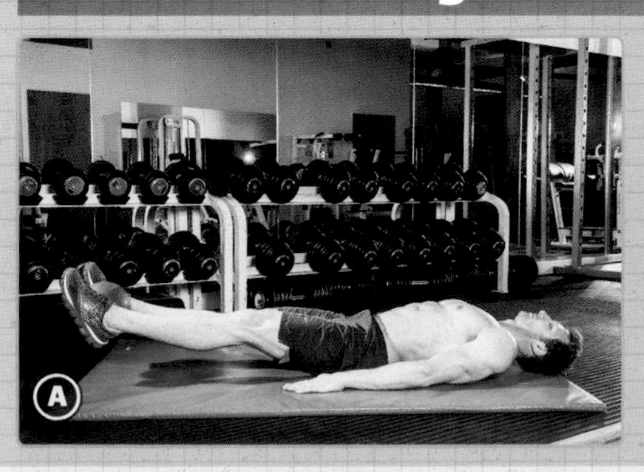

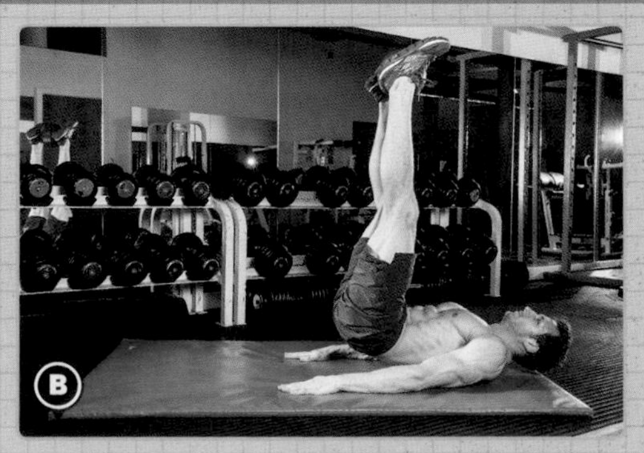

Holding the additional weight of a medicine ball between your feet works your muscles on the way up and the way down.

JACKKNIFE

***Targets** Upper and lower abs*

Test your abs with this advanced move that requires flexibility as well as a strong, tight core

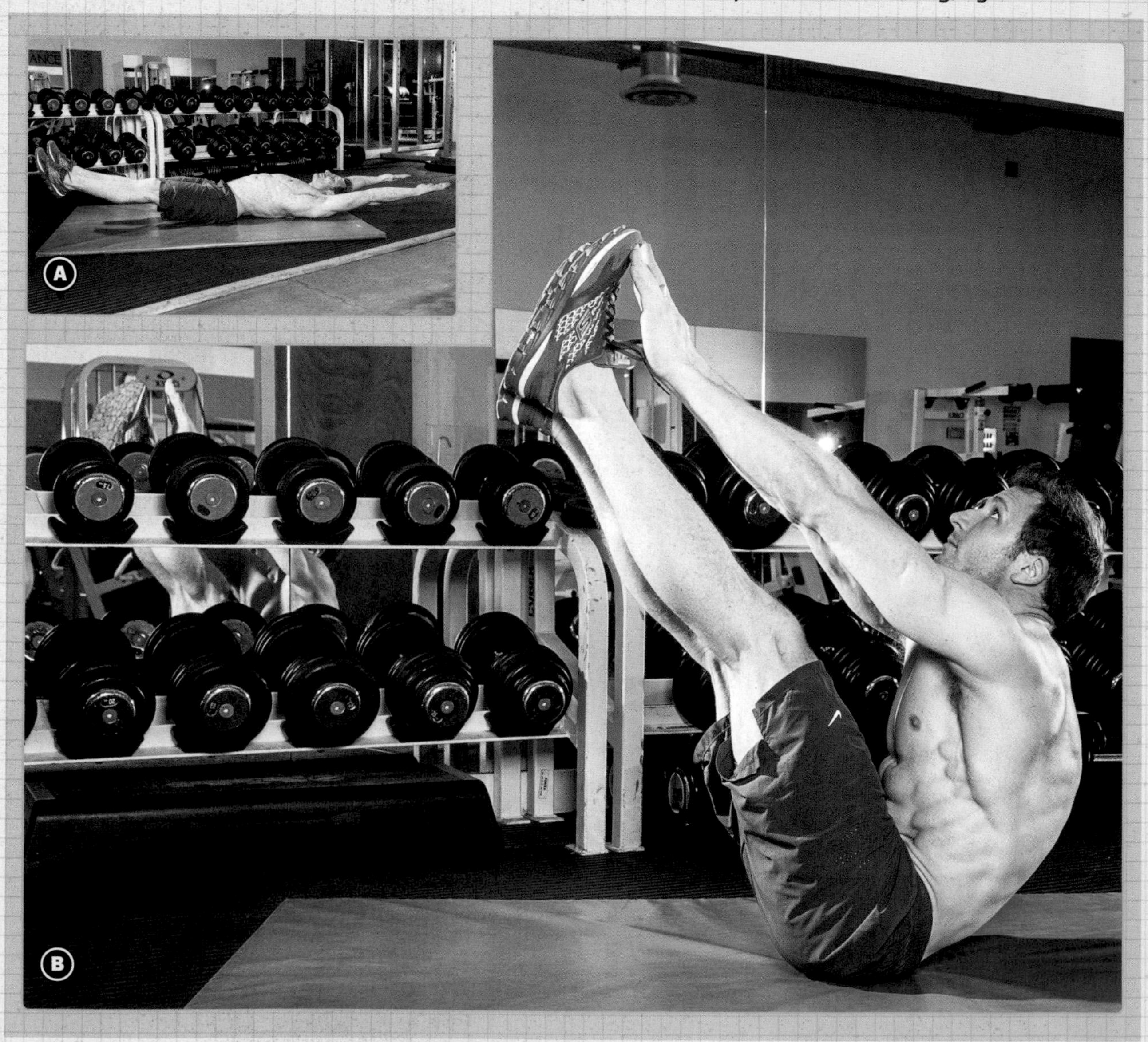

- Lie flat on your back with your arms fully extended and off the floor behind you, and with your legs straight and raised off the ground.
- Contract your abs to raise your arms and legs simultaneously so they meet above your stomach.
- Squeeze your abs in this top position, then slowly lower your arms and legs back down but don't let them touch the ground.

Gym ball jackknife

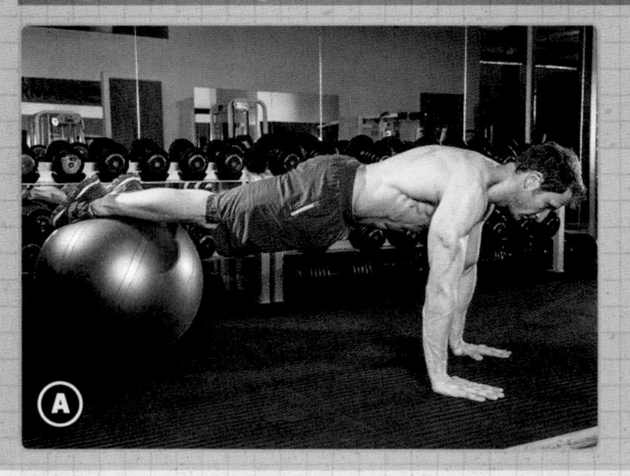

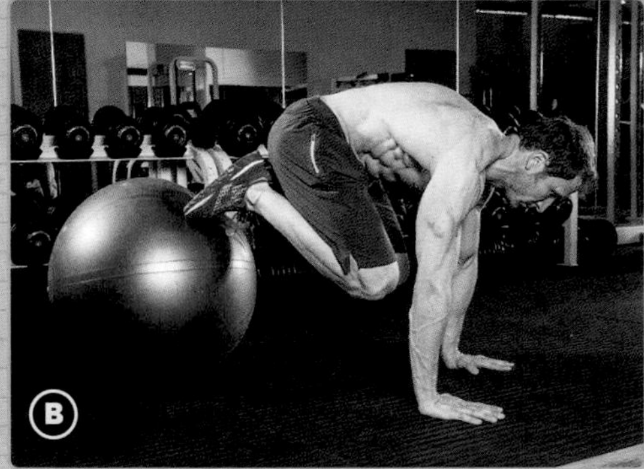

Starting with your feet on a gym ball then using your abs to draw your knees towards your chest forces your core to work hard to maintain balance and stability.

Modified V-sit

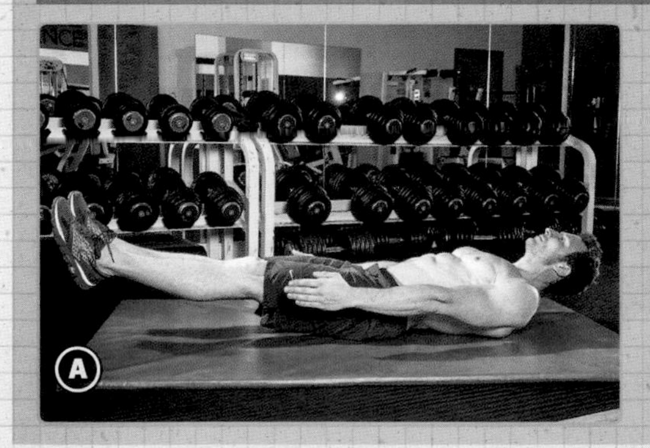

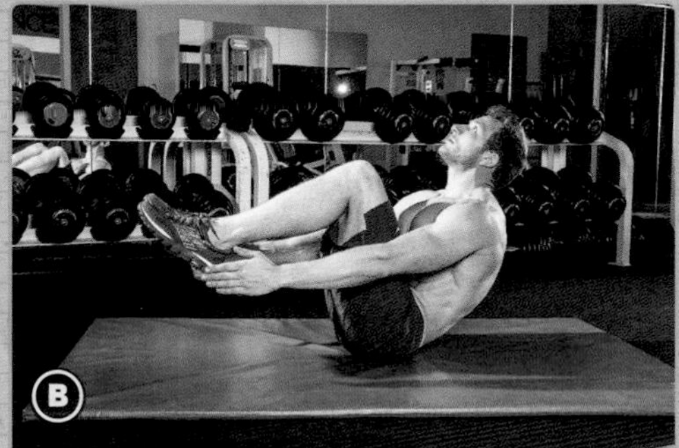

Crunching up while drawing your knees towards your chest is an easier variation of the jackknife but still an effective core-builder.

Gym ball passing jackknife

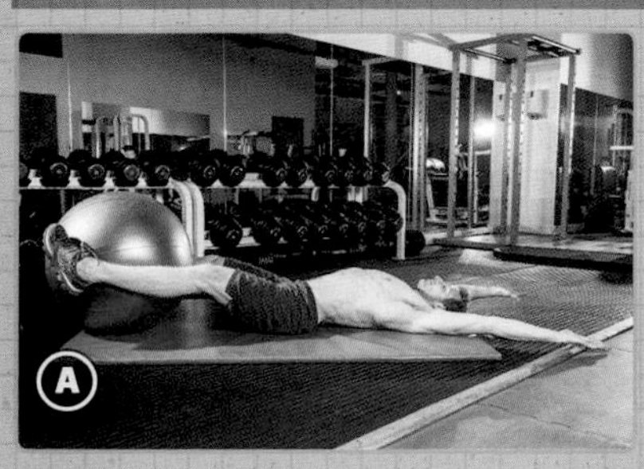

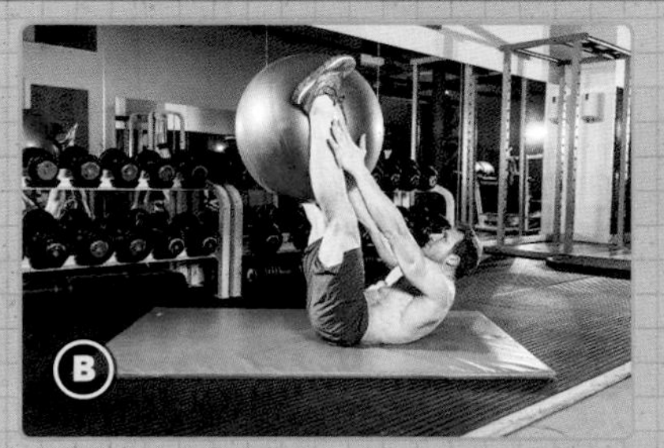

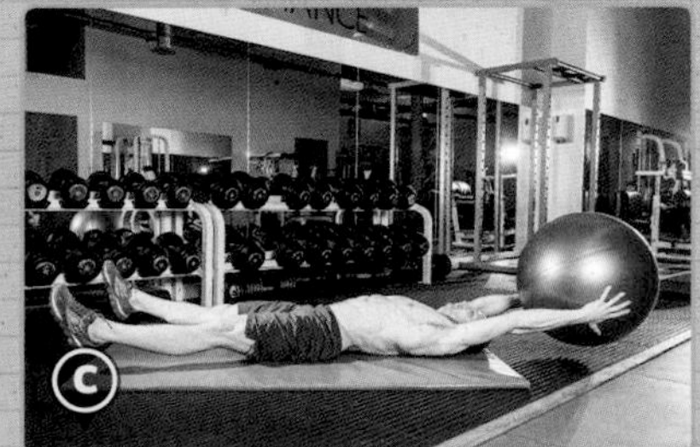

Passing a gym ball from your hands to your feet then back again requires core strength, balance and flexibility.

SEATED RUSSIAN TWIST

***Targets** Abs, obliques*

This rotational move works your entire core with specific emphasis on your obliques as you twist side to side

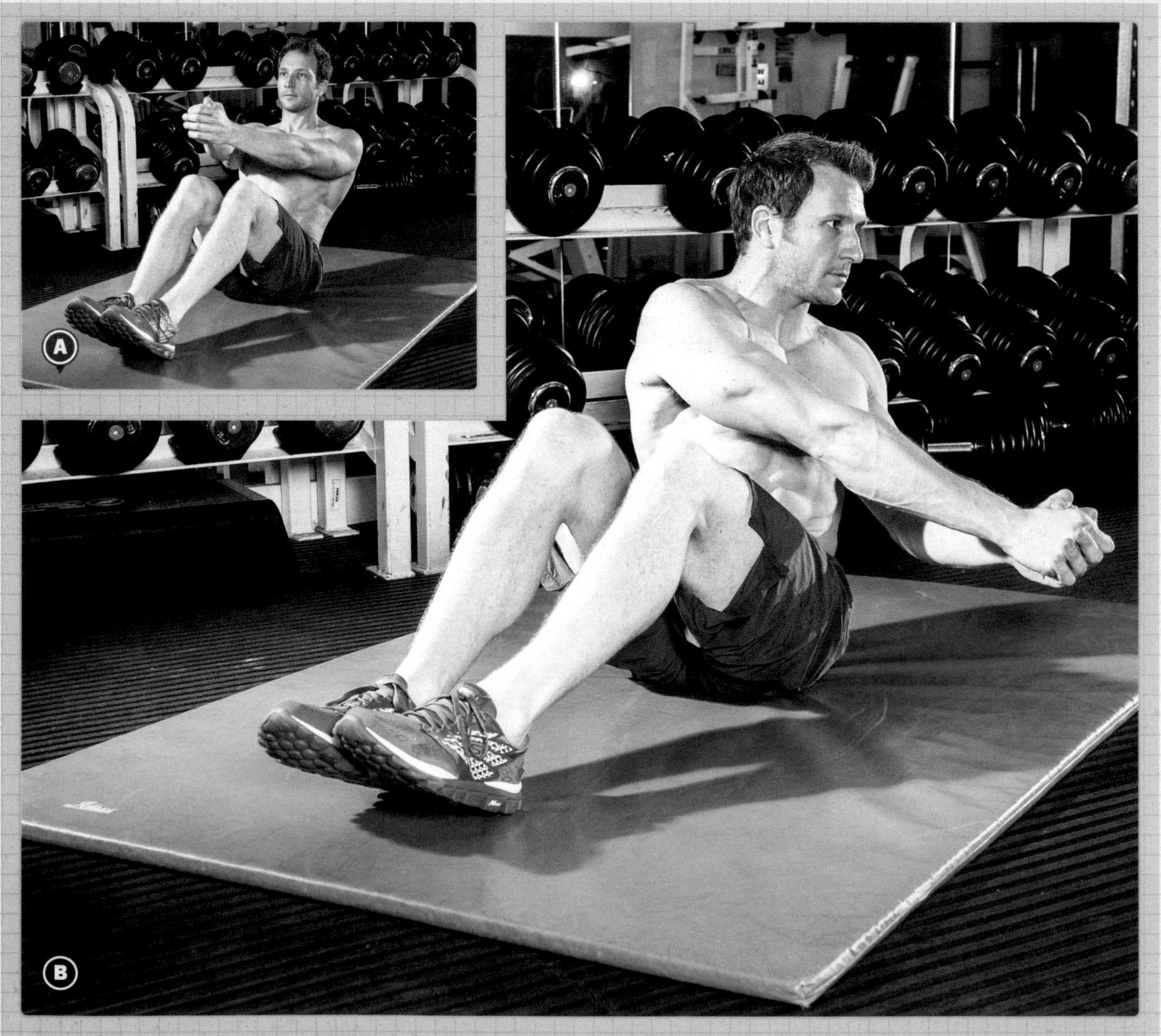

- Sit up with your knees bent, clasping your hands together in front of you at arm's length.
- Twist fully to one side then twist back to the other side, while keeping your torso upright.

Standing cable Russian twist

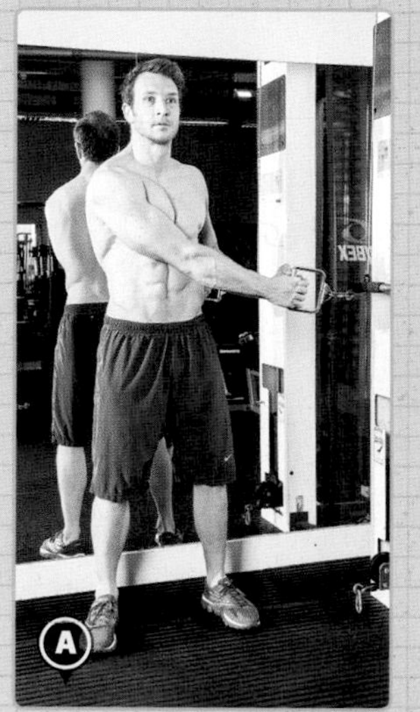

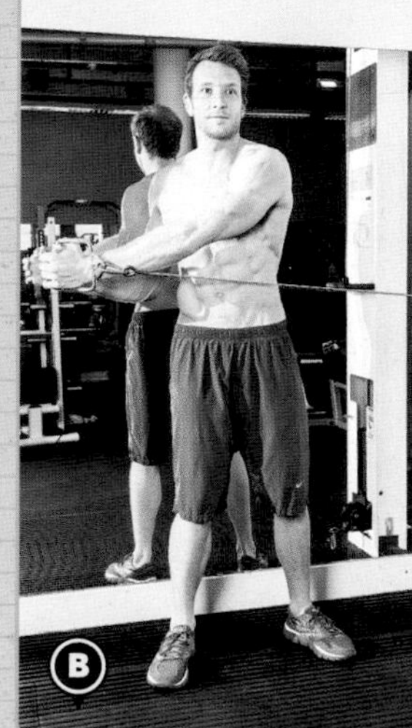

Using a cable places tension on your muscles throughout the move and allows you to increase the weight your muscles must manage.

Gym ball Russian twist

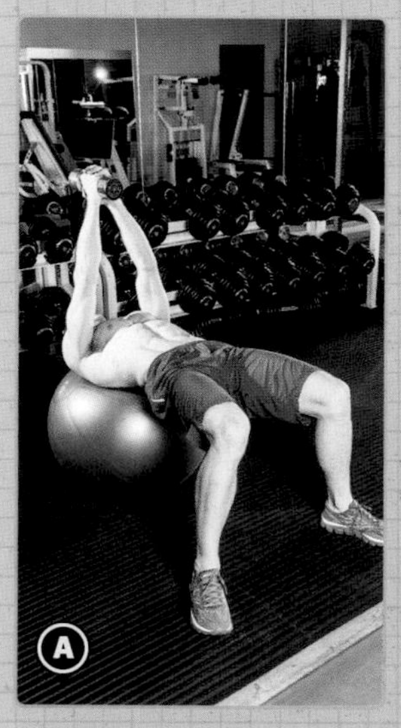

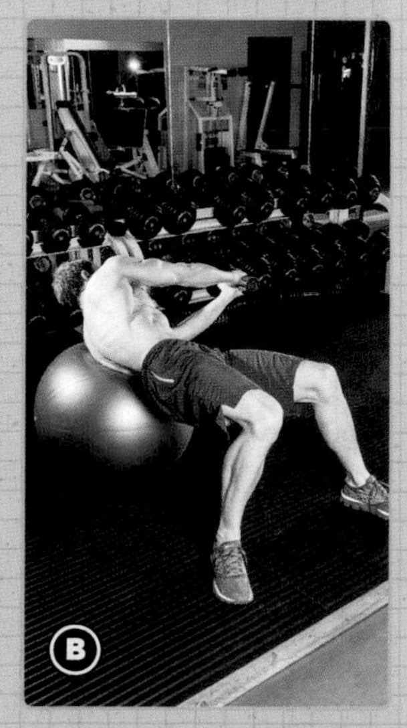

A gym ball makes the move easier on your lower back while allowing for a greater range of motion and the need for your core to work hard to stabilise your body.

Lower-body Russian twist

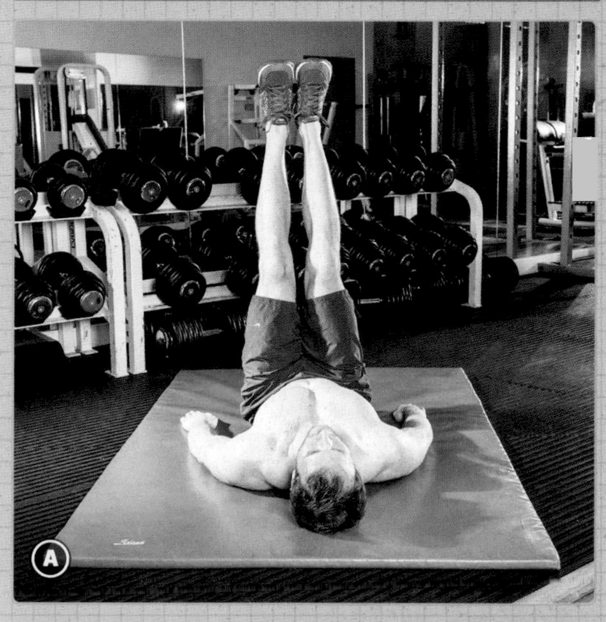

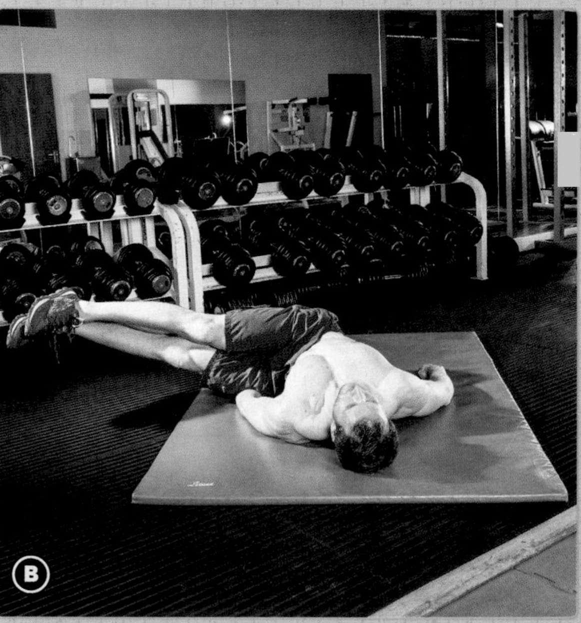

Keeping your back flat on the floor and twisting your straight legs to one side and then the other shifts the emphasis towards your lower abs.

BARBELL ROLLOUT

***Targets* Core**

This tough move works your entire core region, especially those vital deep-lying muscles and your lower back

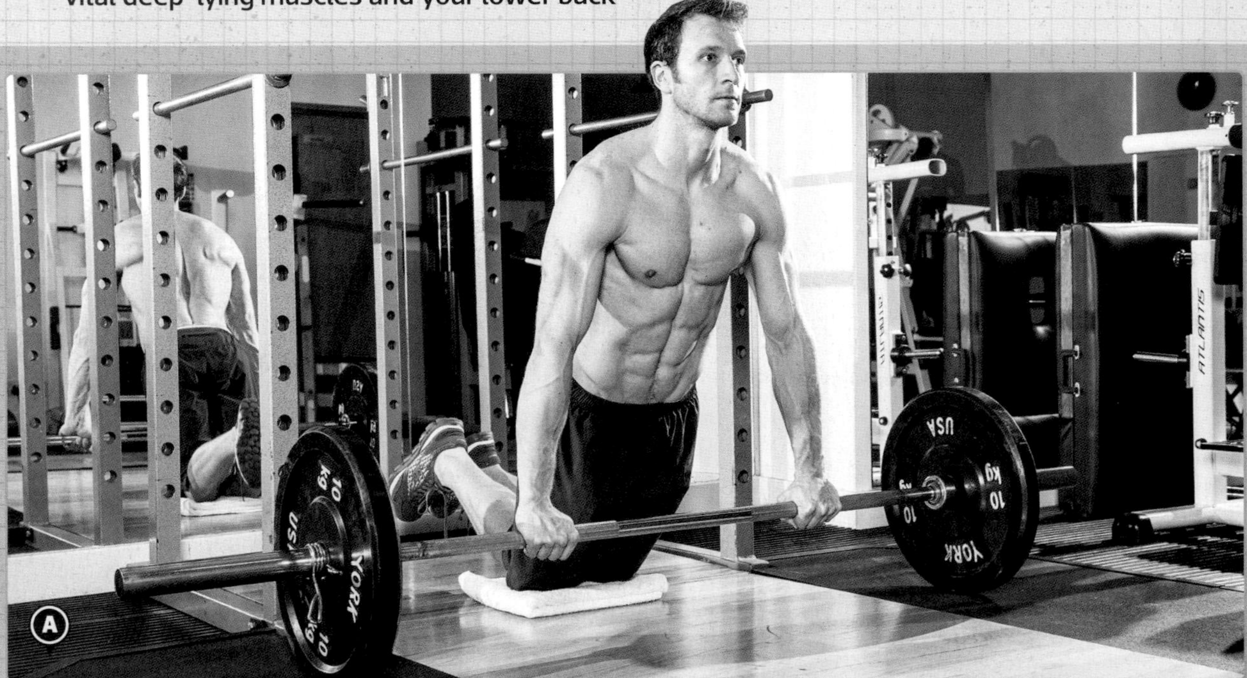

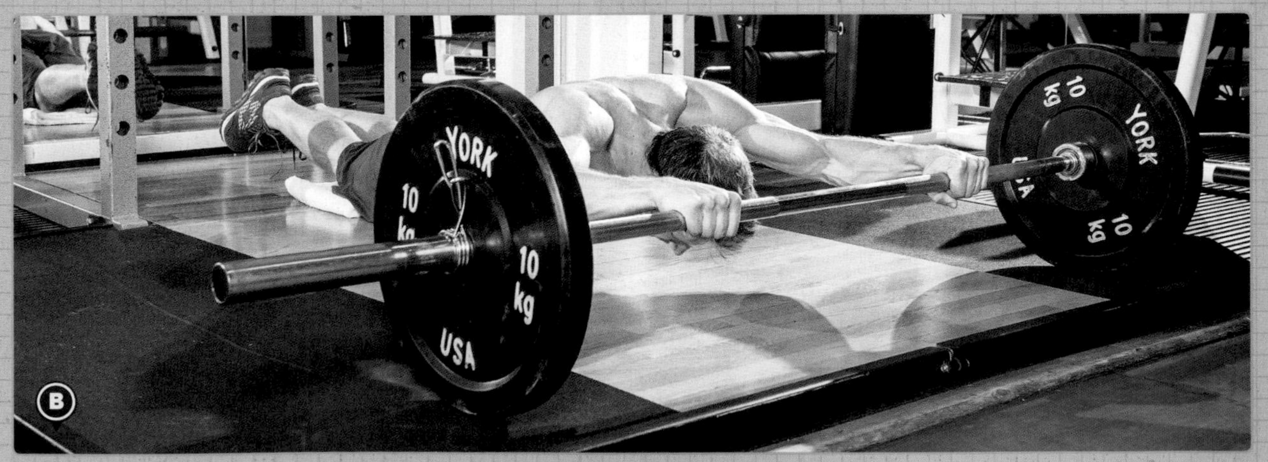

- Get on your knees with your arms extended and your hands holding a barbell with a shoulder-width grip.
- Slowly roll the barbell away from your body, keeping your core braced throughout.
- Slowly roll the barbell back to the start position.

Standing barbell rollout

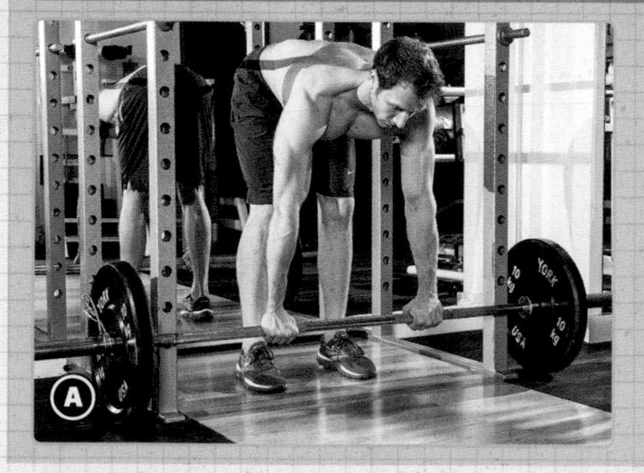

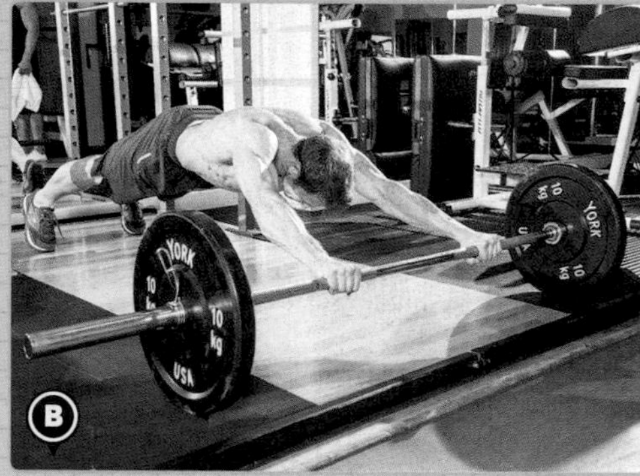

Starting in a standing position then rolling out and back again is one of the hardest, and consequently most effective, moves to work the entire core.

Gym ball rollout

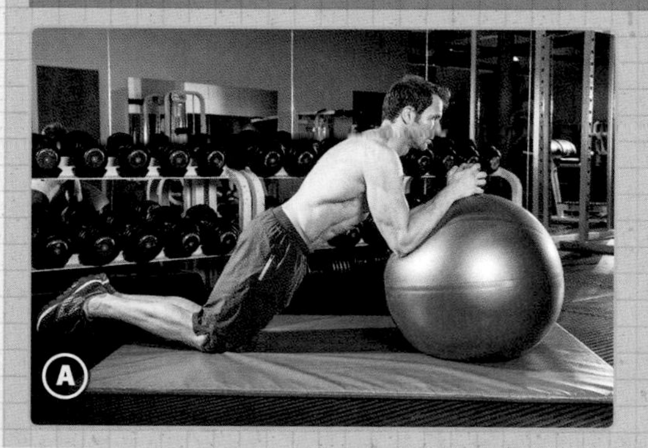

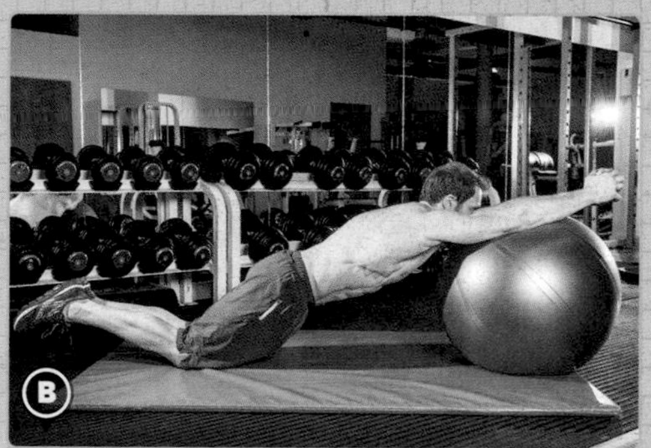

Resting your forearms on a gym ball reduces the strain on your lower back while testing your core to keep your torso stable.

Mountain climber

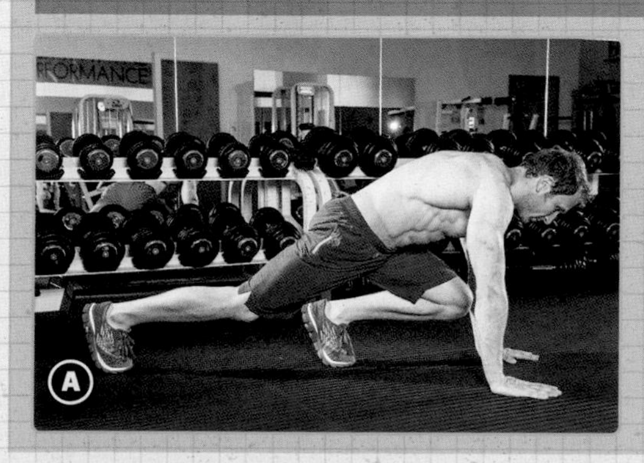

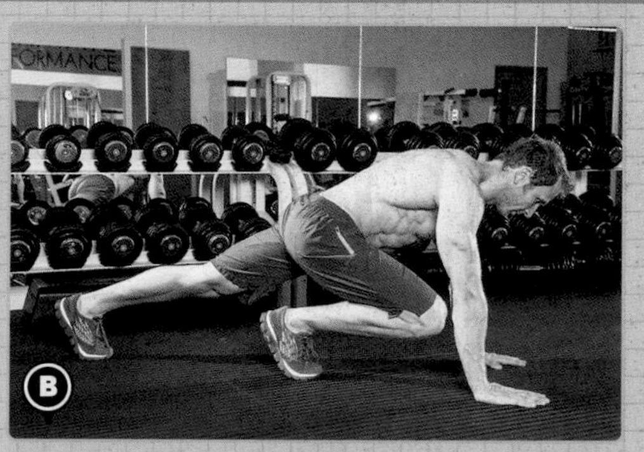

Jumping your feet back and forth quickly is a great beginner's way to build a solid core while sending your heart rate soaring.

WOODCHOP

***Targets** Abs, lower back*

This rotational lift builds a stronger connection between your upper and lower body while also working your legs and shoulders

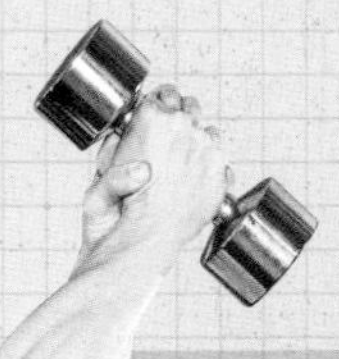

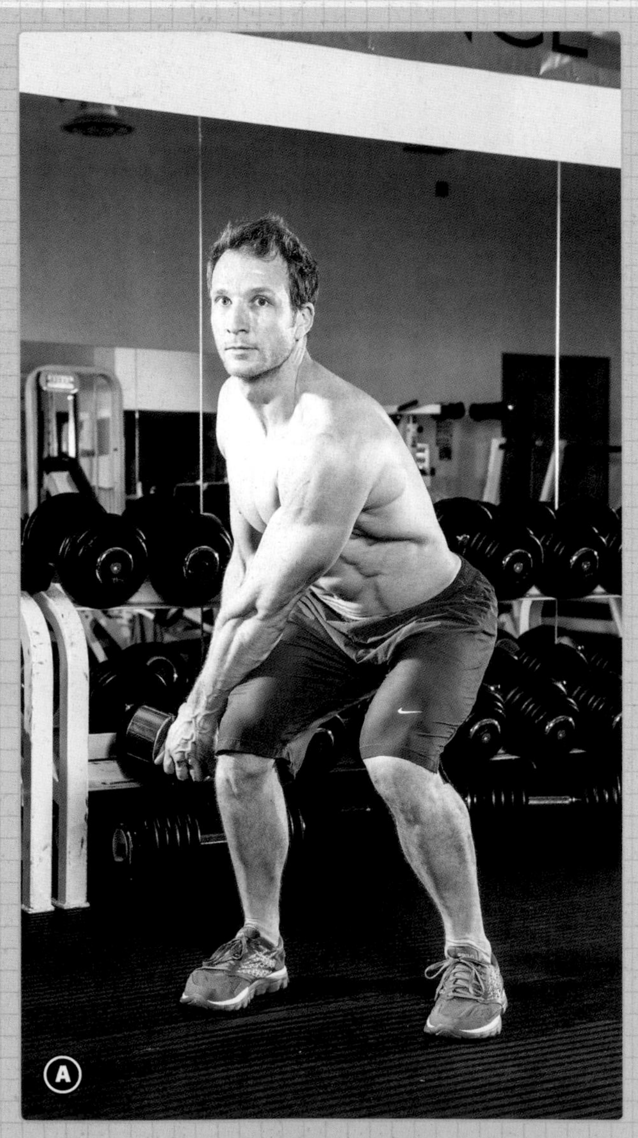

A

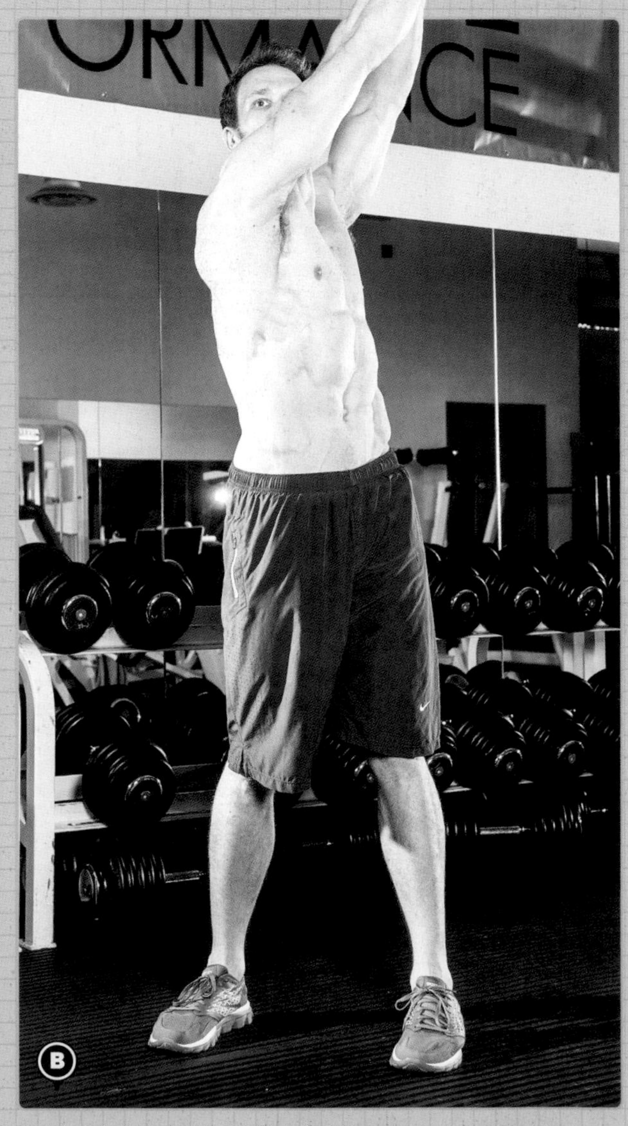

B

- With your feet shoulder-width apart and holding a dumbbell with both hands, squat and swing your arms to one side.
- Stand tall while lifting the weight up and across your body, keeping your arms straight throughout the movement.
- Reverse the move back to the start position.

Low-cable woodchop

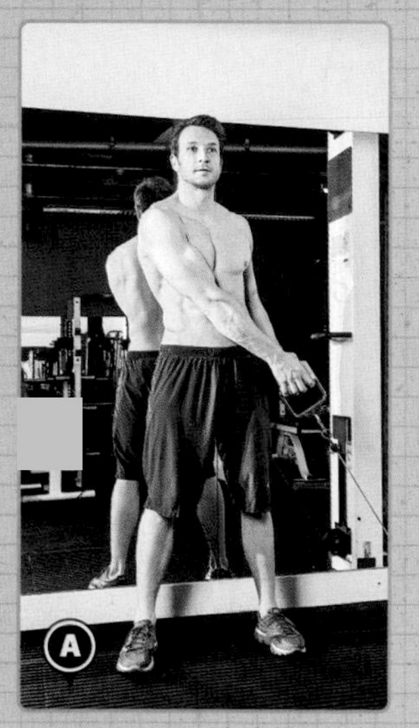
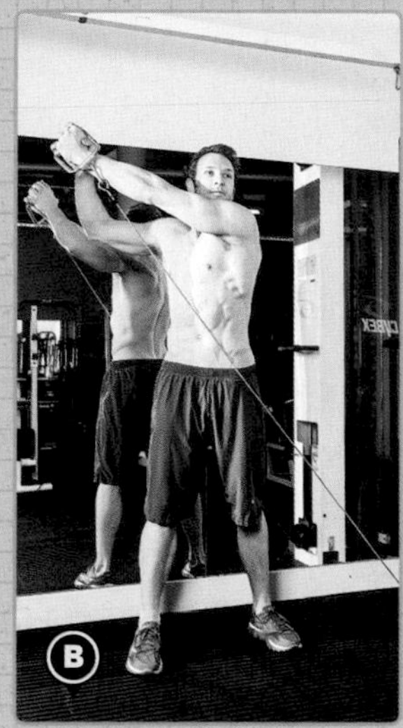

The cable provides constant resistance throughout the move and allows you to lift heavier weights safely.

High-cable woodchop

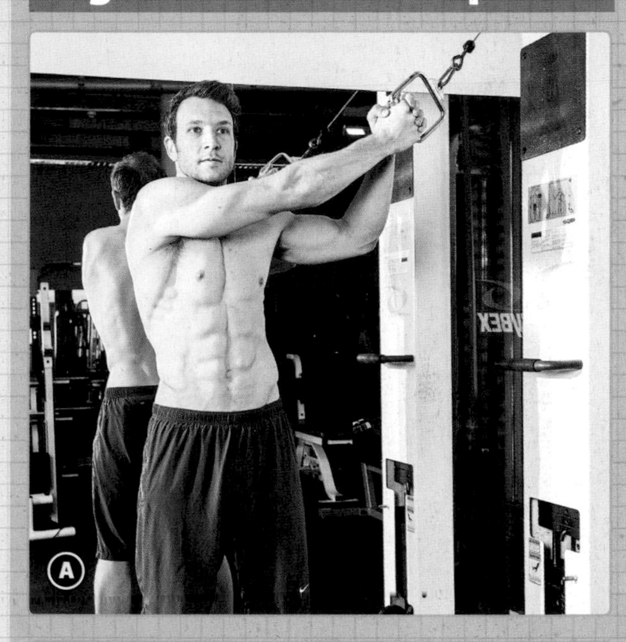
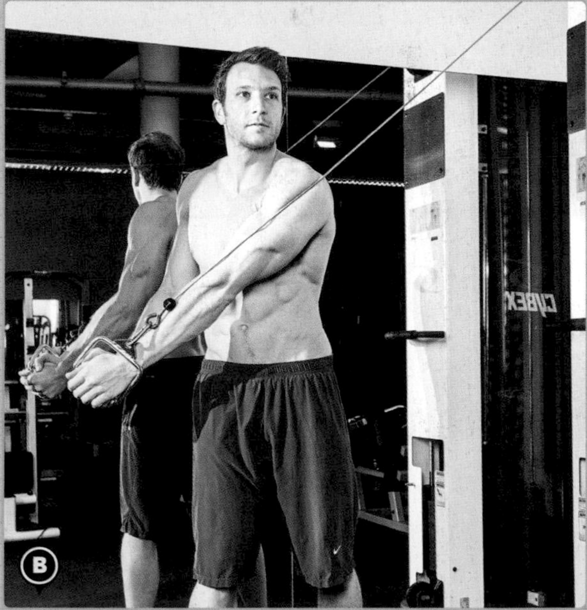

Using the high pulley attachment on the cable works your muscles in the opposite direction to the main move.

Woodchop lunge

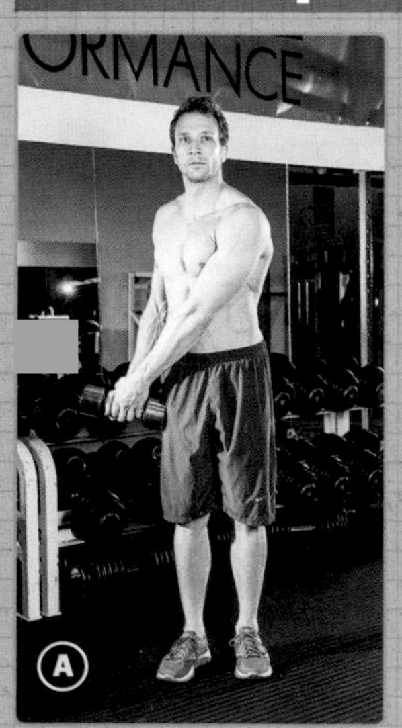
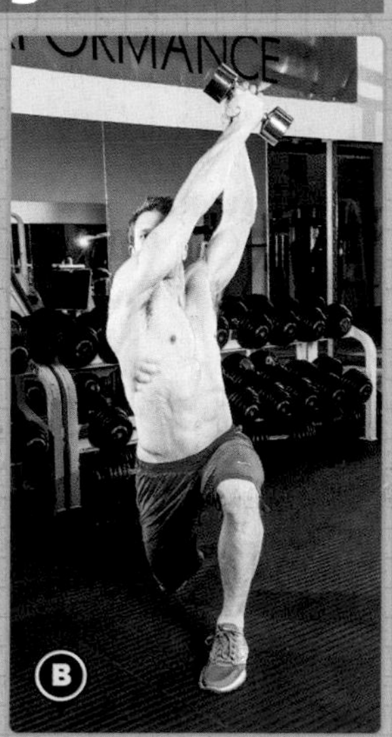

Lunging forwards while rotating the weight up and across your body forces your abs to work harder as you are moving vertically and horizontally at the same time.

ARMS

Build big biceps and thick triceps with these arm moves

Walk into any gym and chances are you'll see a row of men performing barbell or dumbbell curls in an attempt to build bigger biceps. But the key to getting impressive arms is to also work your triceps, the muscle on the back of your upper arm that accounts for about two-thirds of your total arm size.

The biceps and triceps, like many muscle groups paired on the same limb, are called antagonistic muscles, which means they work together to allow joint movement.

Your biceps are made of two different parts, or heads: the long head and the short head. This muscle flexes to bend the elbow joint, which happens every time you bring your hands towards your body, such as in a biceps curl.

Your triceps are made up of three different heads: the long and lateral head combine to form the horseshoe shape at the top of your upper arm, while the medial head runs beneath the long head down to your elbow. They extend your elbow to straighten your arm and are involved in any move that requires you to push away from your body, such as the bench press or press-up.

This chapter looks in detail at the best exercises to improve these muscles.

Arms explained

Here's how your biceps and triceps work

- The biceps and triceps are antagonistic muscles, meaning they work together with one muscle contracting and the other relaxing to allow movement at the elbow joint to bend or straighten your arm.

- The biceps is a two-headed muscle on the front of your upper arm that is responsible for flexing the elbow joint, which bends your arm to bring your hand towards your body. It also allows for supination of the forearm (the motion of turning of your palm upwards).

- The triceps is a three-headed muscle on the back of your upper arm and is responsible for the extension of your elbow joint, which straightens your arm.

- The forearm contains many smaller muscles, such as the brachioradialis, which are responsible for rotating your forearms, controlling your hand and finger dexterity, and grip strength.

The biceps and triceps

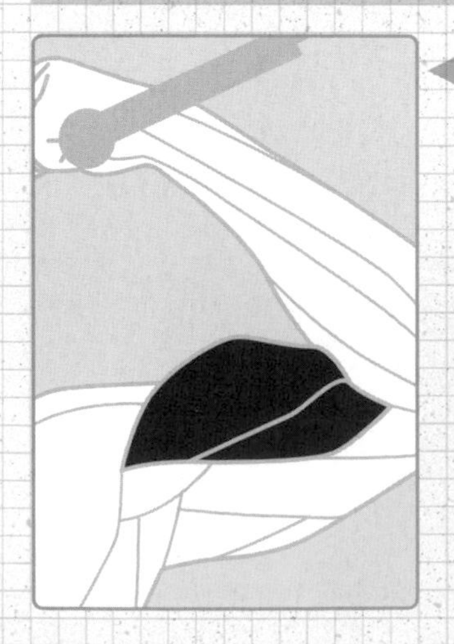

Your biceps muscle shortens, or flexes, to bend your elbow and bring your forearm towards your body. Because they're antagonistic muscles, as the biceps shortens the triceps lengthens.

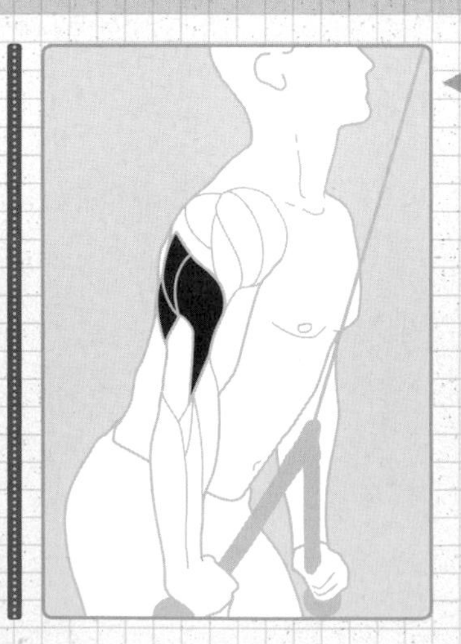

The triceps muscle shortens, or flexes, to straighten your arms. As it shortens, the biceps muscle lengthens.

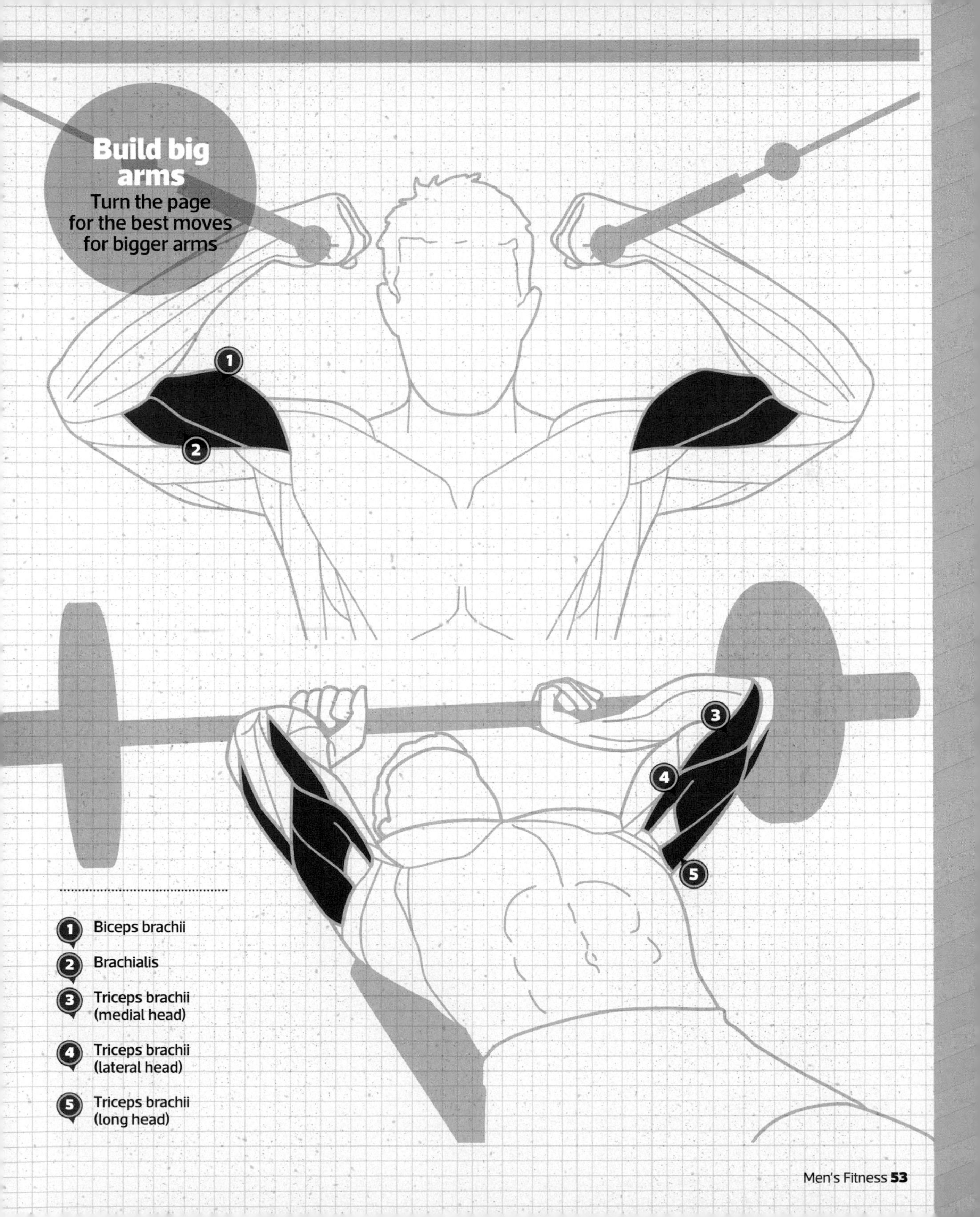
Build big arms
Turn the page for the best moves for bigger arms
1
2
3
4
5
1 Biceps brachii
2 Brachialis
3 Triceps brachii (medial head)
4 Triceps brachii (lateral head)
5 Triceps brachii (long head)

BARBELL BICEPS CURL

Targets ***Biceps***

This classic move allows you to lift heavy to make big muscle gains

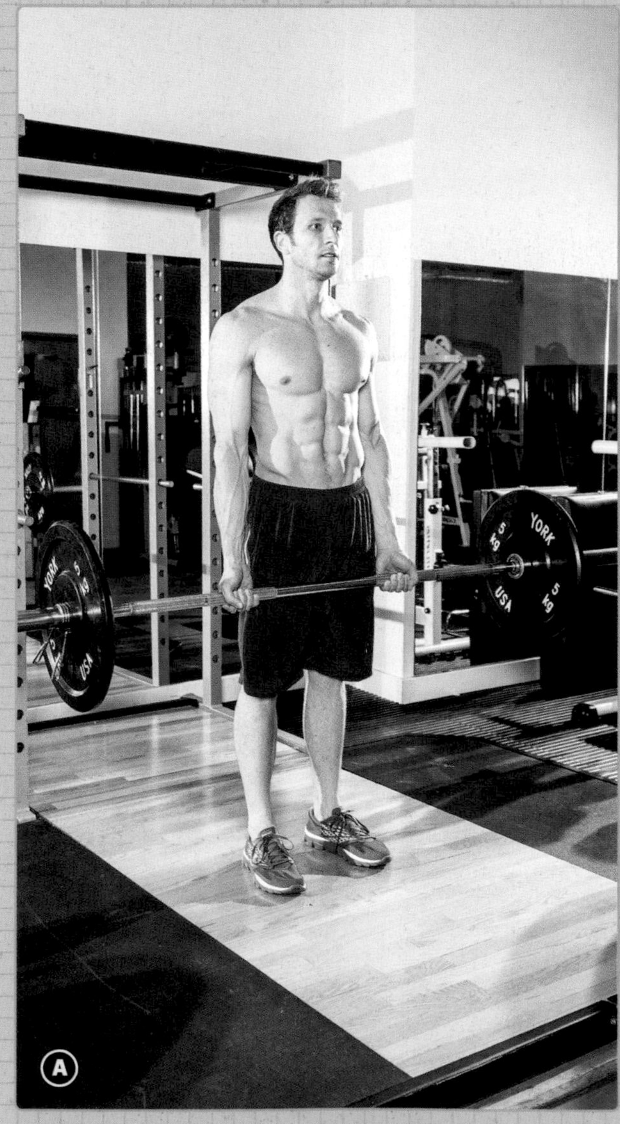

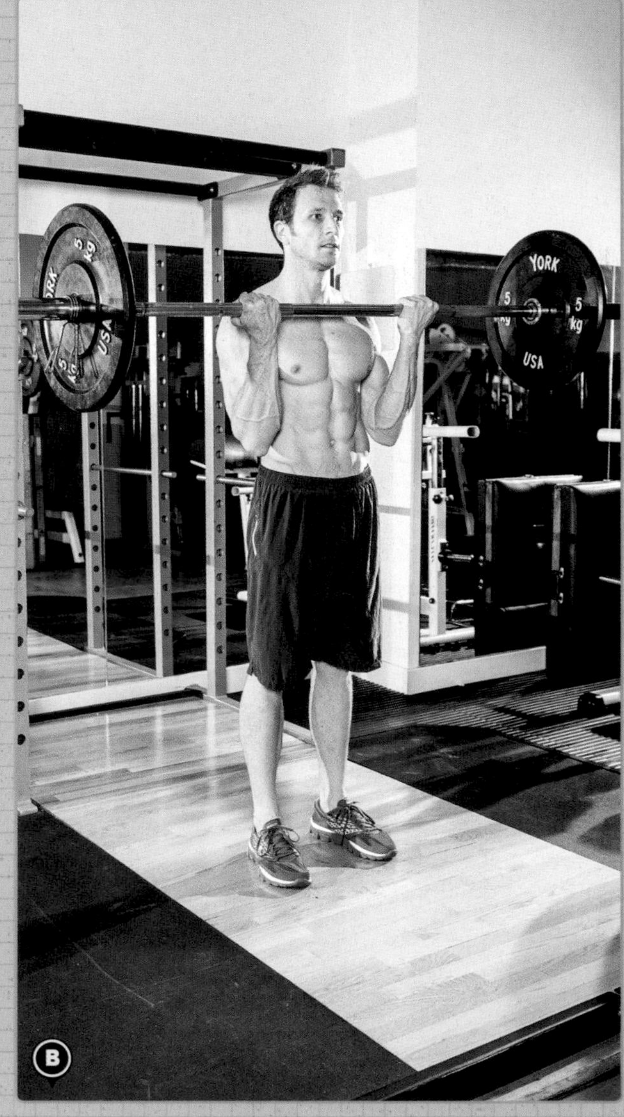

- Stand tall with your shoulders back and feet close together, holding a barbell with an underhand grip with hands just outside your hips.
- Keeping your elbows tucked in to your sides, curl the bar towards your chest, stopping just before your forearms are vertical.
- Lower back slowly to the start.
- Avoid rocking back and forth to generate momentum, which takes the emphasis away from the biceps.

EZ-bar biceps curl

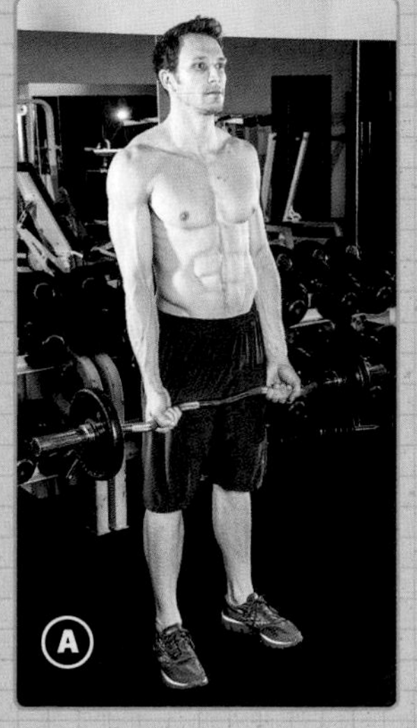

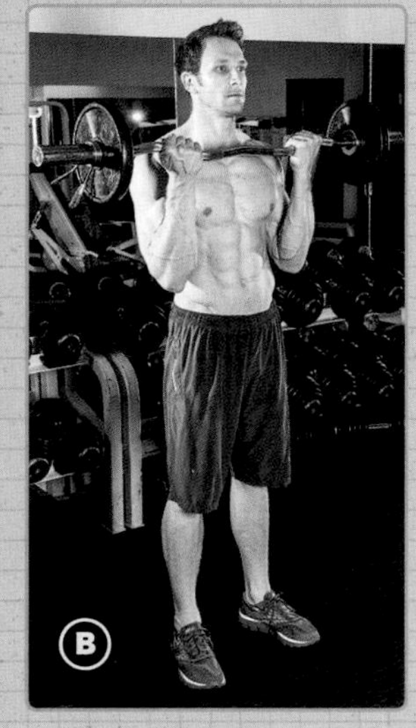

Using an EZ-bar with its inwards grip takes pressure away from the elbow joint to place greater emphasis on the biceps.

Reverse-grip biceps curl

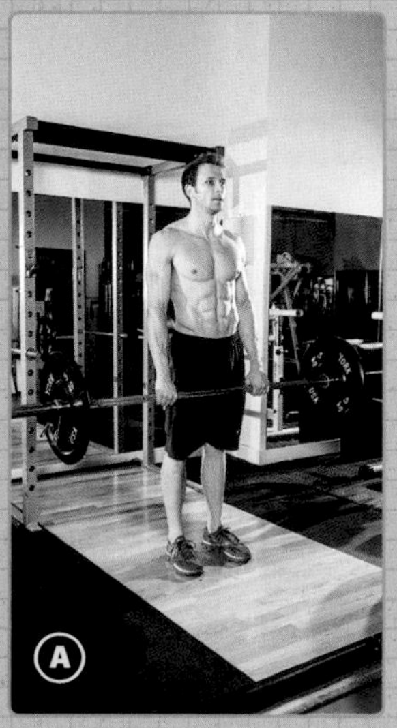

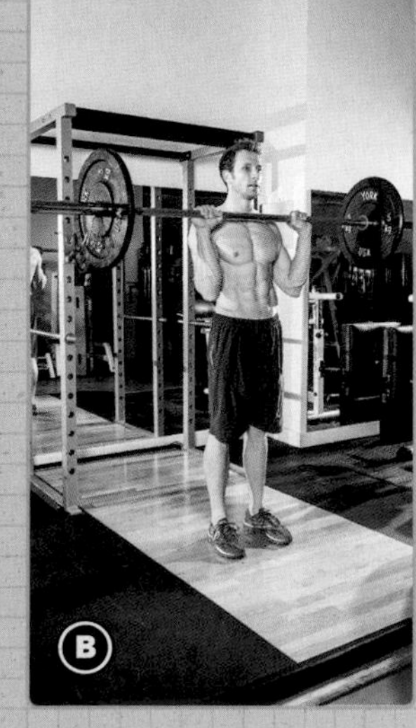

Using an overhand grip shifts focus to the muscles of the forearms while still working your biceps.

Dumbbell biceps curl

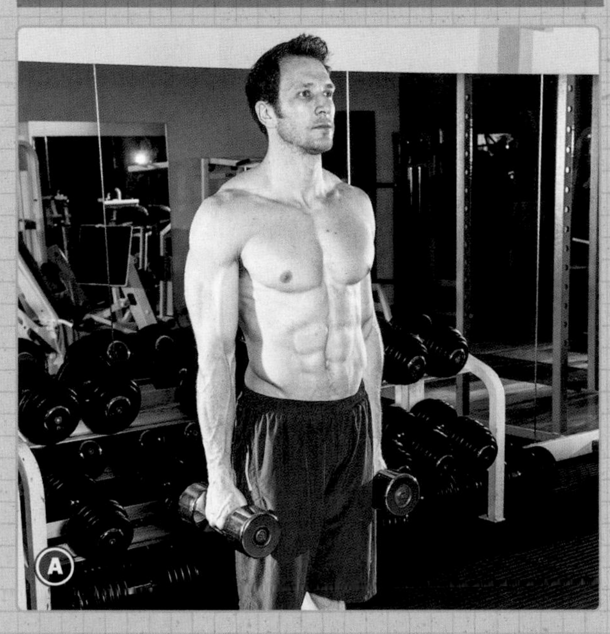

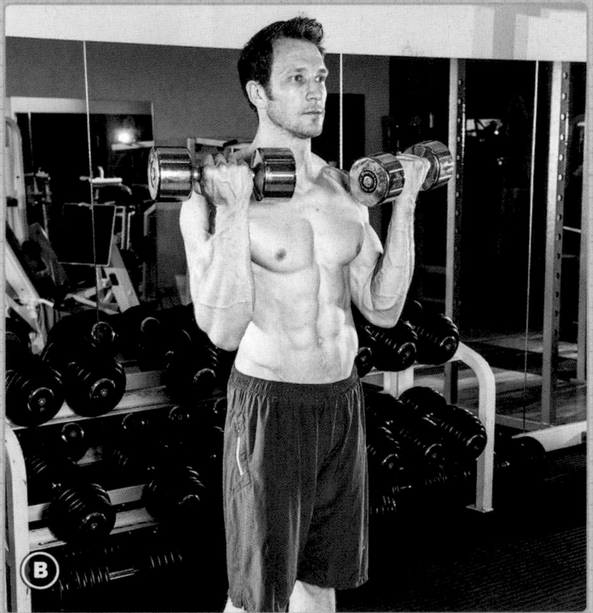

Using dumbbells allows you to work each arm individually, rather than your stronger arm dominating, while also allow for a greater range of motion.

SEATED DUMBBELL CURL

Targets ***Biceps***

The seated position means you can't use other muscles or momentum to start the move so your biceps are forced to lift and control the weight throughout

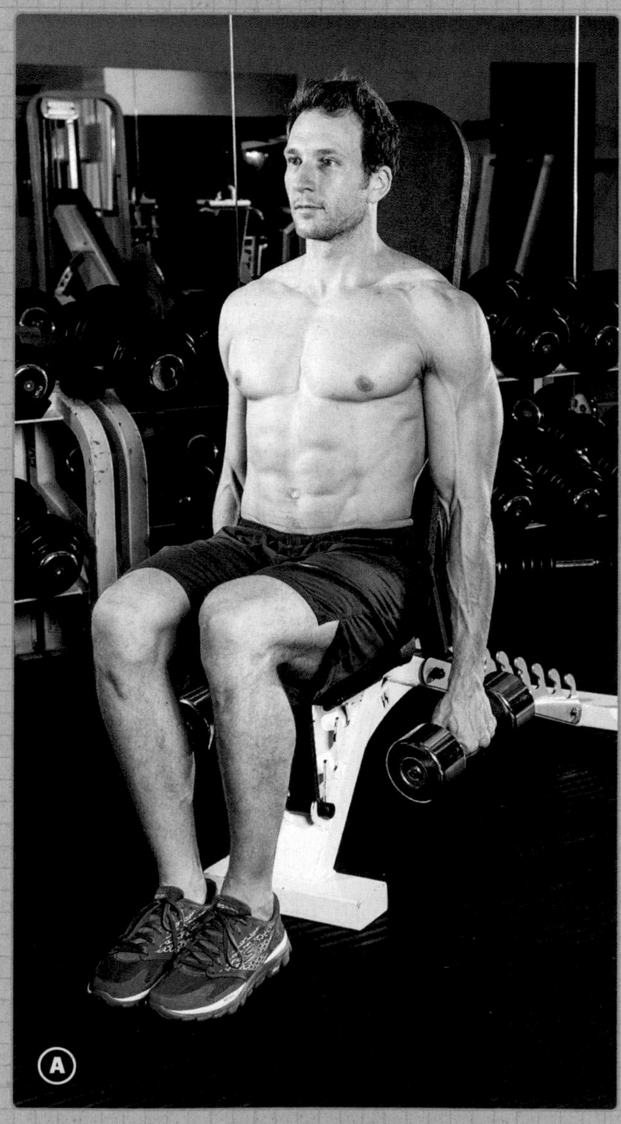

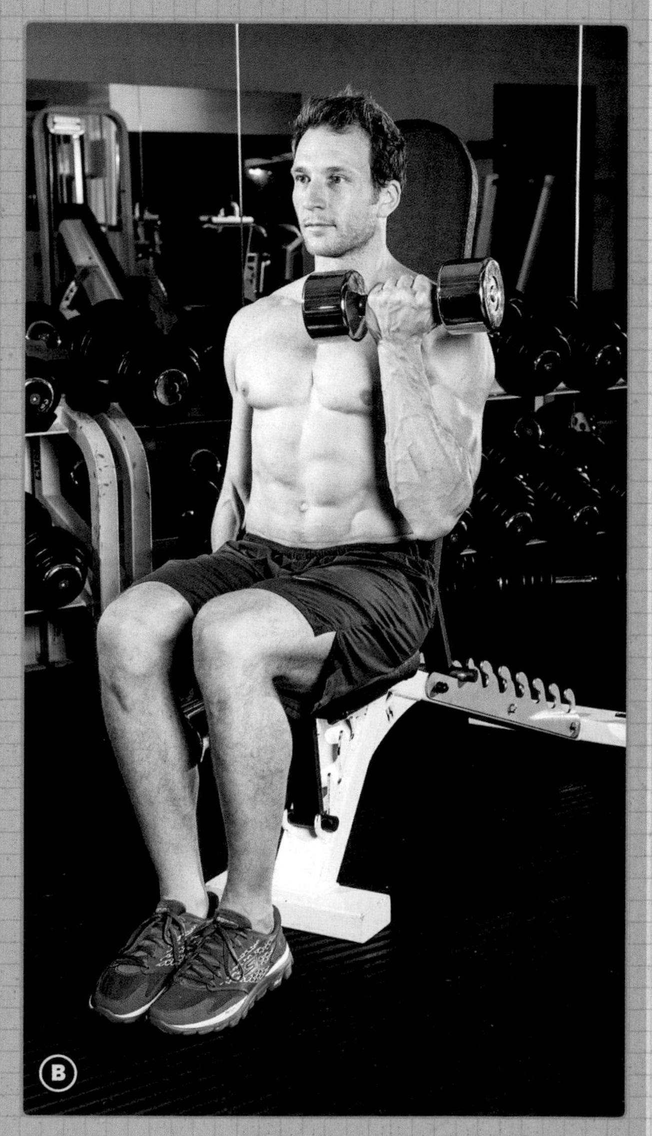

- Sit on an upright bench holding a dumbbell in each hand by your sides.
- Keeping your back flat against the bench and your elbows close to your sides, slowly curl one dumbbell up to shoulder height.
- Squeeze your biceps at the top of the move then slowly return to the start. Repeat on the other side.

Seated hammer curl

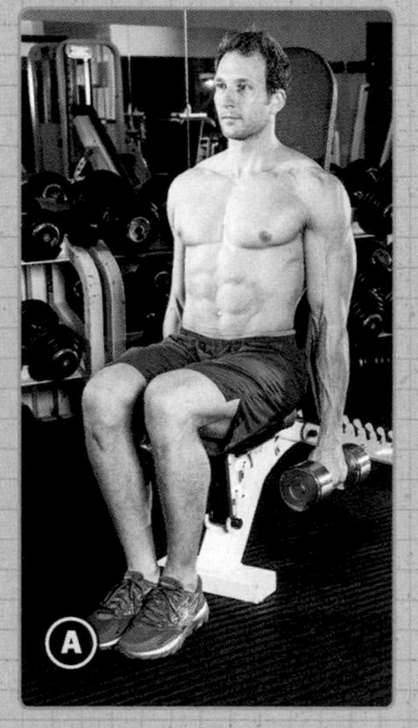

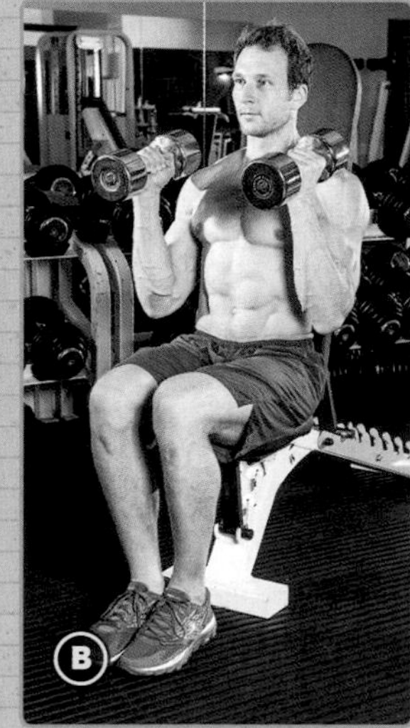

A neutral grip, with your palms facing each other, works the muscles of the forearms harder.

Concentration curl

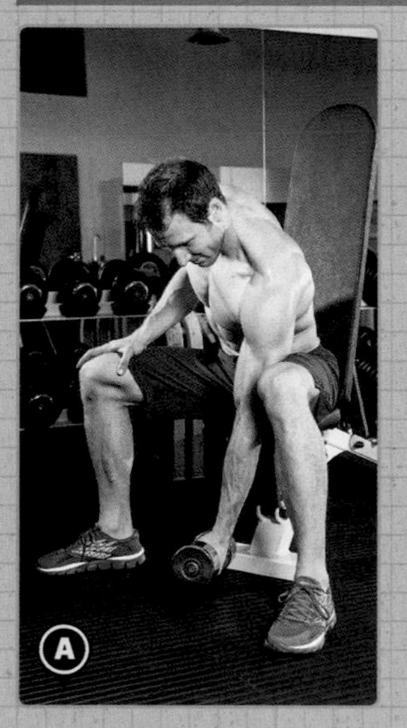

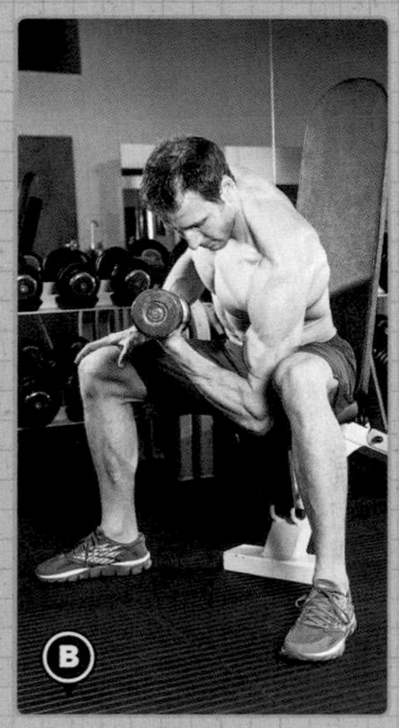

This moves secures your elbow in place so your muscles, rather than momentum, are entirely responsible for lifting and lowering the weight.

Seated incline dumbbell curl

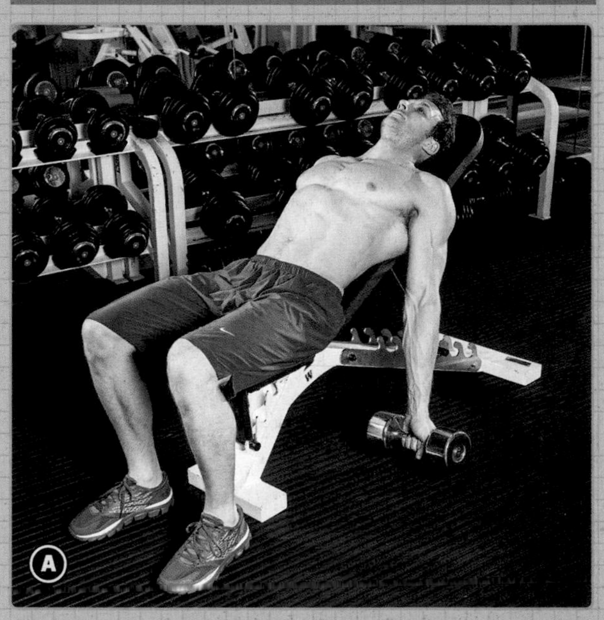

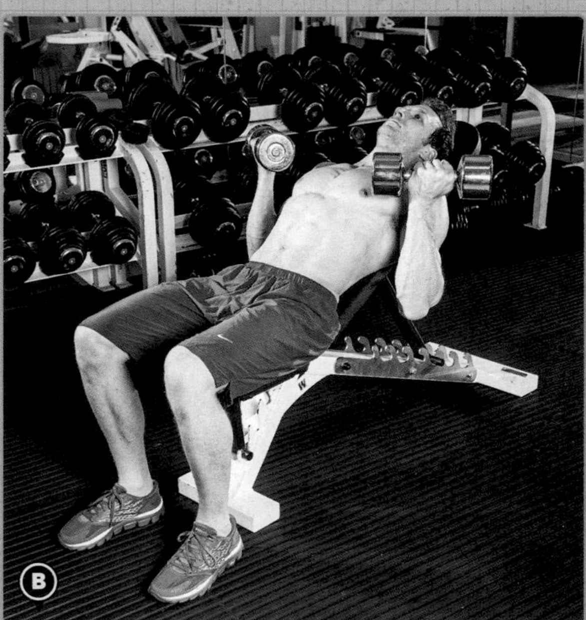

Setting the bench on an incline between 30° and 45° maintains tension on your biceps throughout the move and means you can lift through a greater range of motion.

EZ-BAR PREACHER CURL

Targets ***Biceps***

The preacher bench stabilises your upper arms, removing momentum from the equation so your biceps are fully isolated during the move, while an EZ-bar reduces the strain on your elbows

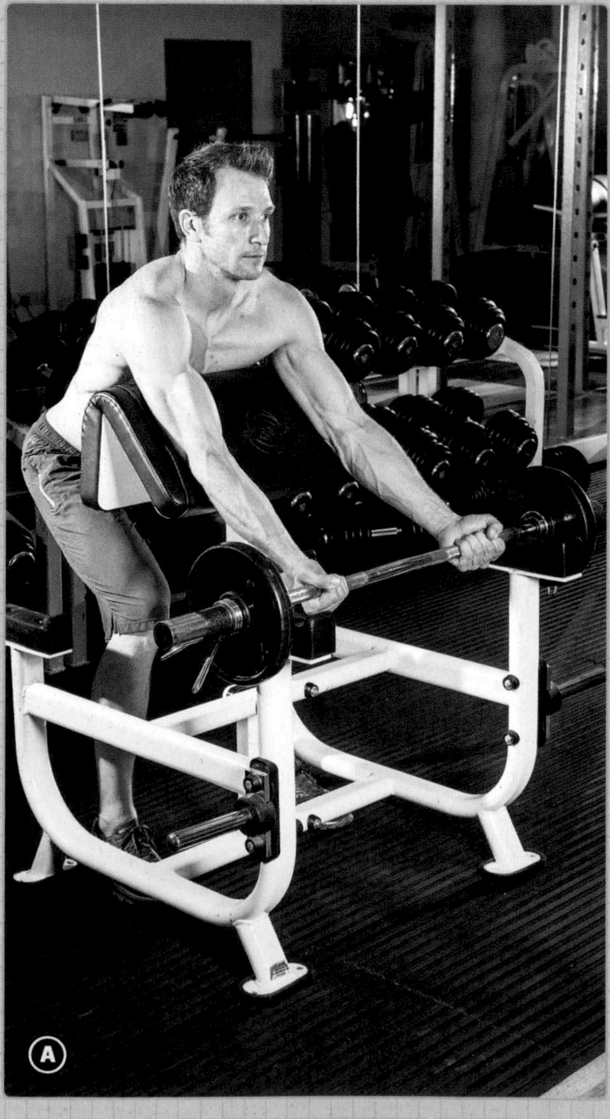

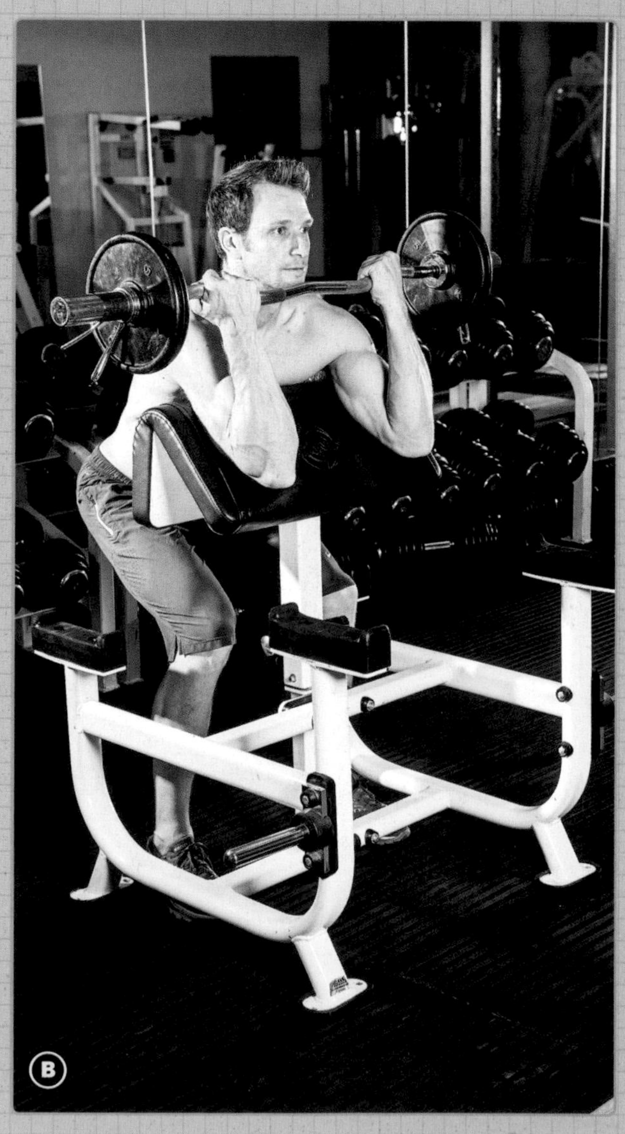

- Sit on a preacher bench with your upper arms flat against the bench, holding an EZ-bar with an underhand grip.
- Keeping your elbows locked in position, curl the bar towards your chin, stopping just before your forearms reach vertical.
- Lower back slowly to the start.

One-arm preacher curl

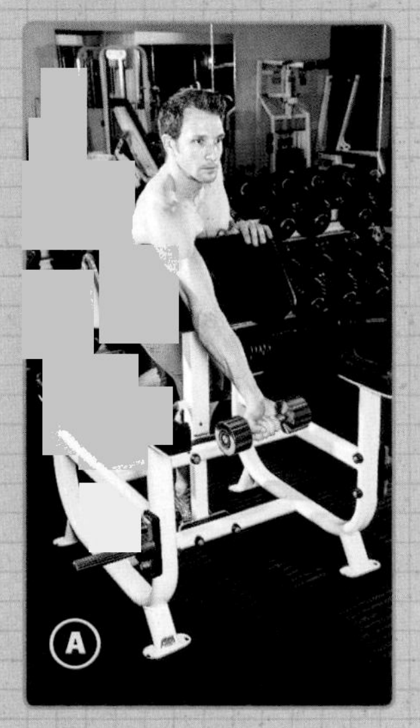

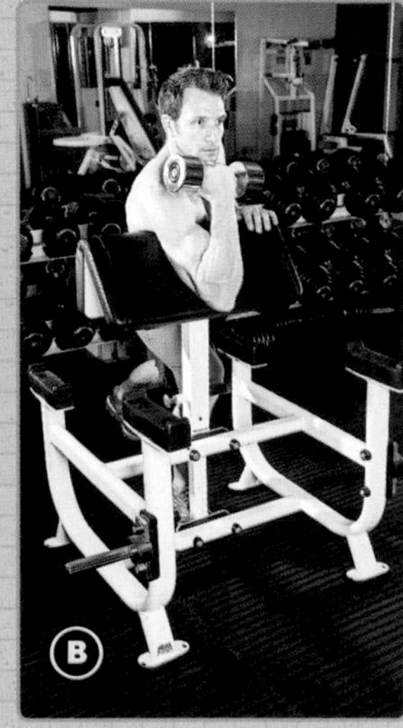

Working each arm individually ensures balanced growth in both biceps.

Reverse-grip preacher curl

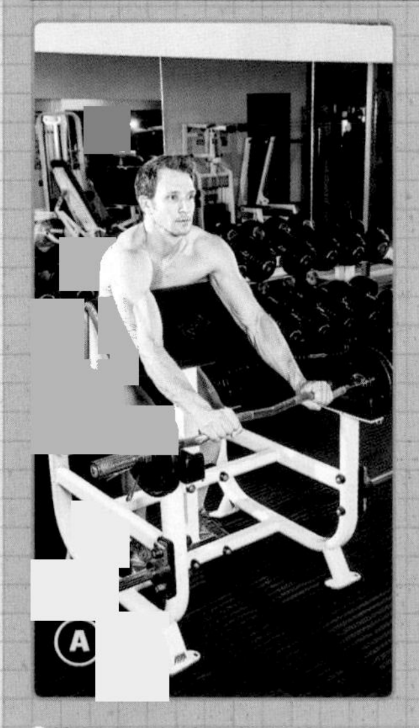

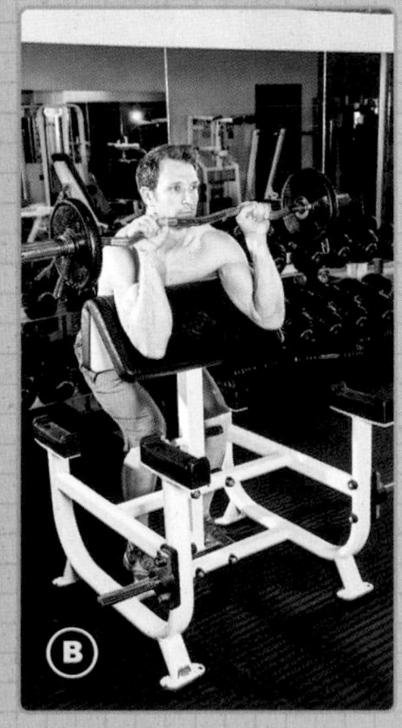

Using an overhand grip places greater emphasis on your lower biceps and forearms.

Spider curl

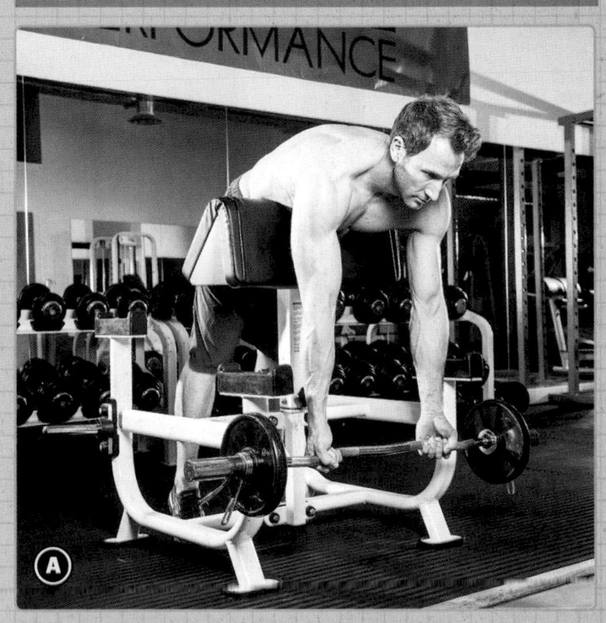

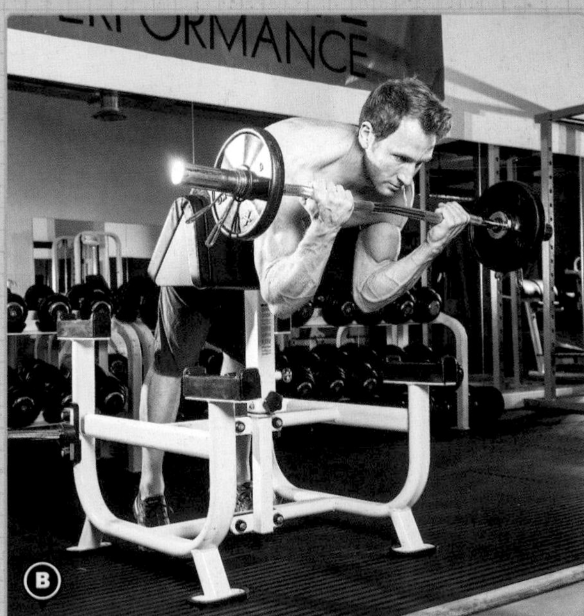

Leaning over the preacher bench still supports your upper body but allows for a greater range of motion.

HAMMER CURL

Targets ***Biceps***

This neutral grip lift still works your biceps but also recruits more muscles from your forearms, making it good for bigger arms

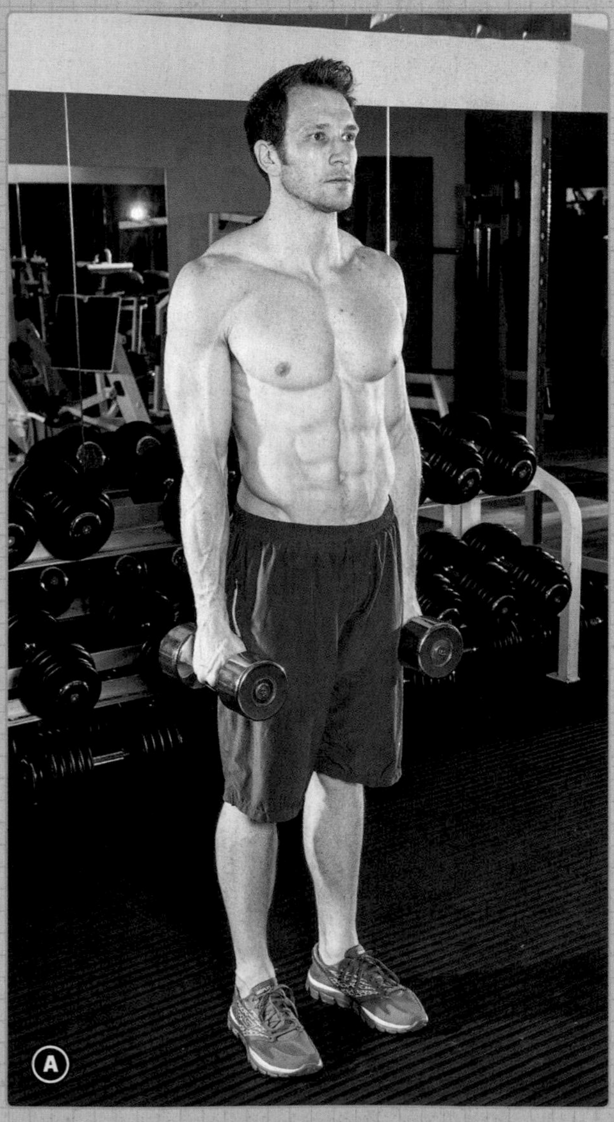

A

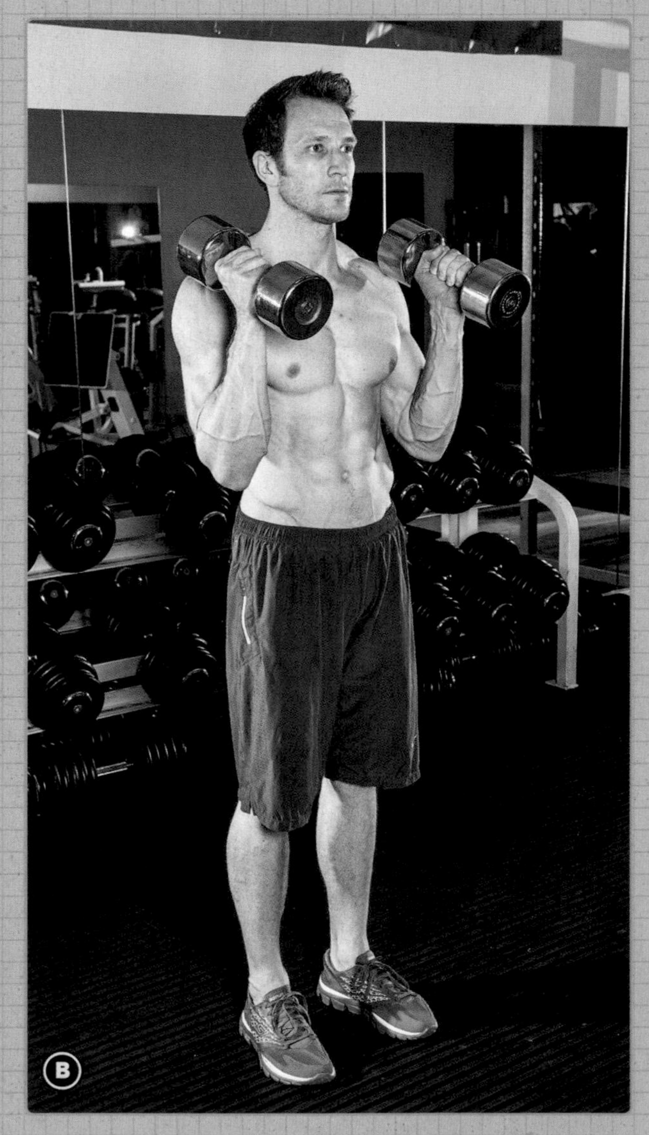

B

- Stand tall with your feet together holding a dumbbell in each hand with your palms facing each other.
- Keeping your elbows close to your sides, raise the weights to shoulder height, squeezing your biceps at the top of the move.
- Slowly return the weights back to the start.

Cable rope curl

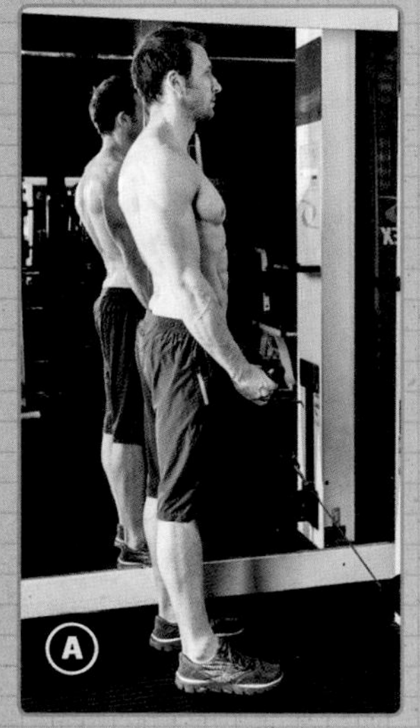

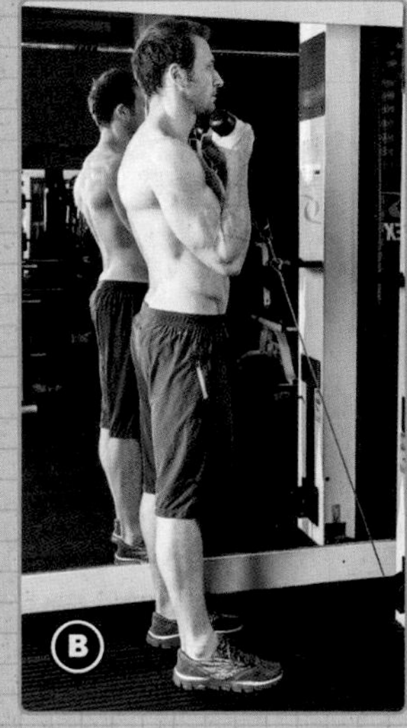

Using a cable ensures there is constant tension on your biceps throughout the move.

Hammer curl with twist

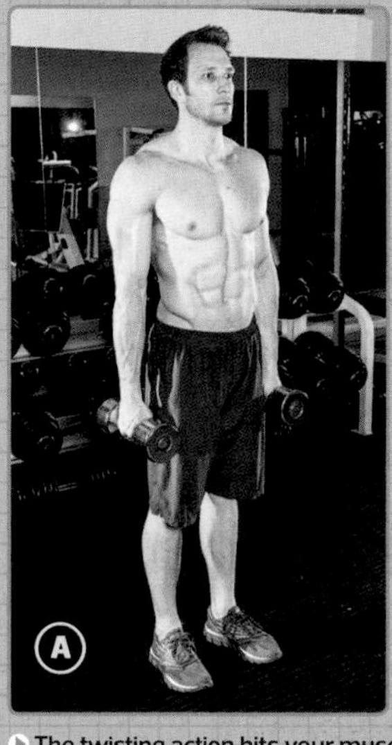

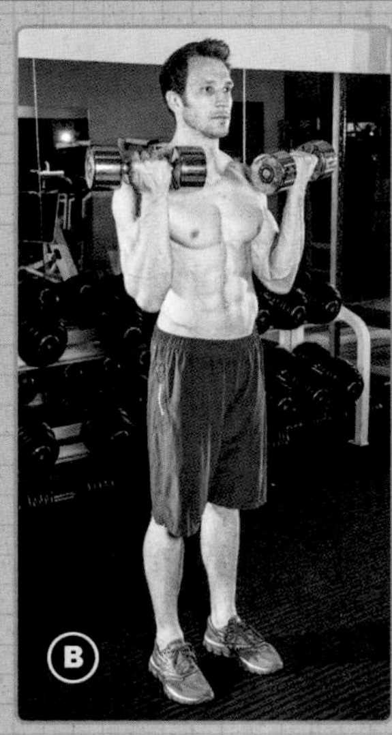

The twisting action hits your muscles from multiple angles and makes them work harder. Keeping your elbows close to your sides makes you less likely to rely on momentum to get the weight moving.

Zottmann curl

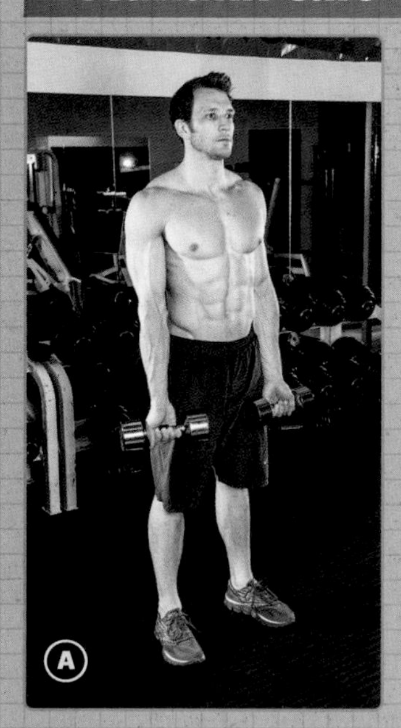

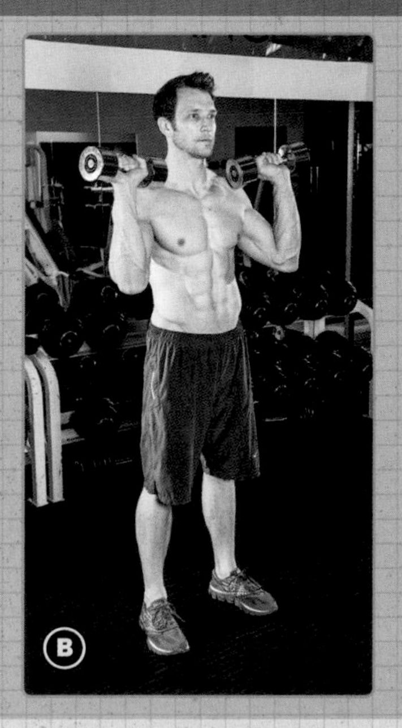

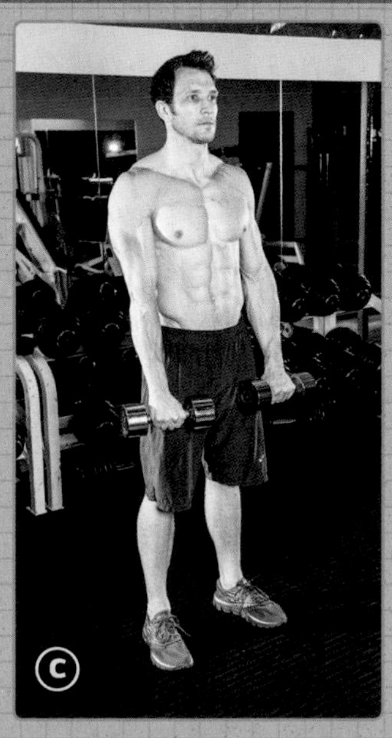

Curling the weights up then rotating your wrists to lower them again hits your forearms harder.

CHIN-UP

Targets *Biceps, upper back*

One of the hardest bodyweight moves there is, this will pack size and strength on your biceps as well as recruiting the major muscles groups of your upper back

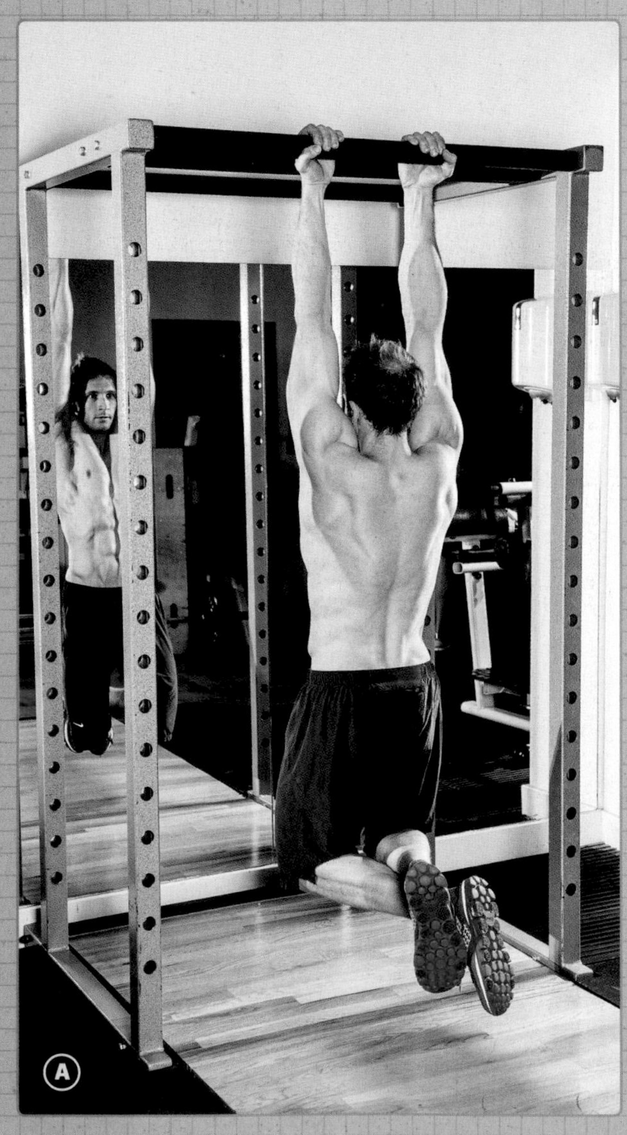

A

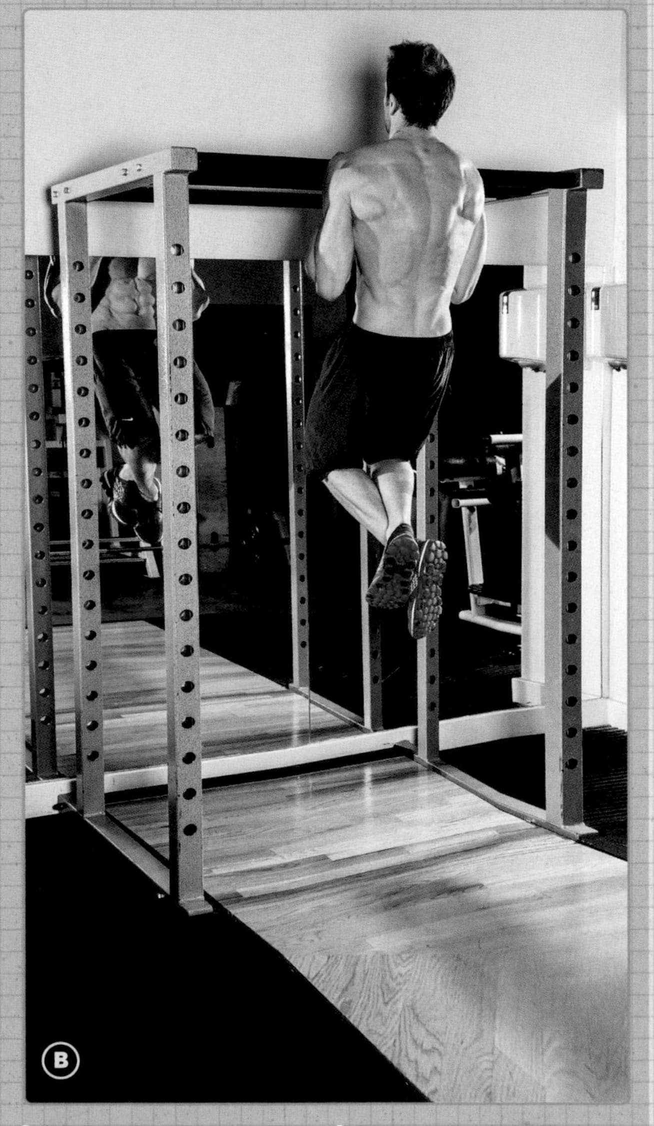

B

- Grab the bar with an underhand grip so your hands are shoulder-width apart.
- Start from a dead hang with your arms fully extended.
- Pull yourself up by squeezing your lats together.
- Once your chin is higher than your hands, lower yourself back to the start.

Neutral chin-up

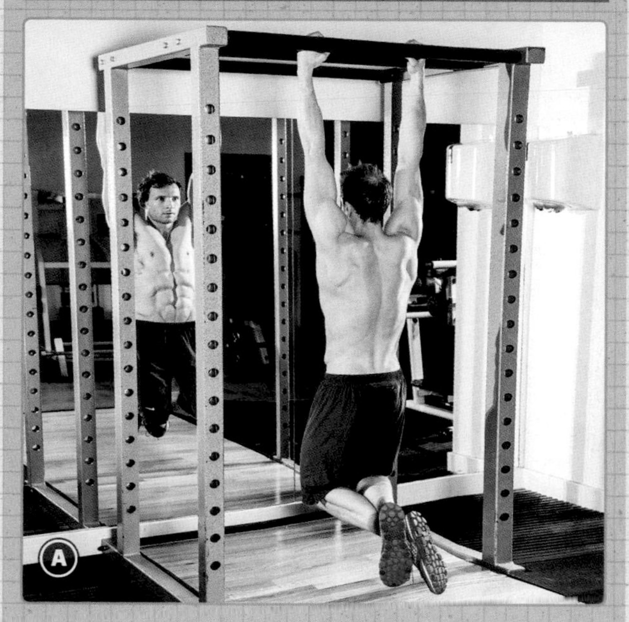

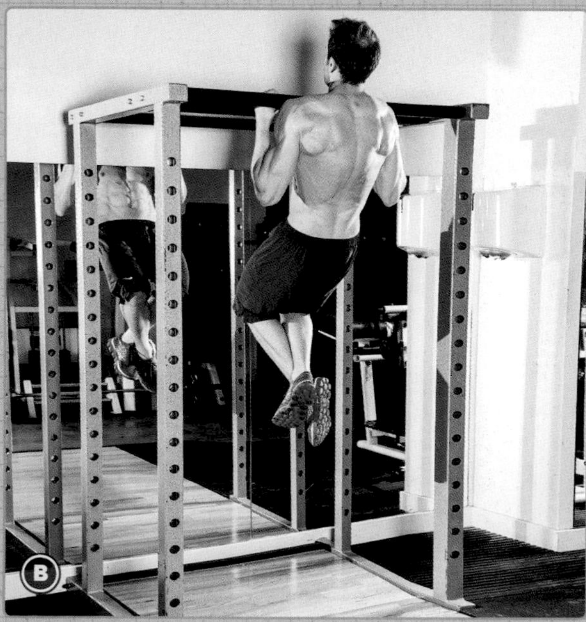

A palms-facing grip recruits the forearms and back muscles more.

Weighted chin-up

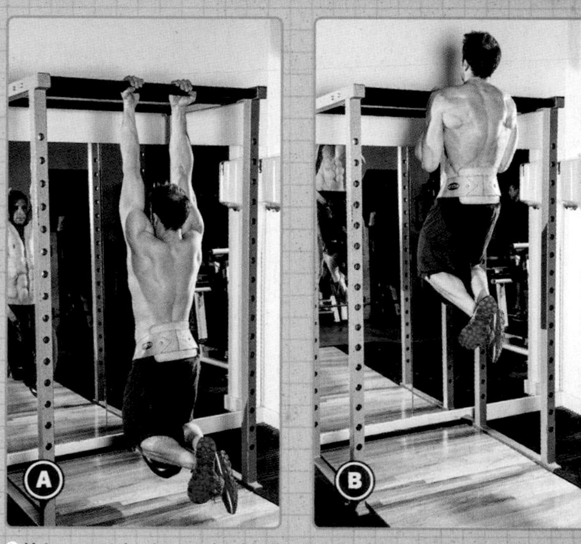

Using a weight plate or dumbbell increases the amount of resistance your muscles must overcome to lift your chin to the bar.

Negative chin-up

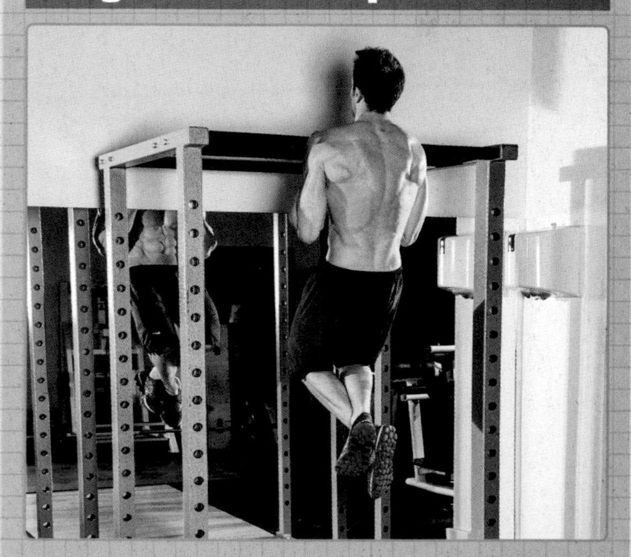

Jumping to the top position then slowly lowering yourself back down is a great way to build the strength to perform full versions of the move.

TRICEPS DIP

Targets ***Triceps, chest, shoulders***

The best move for building big triceps is tough, so ensure your perform it correctly to make safe gains

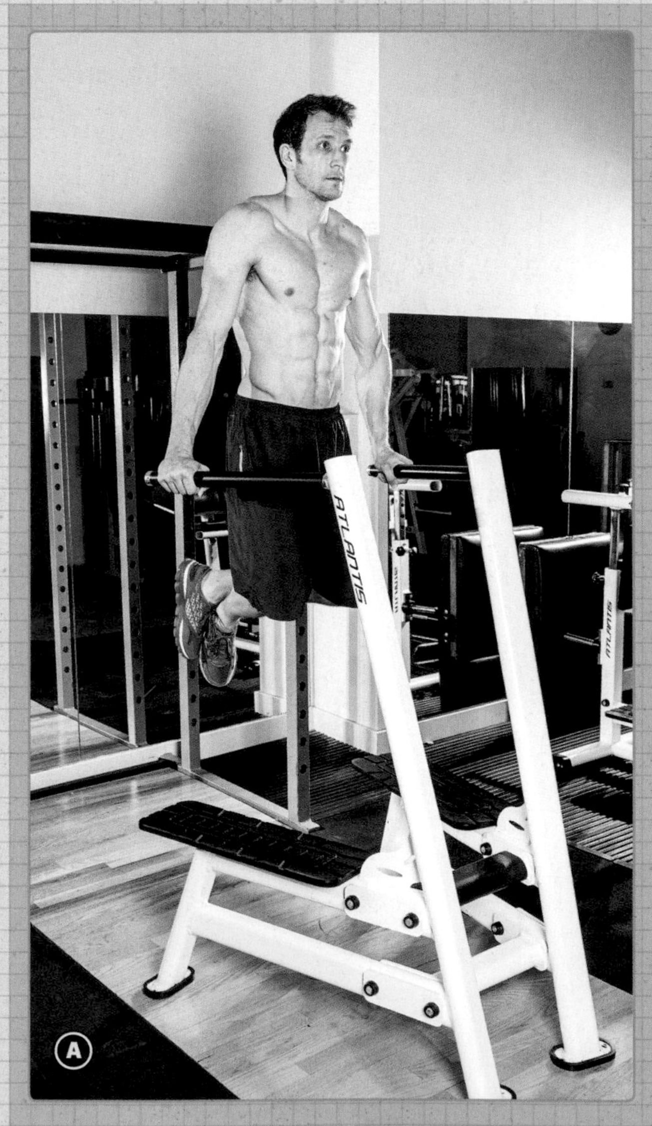

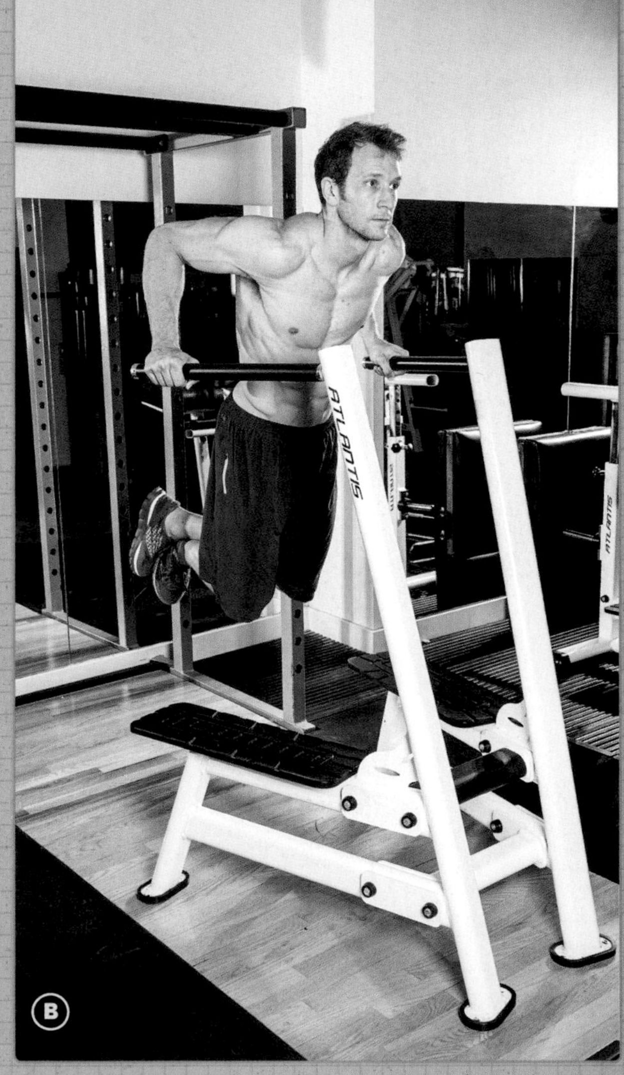

- Grip parallel bars, keeping your body upright.
- With your elbows pointing straight back, lower your body as far down as you can comfortably go without stressing your shoulders.
- Keep your core braced and don't swing your legs for momentum.
- Press back up powerfully but don't lock out your elbows at the top.

Weighted triceps dip

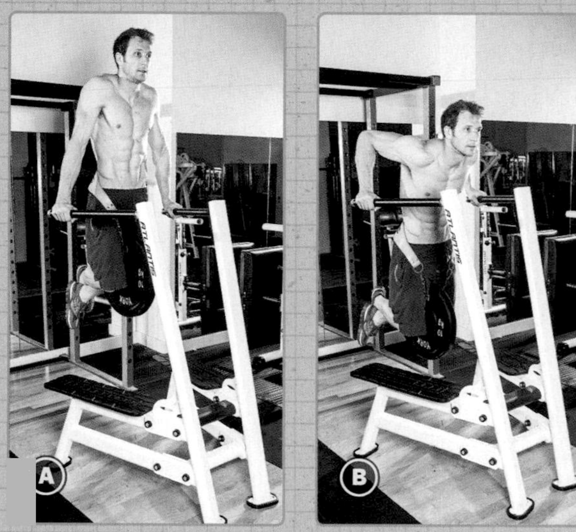

Once you find dips easy you need to add more weight to keep your muscles growing. Holding a weight plate or dumbbell between your knees is the answer.

Negative triceps dip

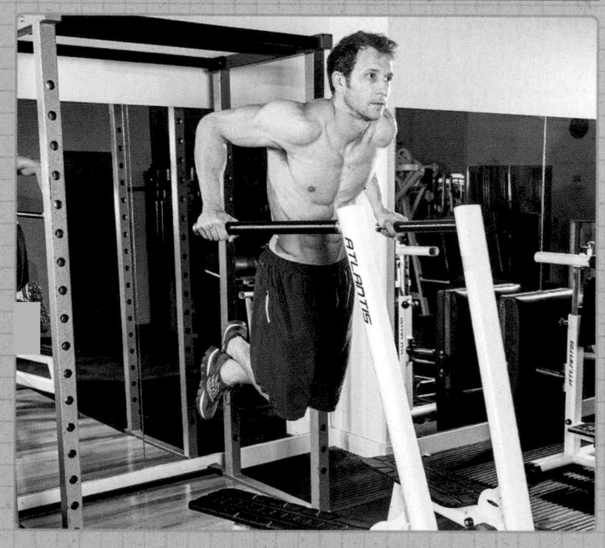

Jumping to the start position then lowering yourself back down slowly is another great way to build triceps strength.

Assisted triceps dip

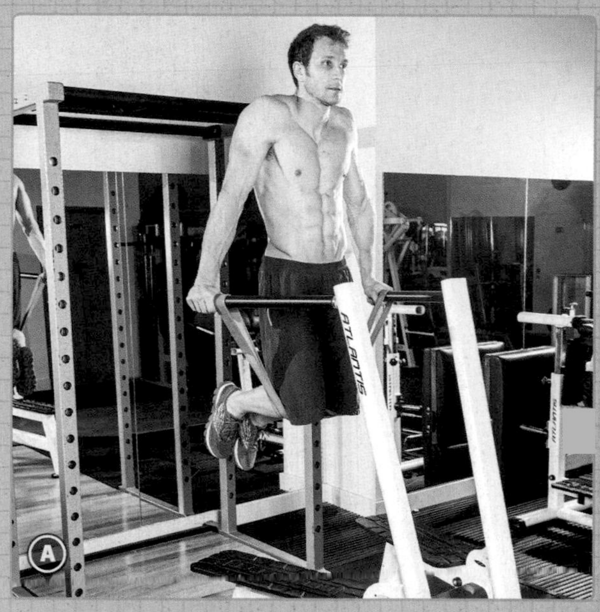

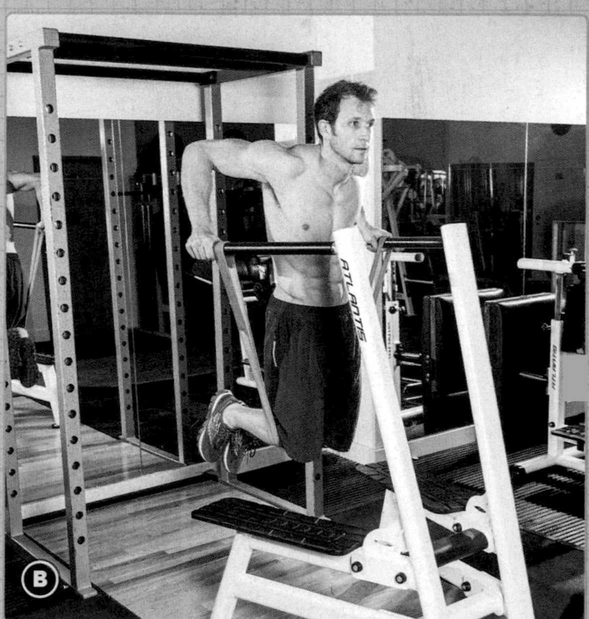

Using a dips machine or a resistance band is a great and safe way to build up the strength to perform the full version of the move.

CLOSE-GRIP BENCH PRESS

Targets Triceps, chest, shoulders

Taking a close grip on the barbell brings your triceps to the fore while still working your chest and the front of your shoulders

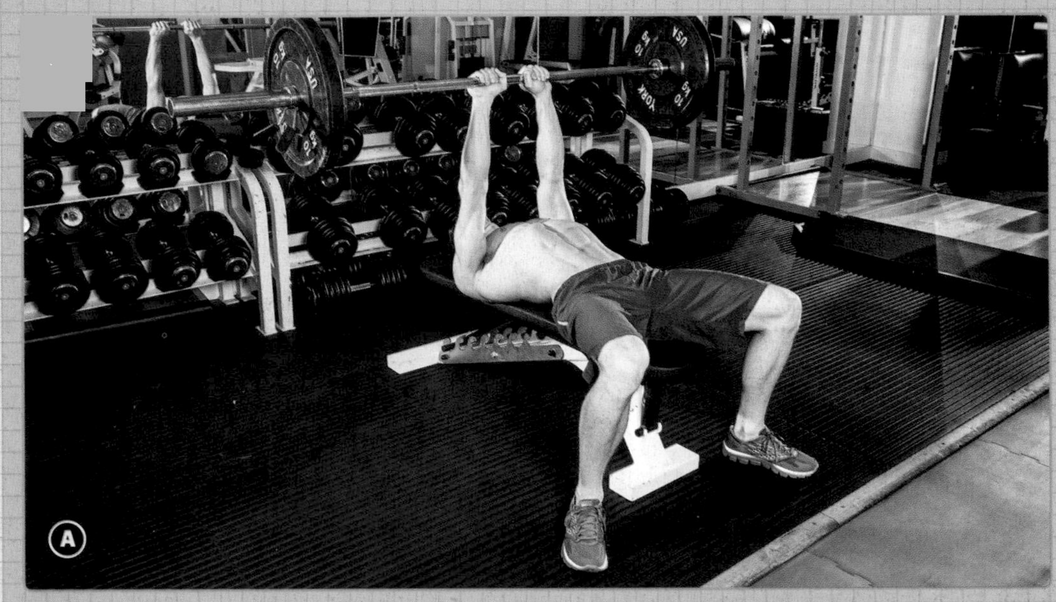

- Lie flat on a bench holding a barbell with a close, overhand grip. Aim for about a fist-sized gap between your hands.
- Keep your head, shoulders and back supported by the bench, with your core braced and feet flat on the floor.
- Lower the bar slowly to your chest, keeping your elbows close your sides to keep the emphasis on your triceps.
- Push back up powerfully but don't lock out your elbows.

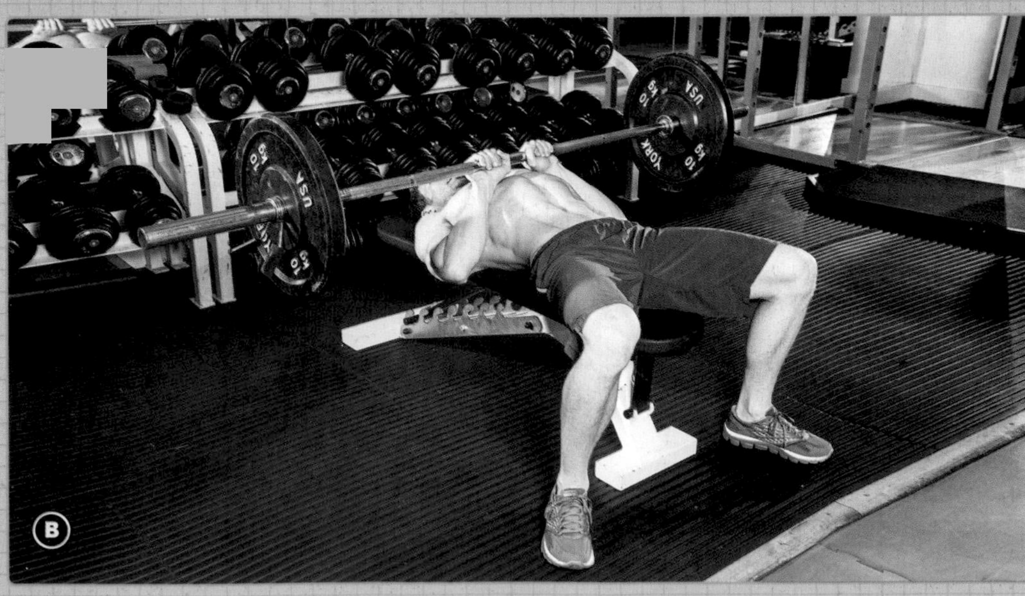

Decline close-grip bench press

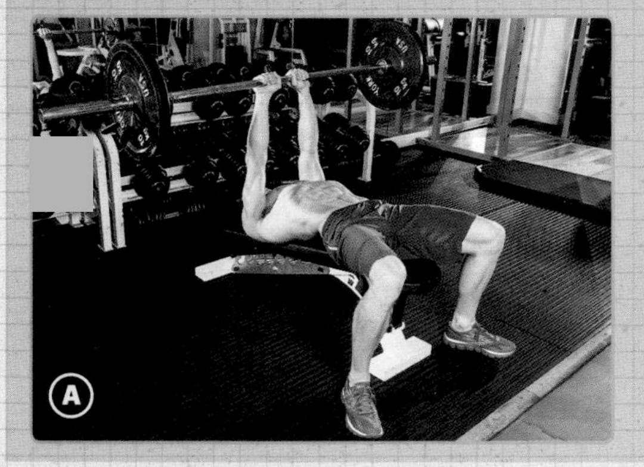

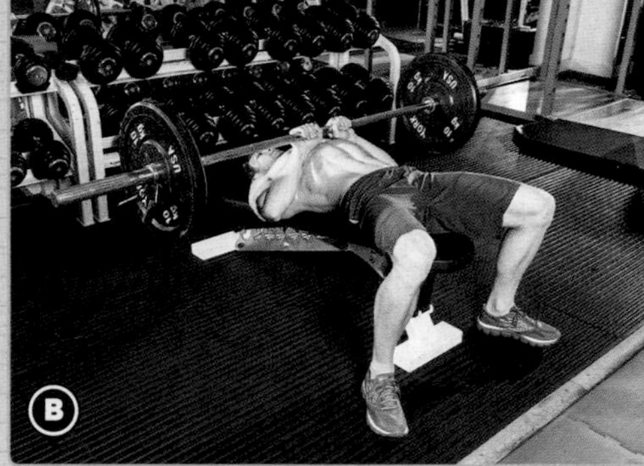

Lying on a decline works your lower chest harder as well as targeting your triceps.

Medicine ball close-grip press-up

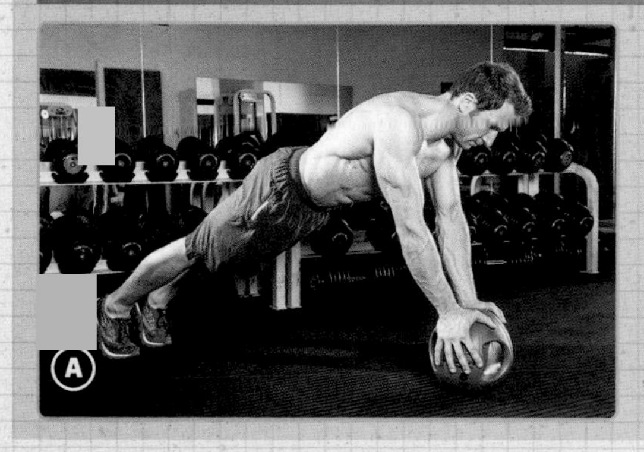

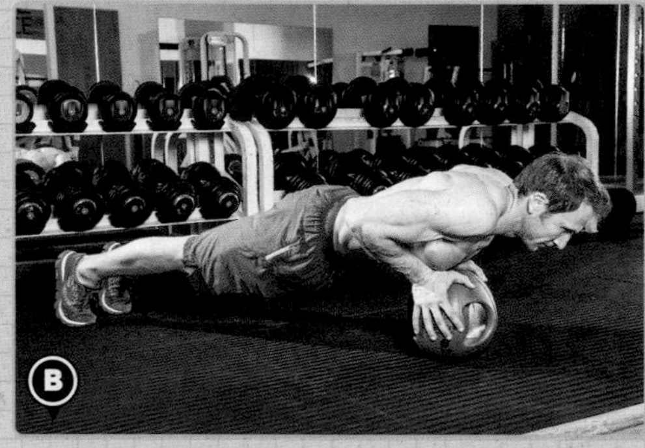

The instability of the medicine ball works your triceps hard and forces your core to engage to provide stability.

Diamond press-up

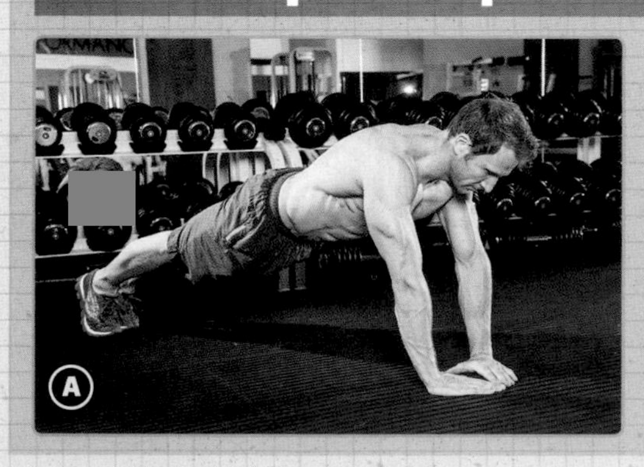

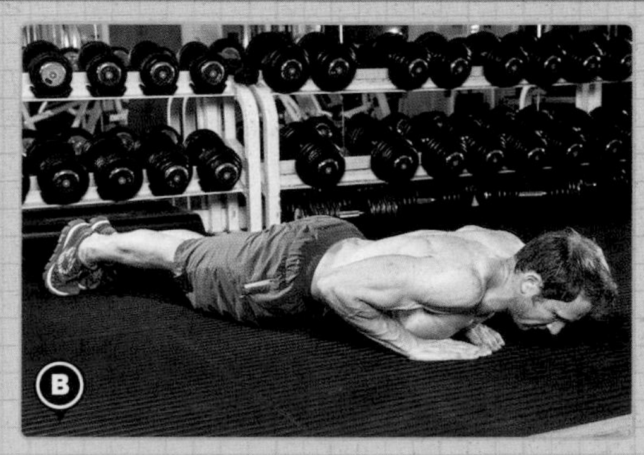

Forming a diamond with your index fingers and thumbs shifts the focus of this press-up from your chest to your triceps.

LYING EZ-BAR TRICEPS EXTENSION

Targets ***Triceps***

This is a classic move for isolating the triceps – using an EZ-bar takes the strain off your joints so your muscles must do all the work

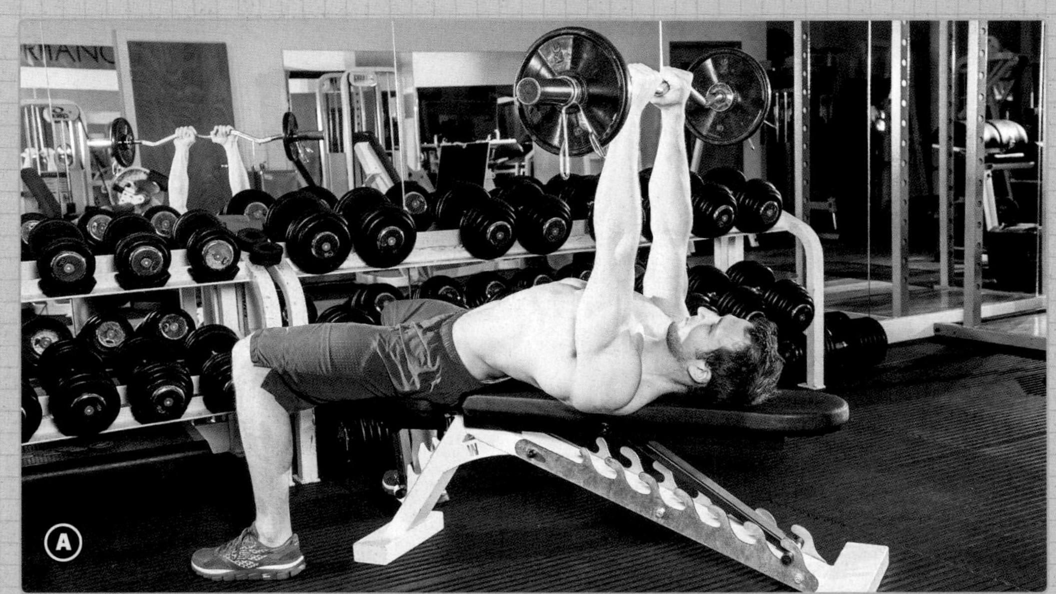

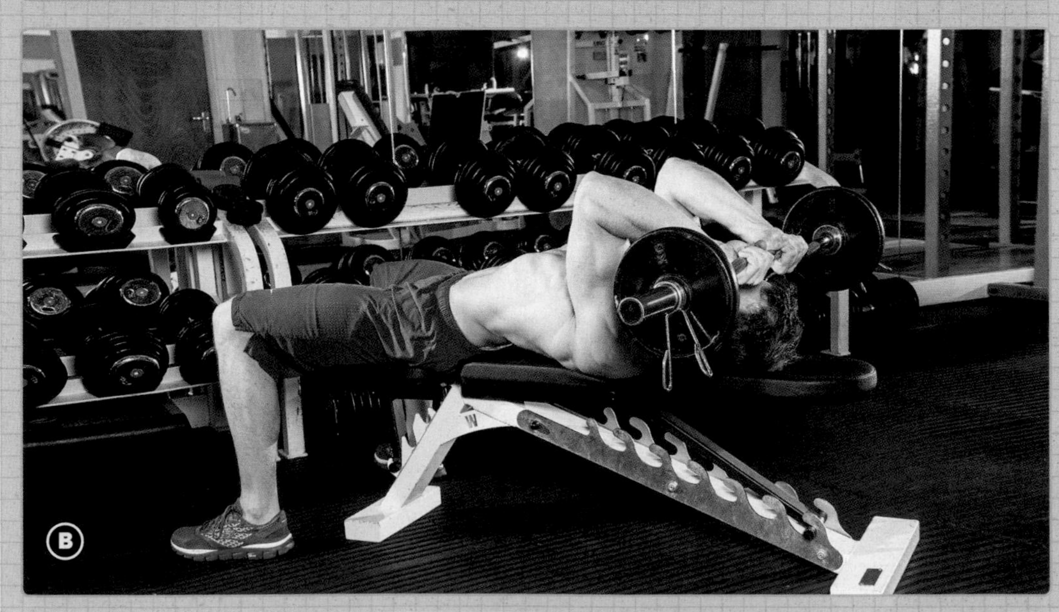

- Lie flat on a bench, holding an EZ-bar above you with straight arms.
- Slowly lower the bar towards the top of your head by bending your elbows, which should stay pointing to the ceiling.
- Without arching your back, slowly return the bar to the start position by straightening your arms.

Standing EZ-bar triceps extension

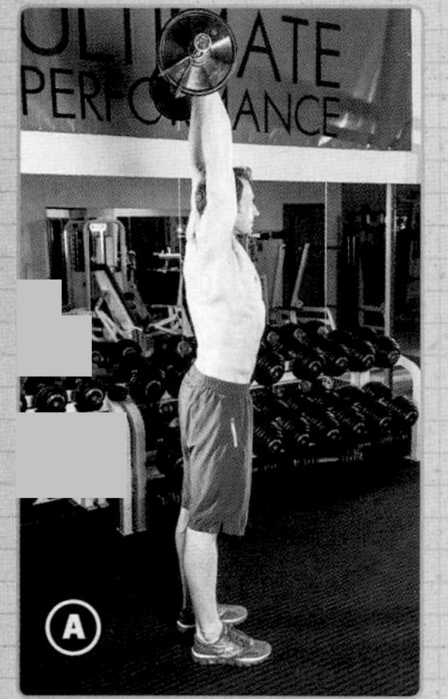

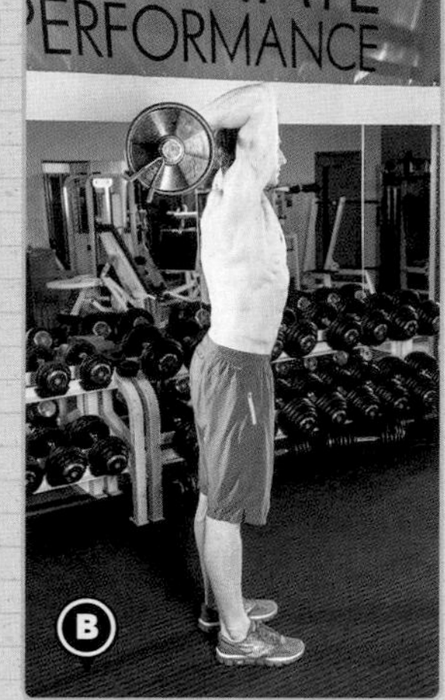

Standing engages your core and allows you to lift heavier weights safely.

Reverse-grip lying triceps extension

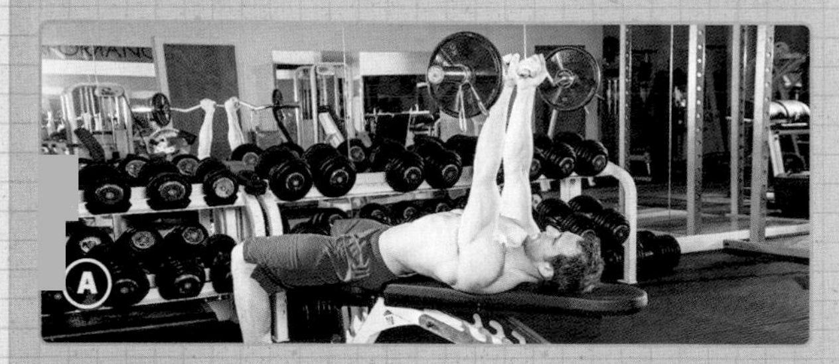

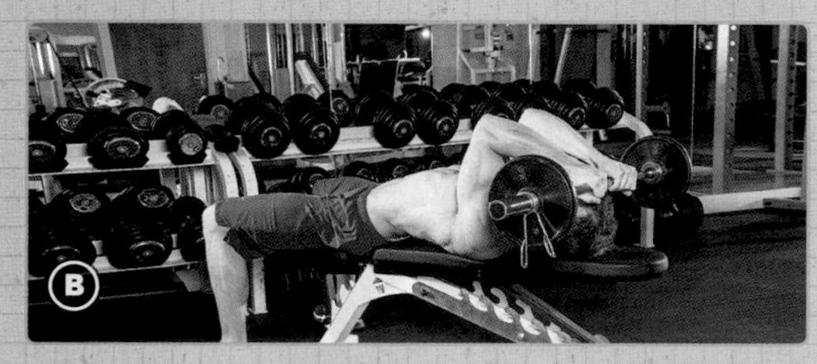

Holding the bar with an underhand grip shifts the focus to the lateral head of your triceps muscle.

Lying triceps extension and pull-over

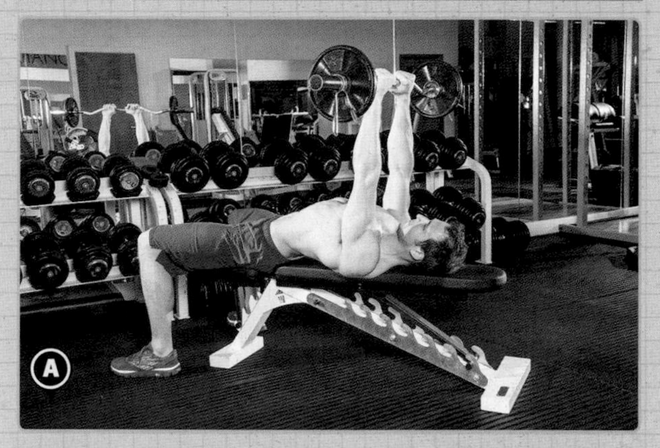

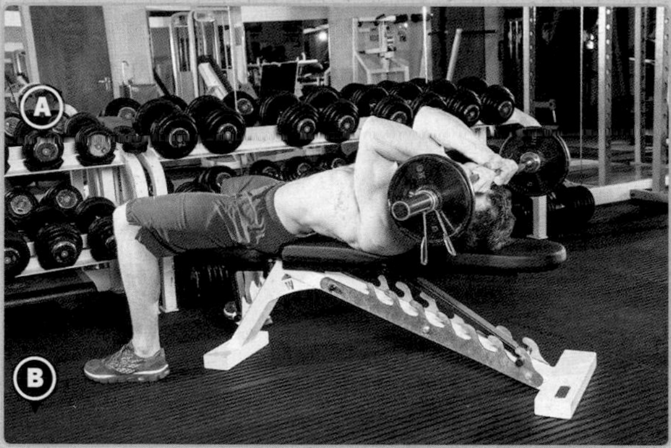

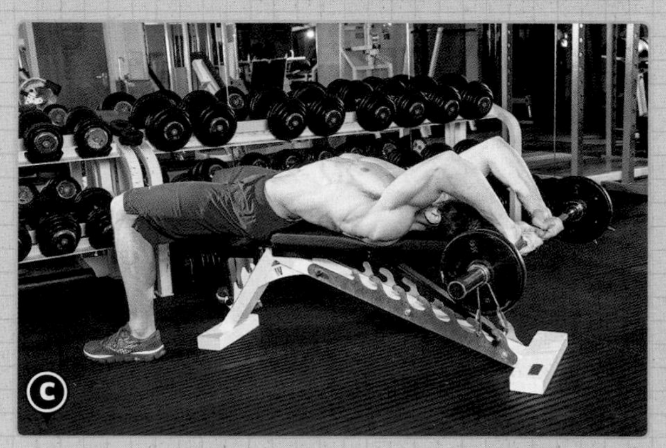

Extending your arms behind your head, rather than just down towards it, makes this move harder and recruits your back and chest muscles.

ONE-ARM TRICEPS EXTENSION

Targets ***Triceps***

Add size and strength to your triceps by working each arm independently

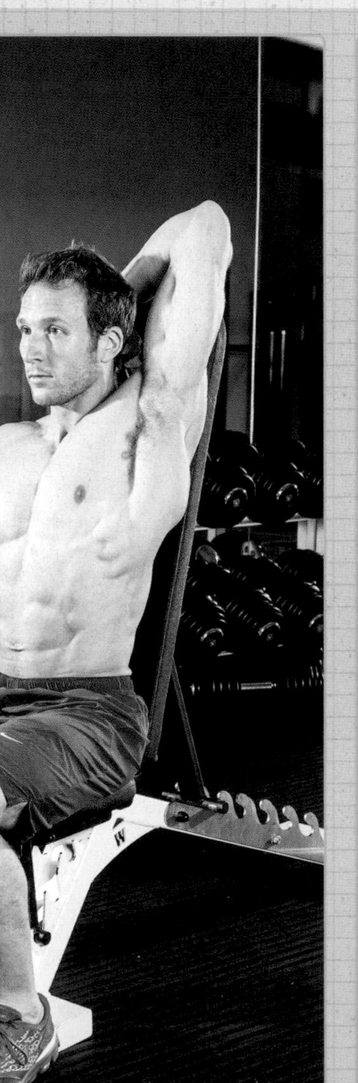

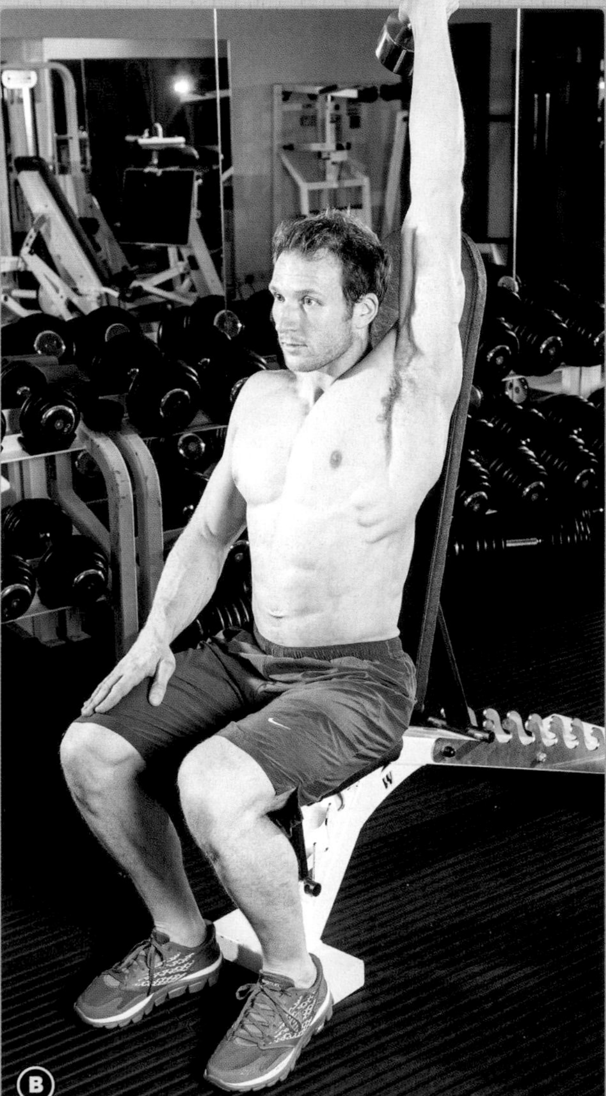

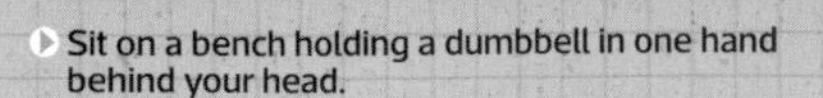

Sit on a bench holding a dumbbell in one hand behind your head.

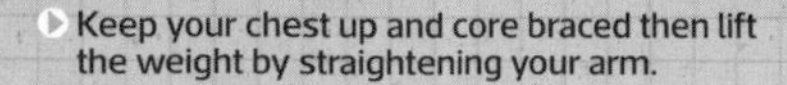

Keep your chest up and core braced then lift the weight by straightening your arm.

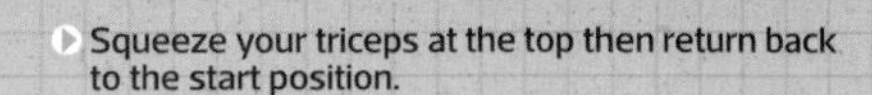

Squeeze your triceps at the top then return back to the start position.

Seated EZ-bar overhead triceps extension

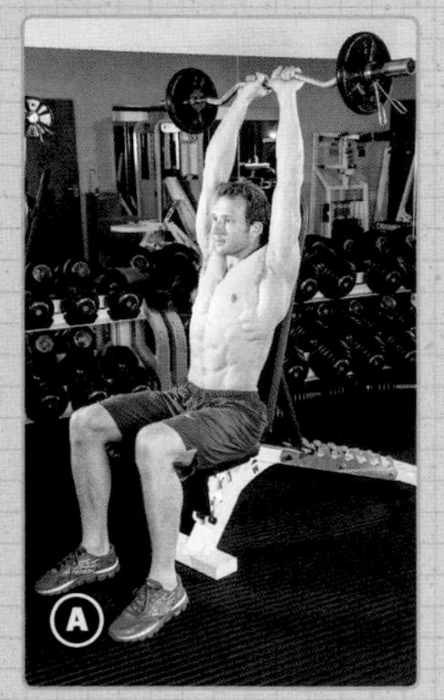
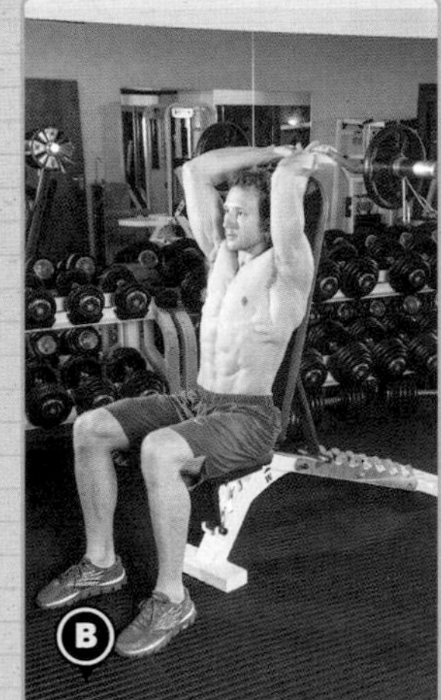

Using an EZ-bar works both arms at the same time and allows you to lift heavier weights.

Gym ball one-arm overhead triceps extension

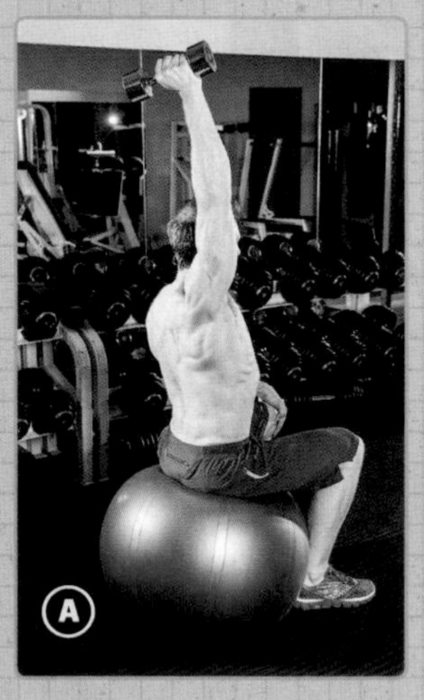
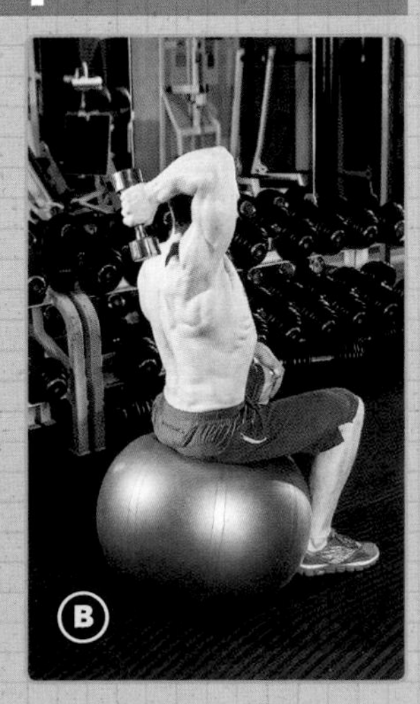

Sitting on the unstable gym ball forces your core to work hard to balance your body as you lift and lower the weight.

Dumbbell overhead triceps extension

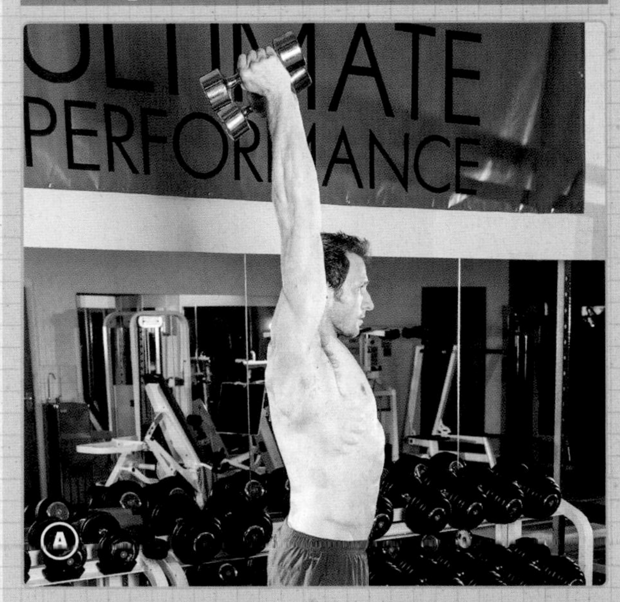

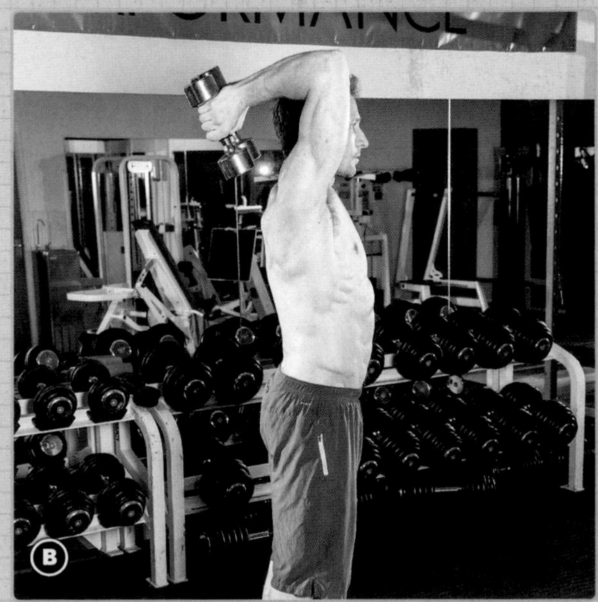

Using both hands to hold the dumbbell makes this a foundation move for building up your triceps.

CABLE TRICEPS PRESS-DOWN

Targets *Triceps, lower chest*

Working your triceps with the cable keeps constant tension on the muscle throughout every rep, while the double rope handles enable you to move through the complete range of motion

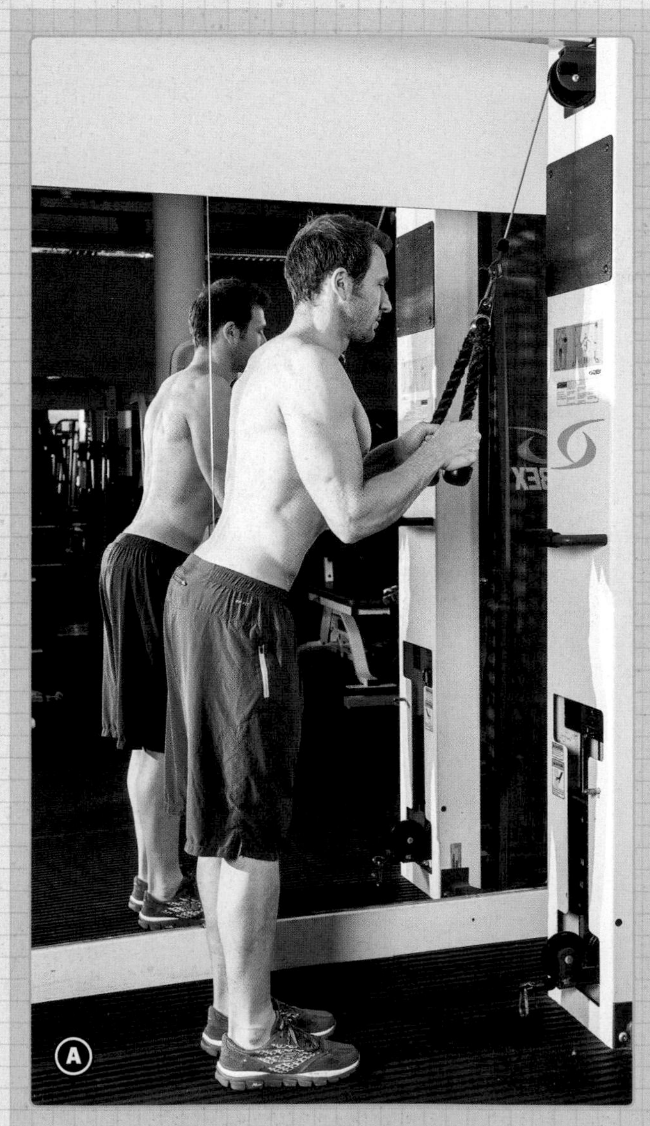

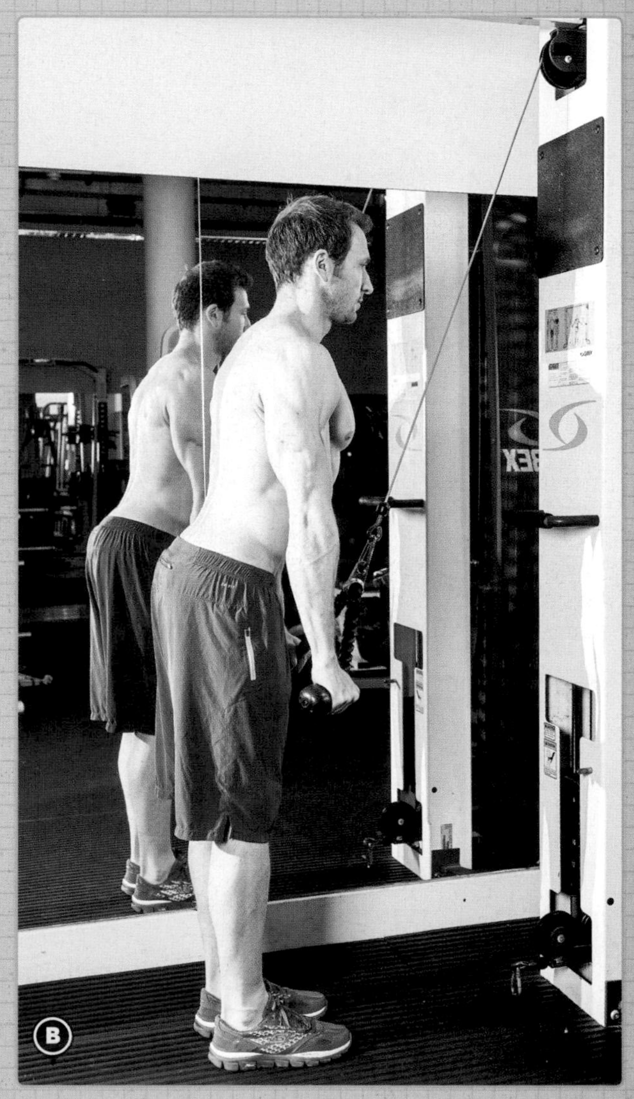

- Stand tall, holding a double-rope cable handle attached to the high pulley of a cable machine.
- Keeping your elbows next to your body, press your hands down to straighten your arms.
- Take the handles to either side of your legs to complete the full range of motion.
- At the bottom squeeze your triceps then return to the start, flexing your biceps when back at the very top.

Standing cable overhead triceps extension

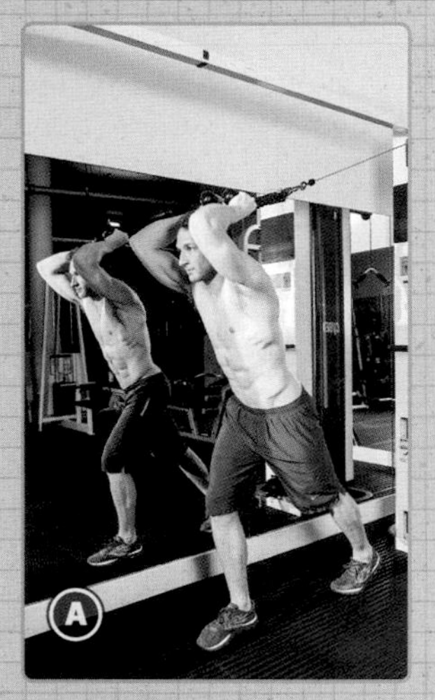

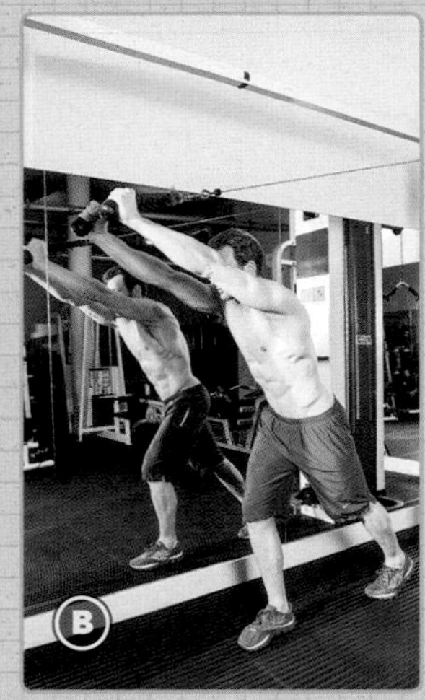

Facing away from the cable and extending your arms over your head works the target muscles from a different angle.

One-arm triceps press-down

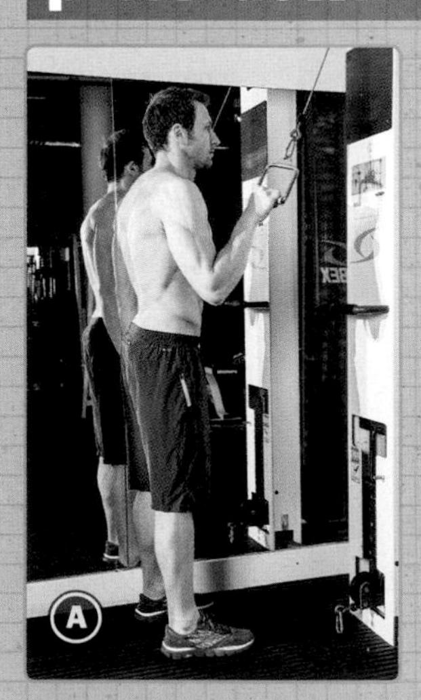

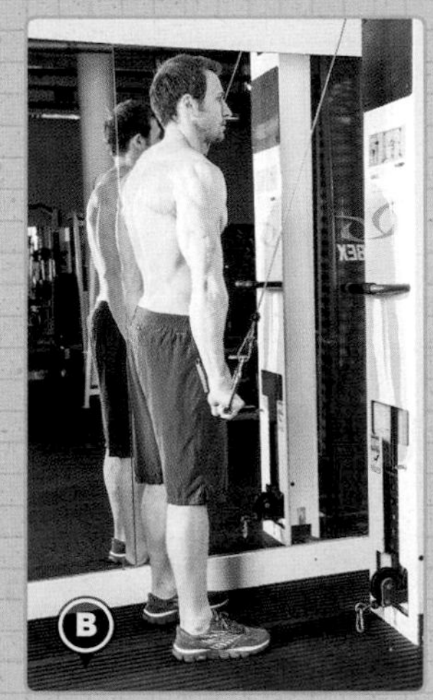

Working one arm at a time enables you to work your non-dominant arm independently of your stronger one, ensuring even muscle gains.

Cable EZ-bar triceps press-down

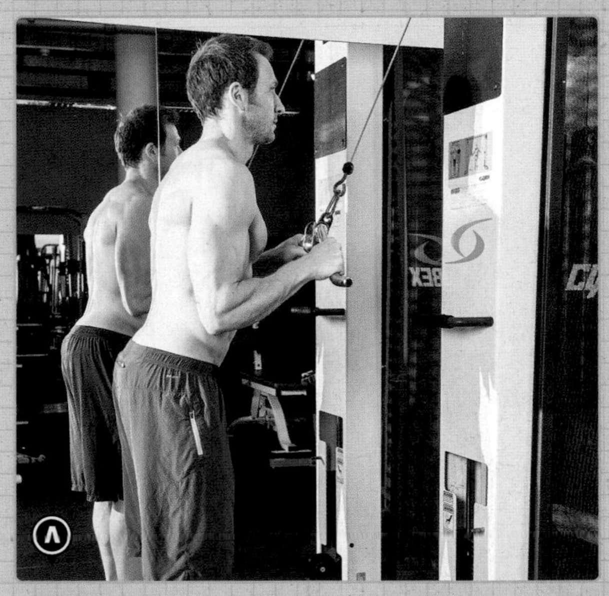

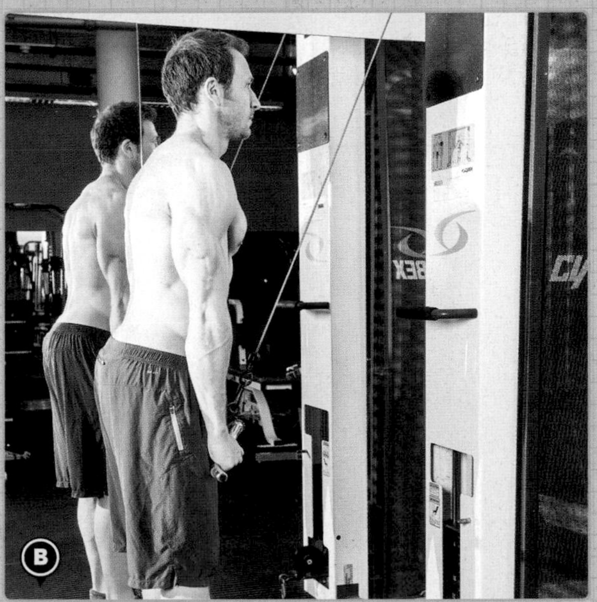

Using an EZ-bar works both arms together while minimising stress on your elbow joints.

DUMBBELL TRICEPS KICKBACK

Targets *Triceps*

This simple but effective move hits your triceps from a fresh angle and will build bigger triceps for beginners and experts

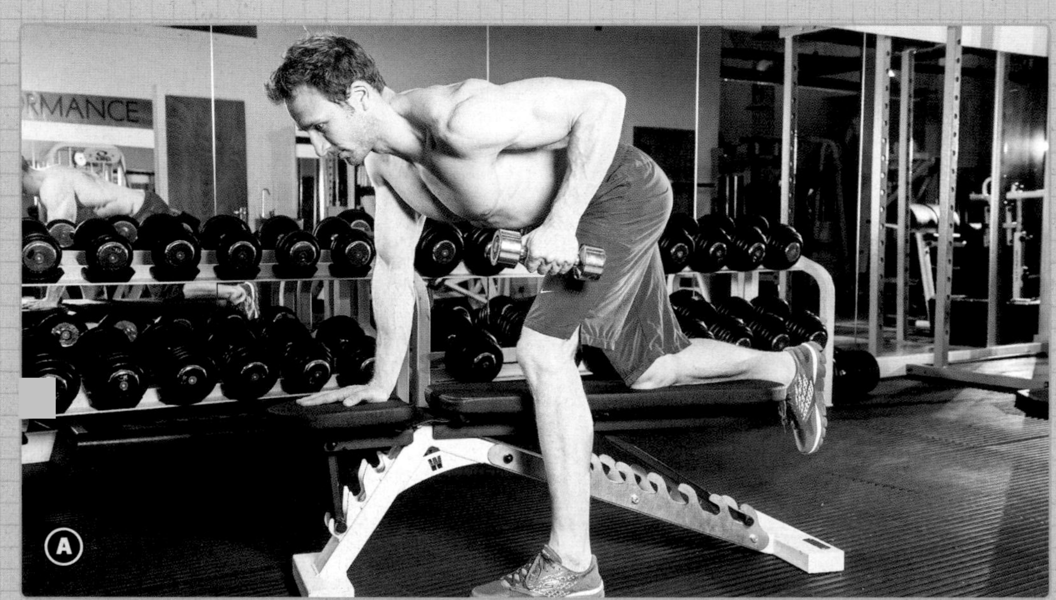

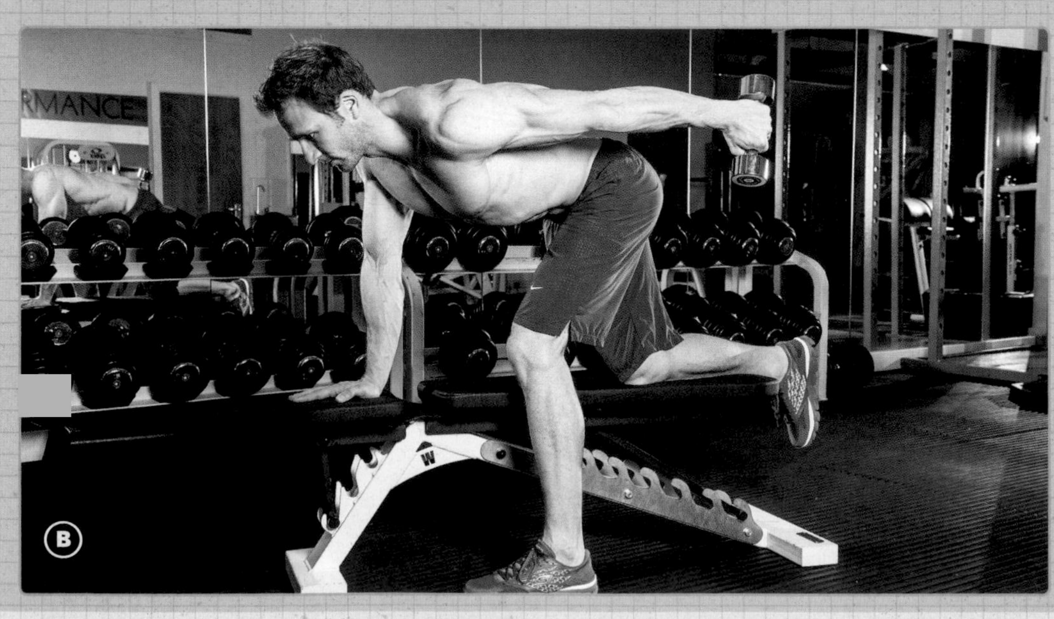

- Kneel on a flat bench with one arm straight to support your torso, holding a dumbbell in the other, which is bent at the elbow.
- Keeping your core braced, raise the weight by straightening your arm until your elbow is locked out.
- Return to the start.

Two-arm kickback

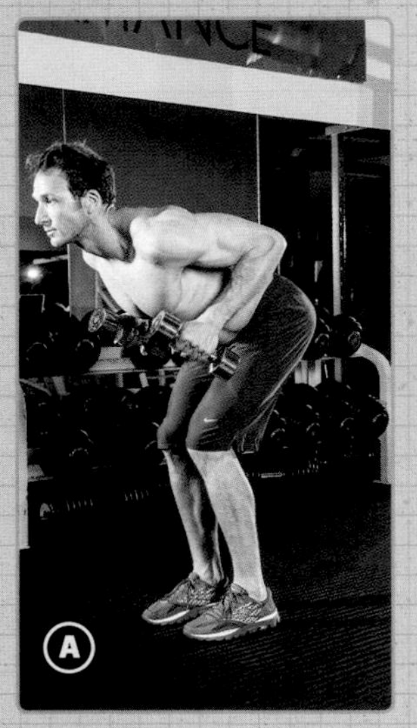

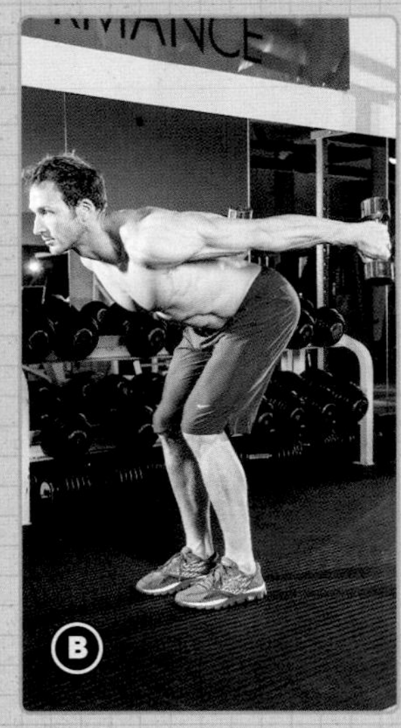

This works both arms at the same time, but requires strong stabilising muscles in your back and core to keep your torso in the correct position

Cable kickback

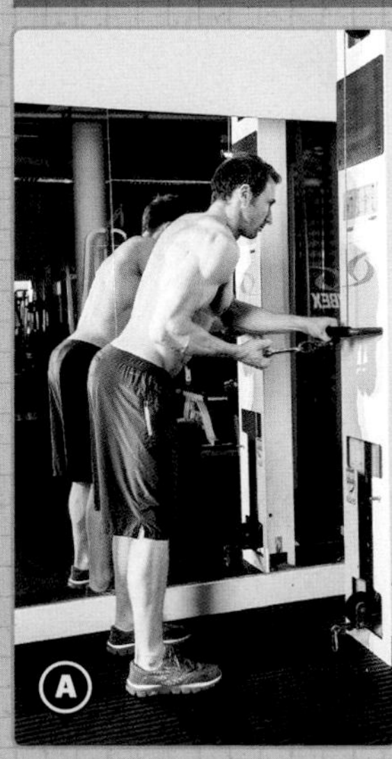

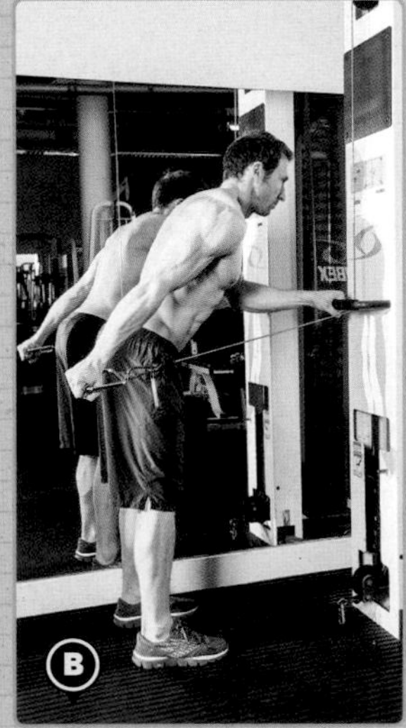

Using a cable machine places your muscles under greater tension throughout the entire rep.

Dumbbell kickback with lift

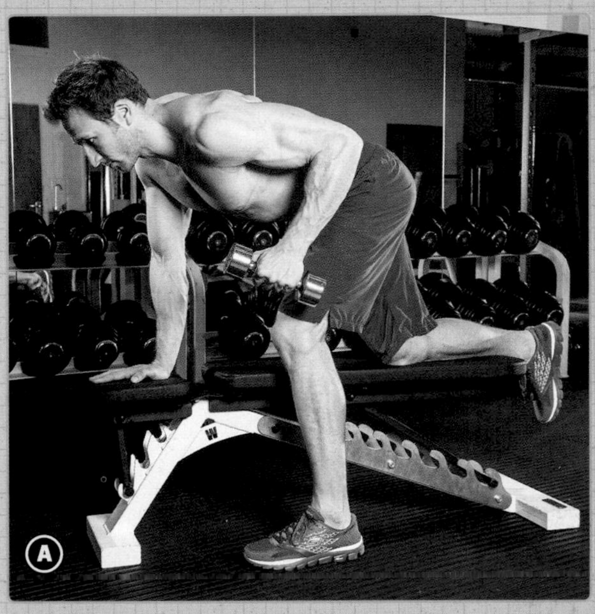

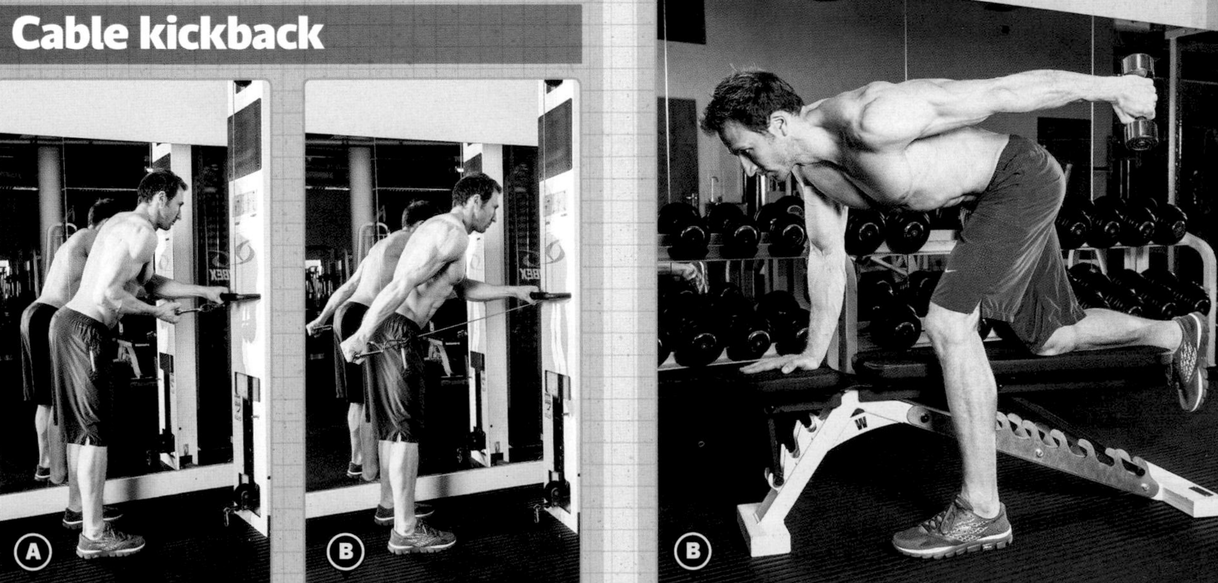

Raising the weight higher than your back recruits the upper back and shoulder muscles.

BACK

Build a big, strong and wide back with these key lifts

It's easy to discount the importance of a strong upper back. It's a major muscle group but because you can't see it in the mirror, it's easy to dedicate more of your training time to your chest, shoulders and arms, and other muscles on the front of your body.

This is a big mistake. A strong, powerful back improves your physique, corrects your posture and prevents injury, especially if you spend a lot of time working on your chest. A weak back in relation to a strong chest, on the other hand, will pull your shoulders forwards, which not only looks bad but also, as with any muscular imbalance between antagonistic muscles, will inevitably result in pain and injury.

Anatomically your back runs from the bottom of your neck to the top of your buttocks, and is a complex muscular structure. The upper half is primarily involved in the movement of the shoulder blades, while the lower part works with your abs to provide support, stability and posture.

> **"A strong, powerful back improves your physique, corrects your posture and prevents injury"**

Back explained

Here's how back muscles work

- The trapezius, or traps, is a diamond-shaped muscle that runs from your neck to your mid-back, and out to each shoulder joint. Its major role is to elevate and retract your scapula (shoulder blades).
- The rhomboid is a small, two-part, deep-lying muscle that is responsible for the retraction of the shoulder blades.
- The latissimus dorsi, or lats, is a larger, flat muscle partly covered by the traps. It is responsible for the extension, adduction, flexion and internal rotation of the shoulder joint.
- The teres major is a thick, flat muscle that assists the lats in moving your arms down towards your sides.
- The erector spinae is a group of muscles and tendons responsible for straightening the back and, with the abdominals, makes up the core that provides postural support and stability.

The back muscles

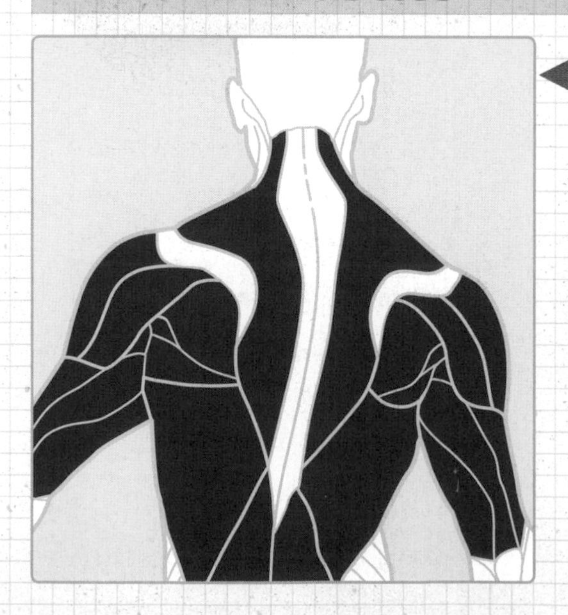

Training your back muscles is essential to getting a strong, balanced and injury-proof body. Working these muscles, especially your traps and lats, is also crucial to building a desirable V-shape torso, so never neglect back training if you want a bigger and stronger torso.

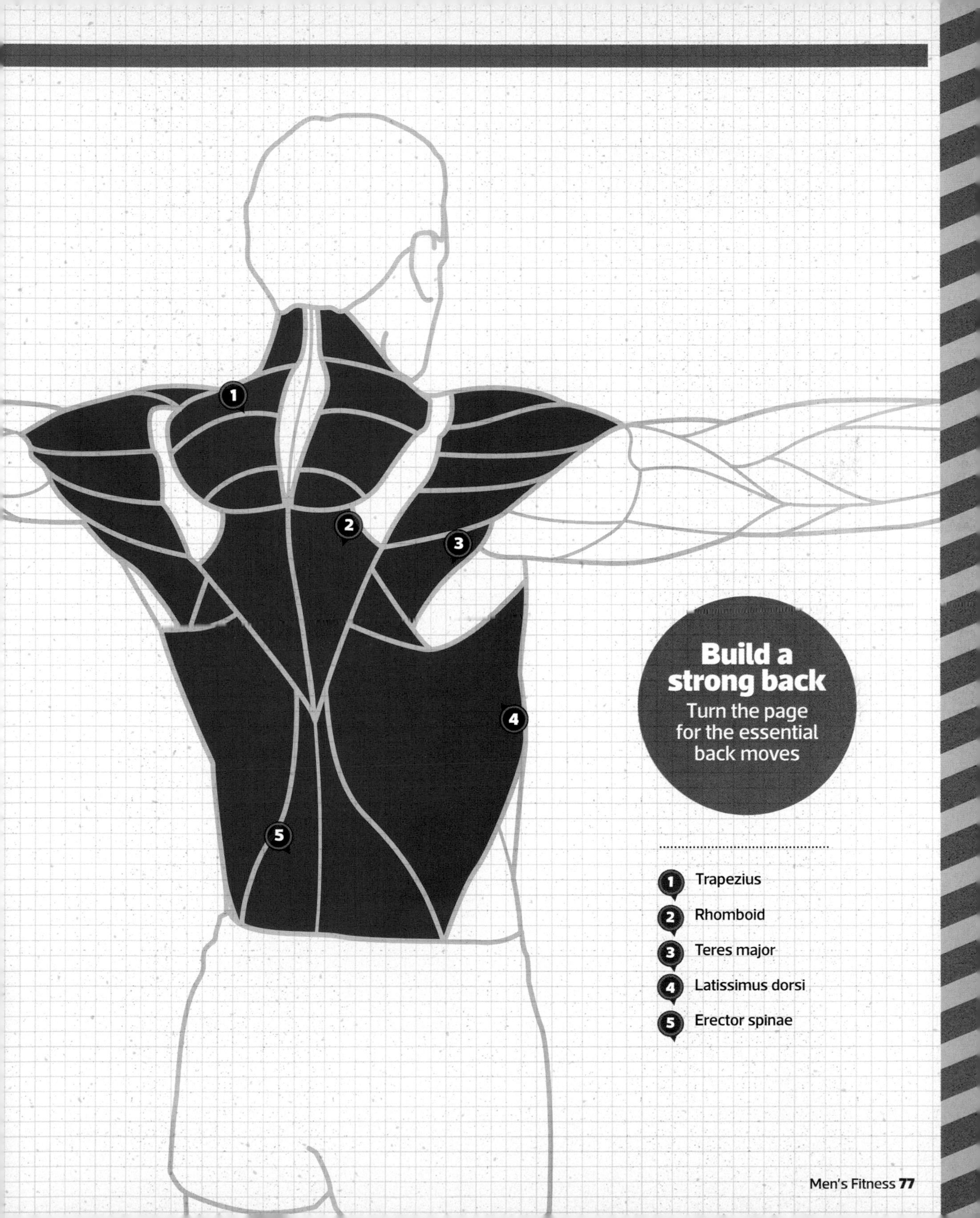
1
2
3
4
5
Build a strong back
Turn the page for the essential back moves
1 Trapezius
2 Rhomboid
3 Teres major
4 Latissimus dorsi
5 Erector spinae

PULL-UP

***Targets** Lats, traps, rhomboids*

The classic test of strength requires you to lift and control your entire bodyweight to hit all the major muscles of your upper back

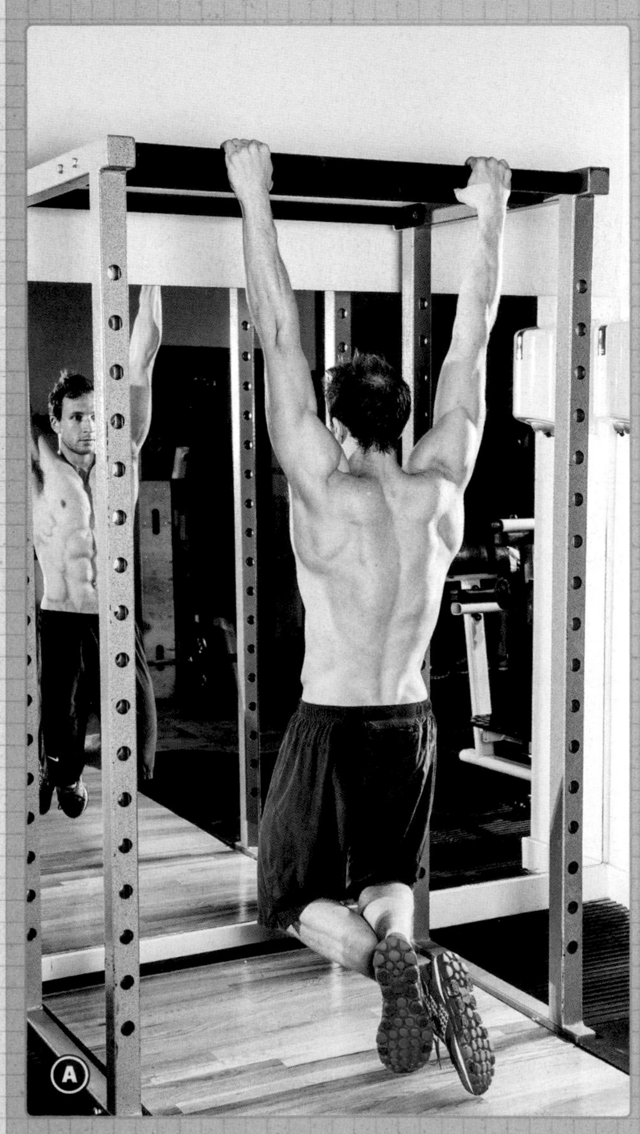

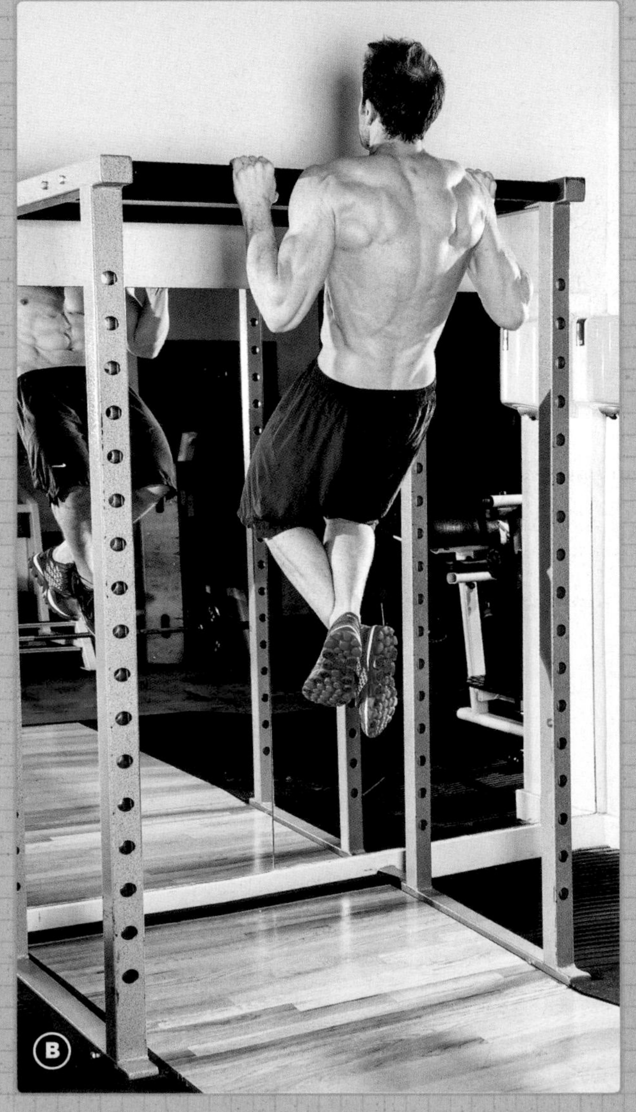

- Grab the bar with an overhand grip with your hands shoulder-width apart.
- Start from a dead hang with your arms fully extended.
- Pull yourself up by squeezing your lats together.
- Once your chin is higher than your hands, slowly lower back to the start.

Negative pull-up

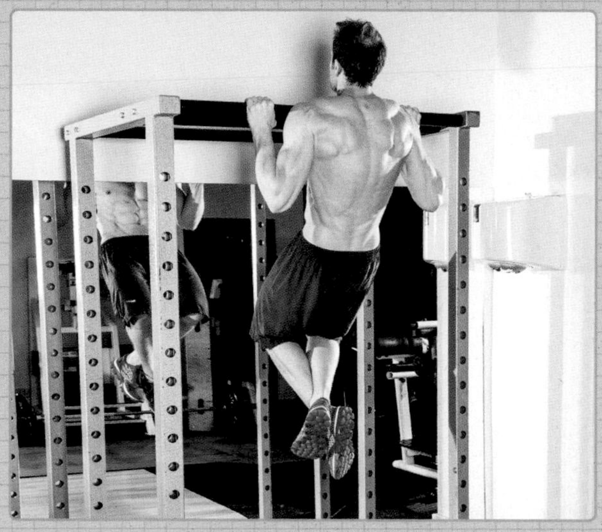

Jumping to the top position then slowly lowering yourself back down is a great way to build up the strength to perform full versions of the move.

Weighted pull-up

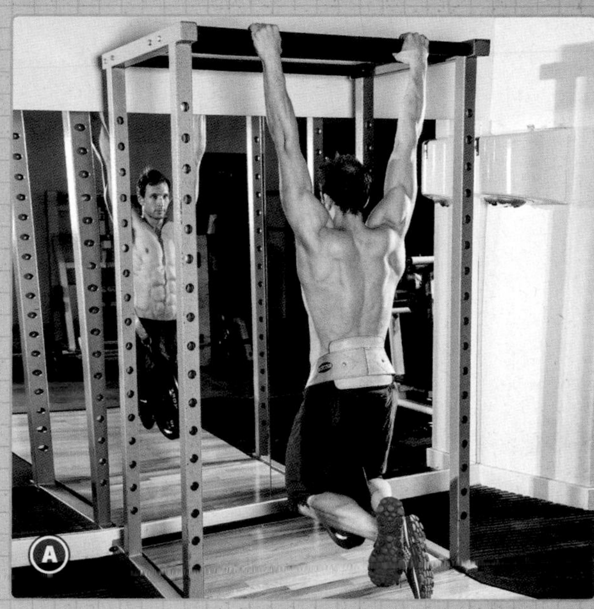

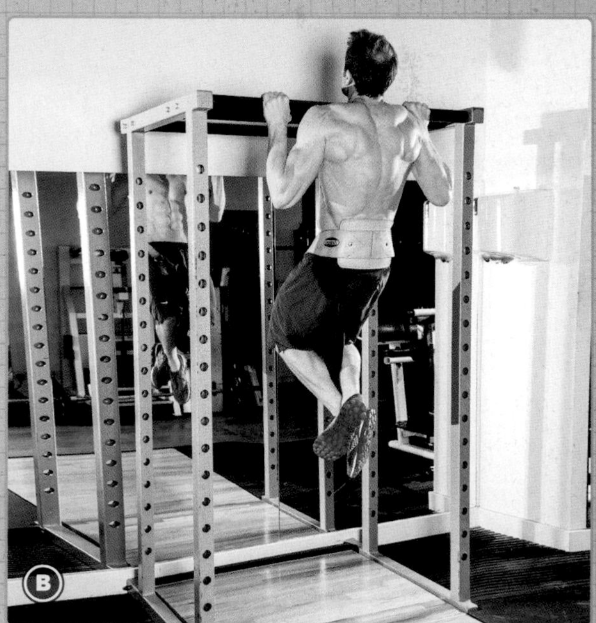

Adding extra weight to this move makes it far harder and far more effective at building size and strength.

Wide-grip pull-up

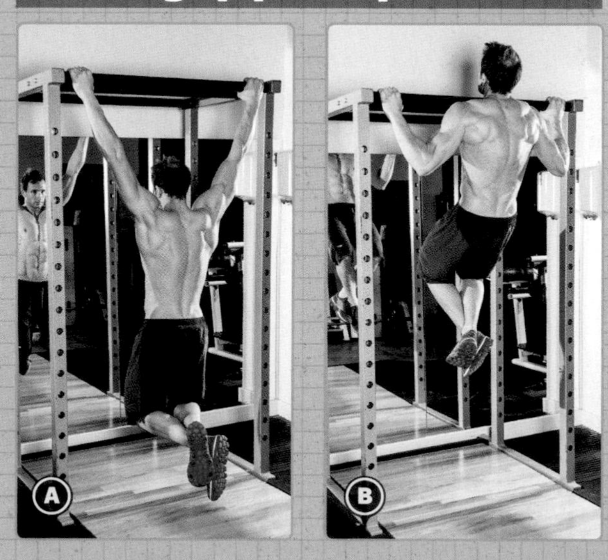

The wider the grip, the harder your upper back muscles have to work to raise you to the top position.

BENT-OVER ROW

***Targets** Traps, lats, rhomboids*

One of the key moves for targeting your entire back, while also working your core, biceps and shoulders

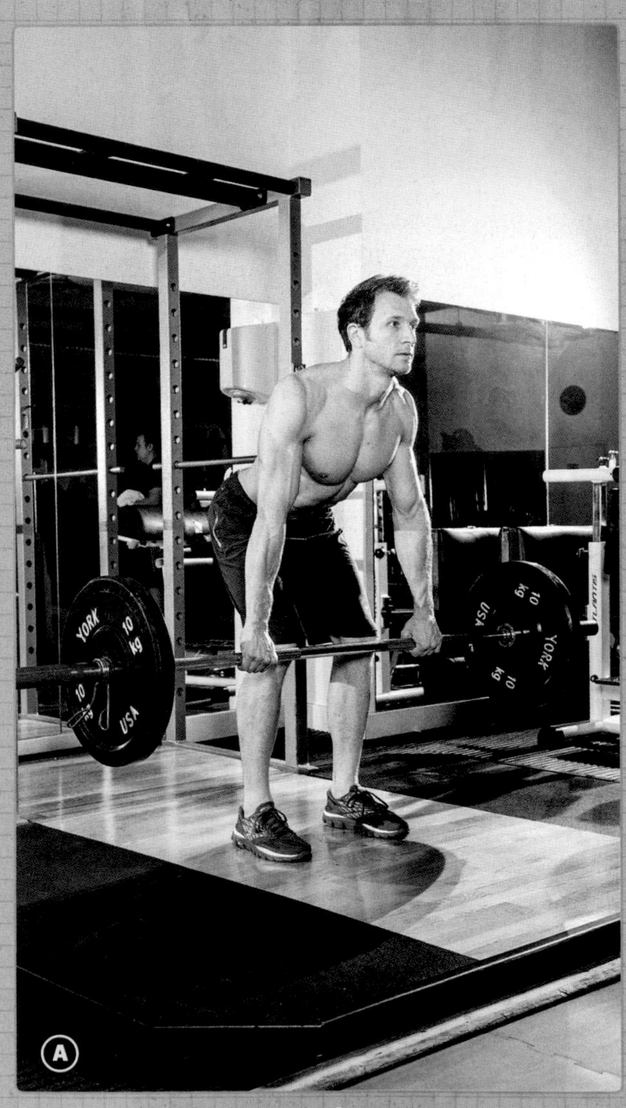

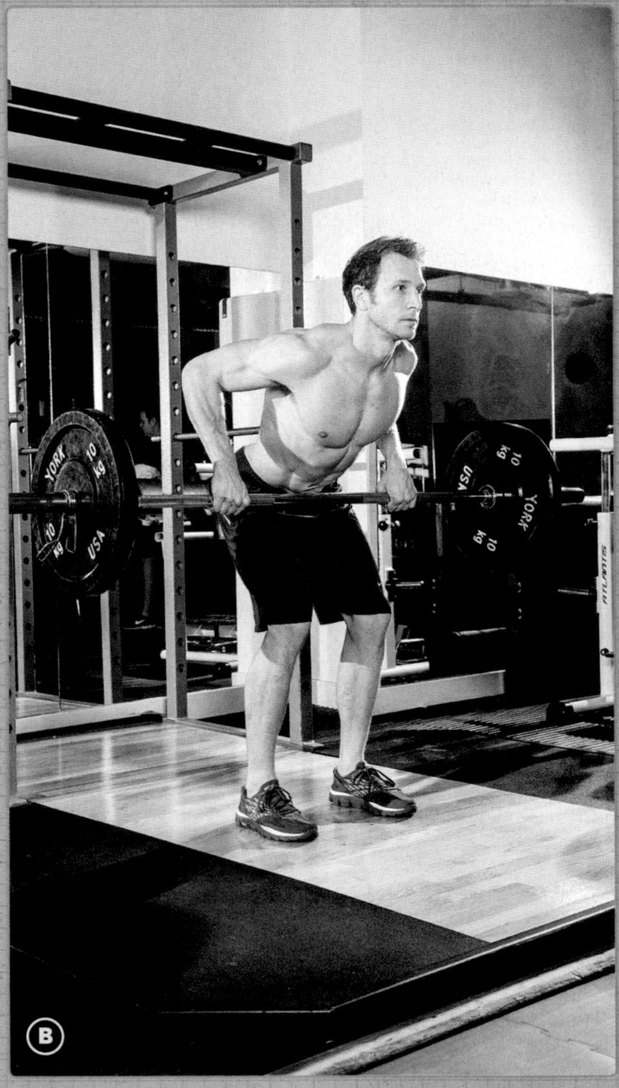

- Start with your core braced, your back straight and your shoulder blades retracted.
- Bend your knees slightly and lean forwards from the hips.
- Grip the bar with your hands just wider than shoulder-width apart, letting them hang at knee level.
- Pull the bar up to your lower sternum, retracting your shoulder blades to allow the bar to come up to your chest, then lower the bar slowly to the start.

Reverse-grip bent-over row

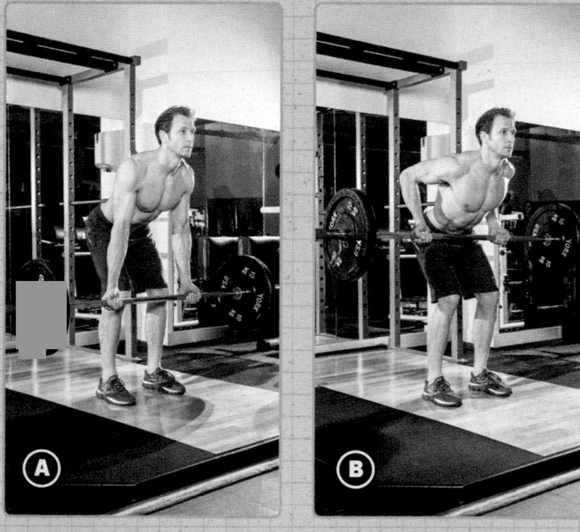

Taking an underhand grip places more emphasis on your biceps.

Bent-over flye

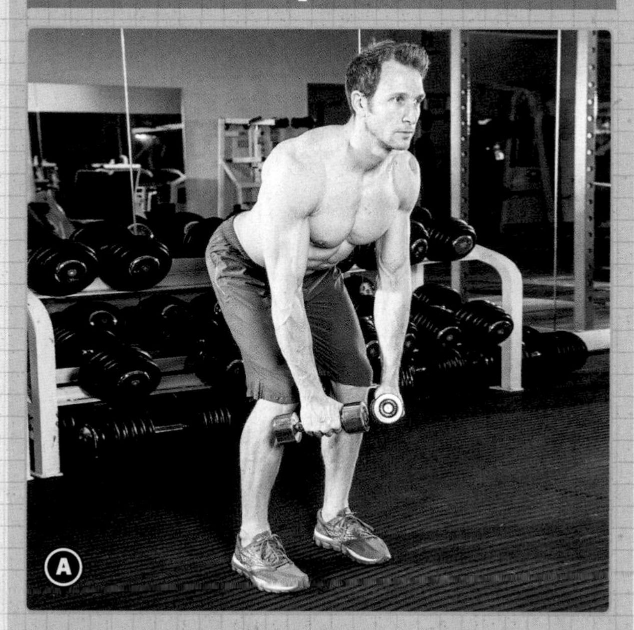

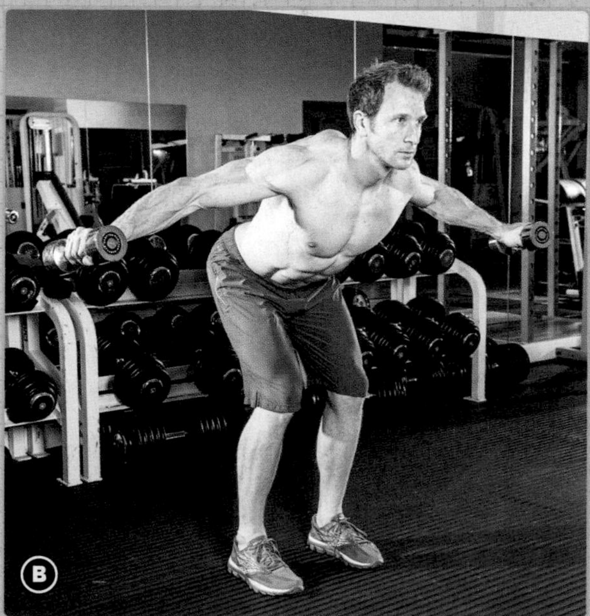

Keeping a slight bend in your elbows as you raise your arms to the sides works your shoulders as well as upper back and core.

Dumbbell bent-over row

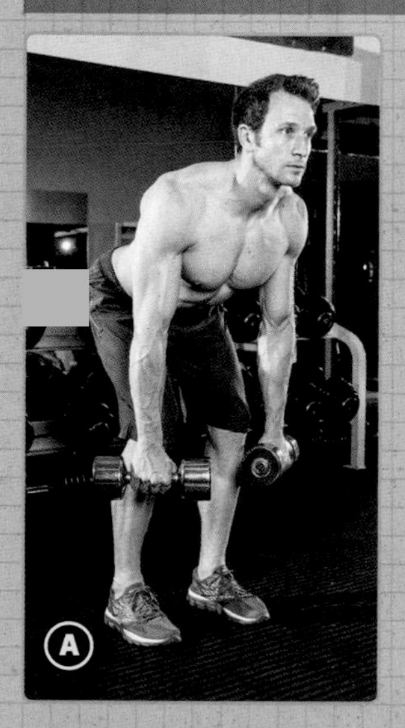

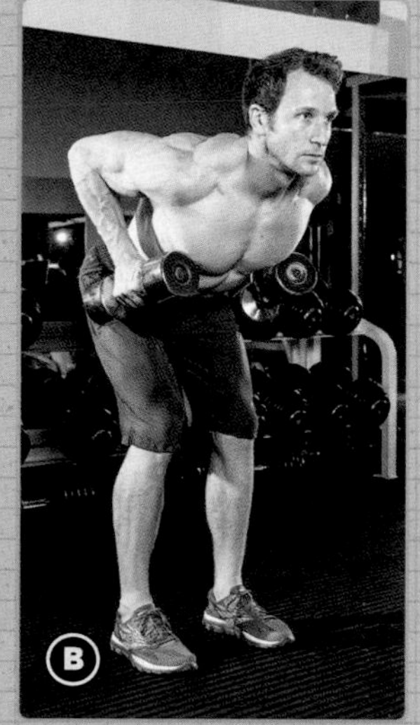

Using dumbbells involves the same target muscles while preventing the stronger side of your body doing more than its share of the work.

LAT PULL-DOWN

***Targets** Lats, traps, rhomboids*

This works the same muscles as the pull-up but the machine allows you to adjust the resistance to lift lighter or heavier than your bodyweight to build strength and muscle mass

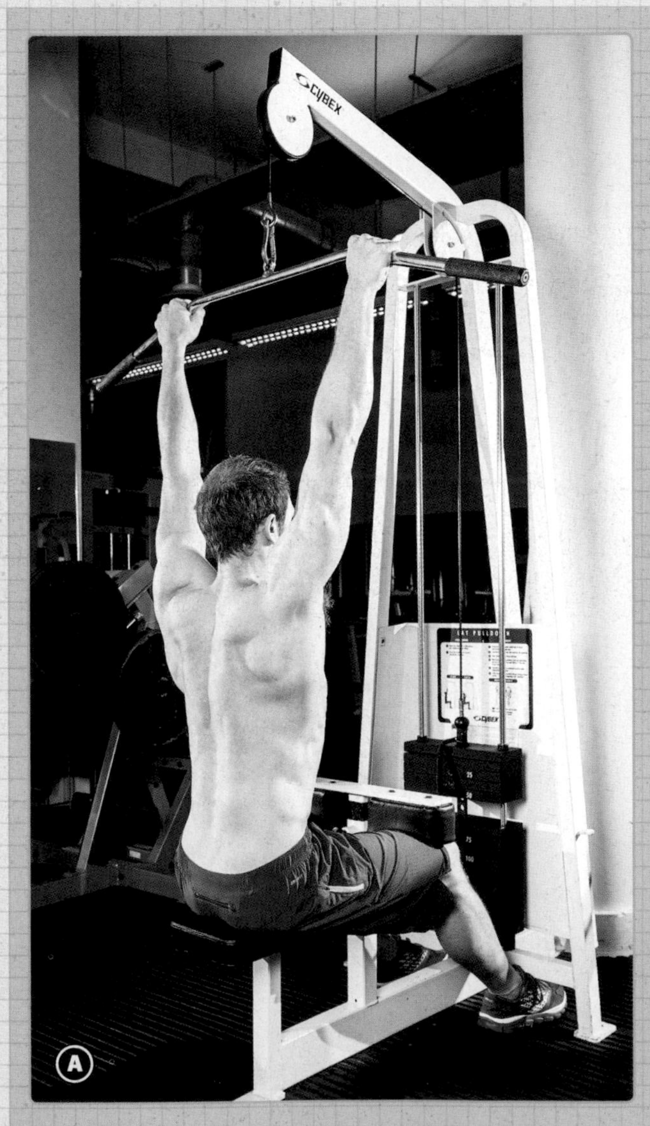

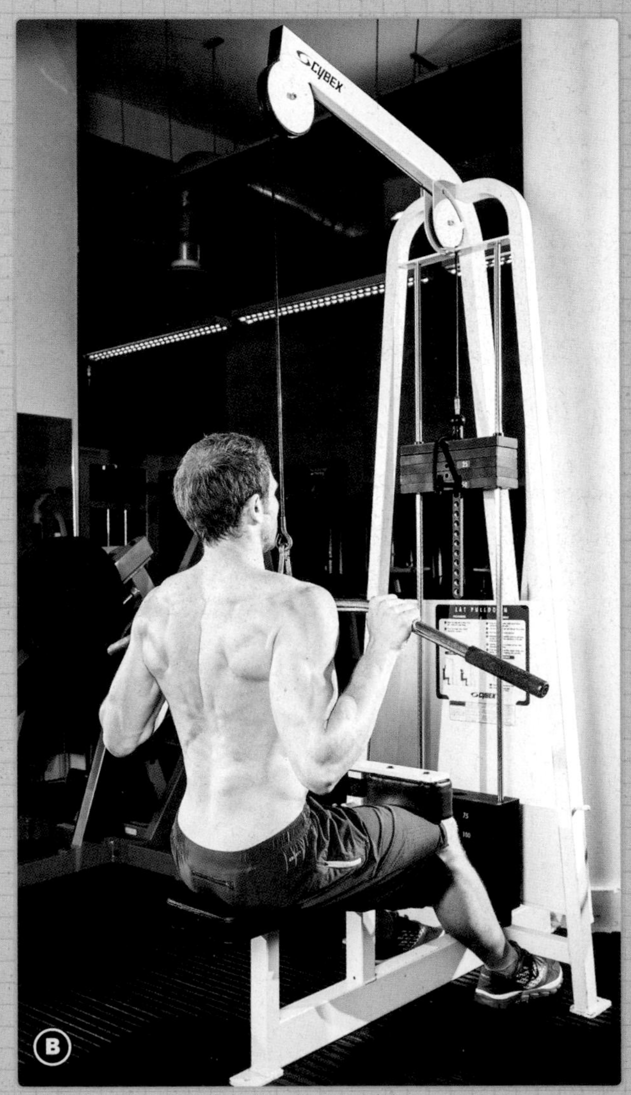

- Sit on the seat and take an overhand, wide grip on the bar.
- Look forwards, retract your shoulder blades and keep your torso upright.
- Pull the bar down in front of you until it reaches your upper chest. Don't lean back to aid the movement.
- Squeeze your lats at the bottom of the move and return the bar slowly to the top.

Underhand lat pull-down

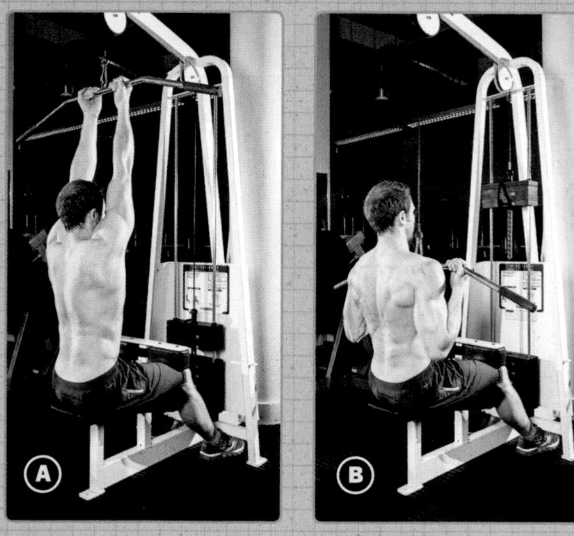

Gripping the bar so your palms are facing your body brings your biceps into play more.

One-arm lat pull-down

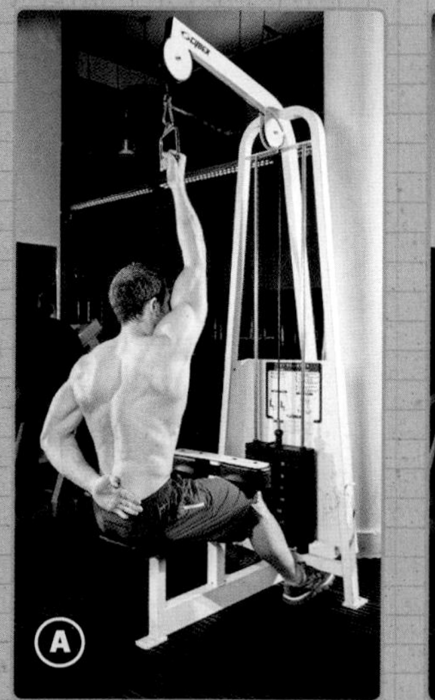

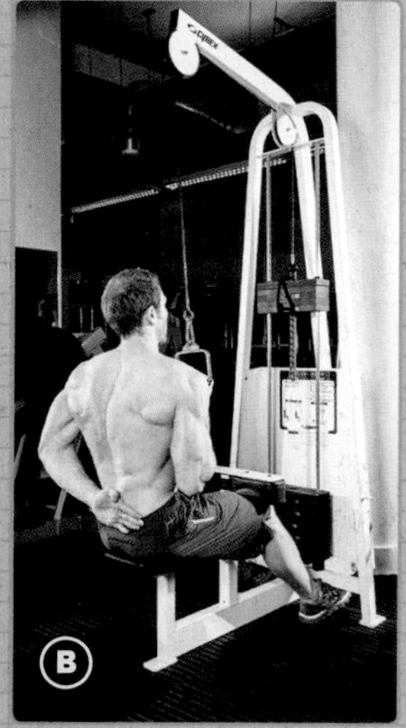

Working each arm individually promotes balanced growth and prevents your stronger side from dominating the move.

Close-grip lat pull-down

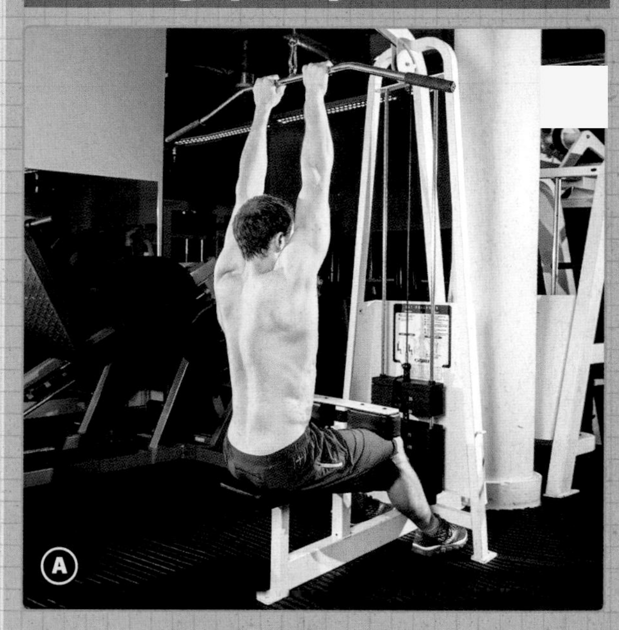

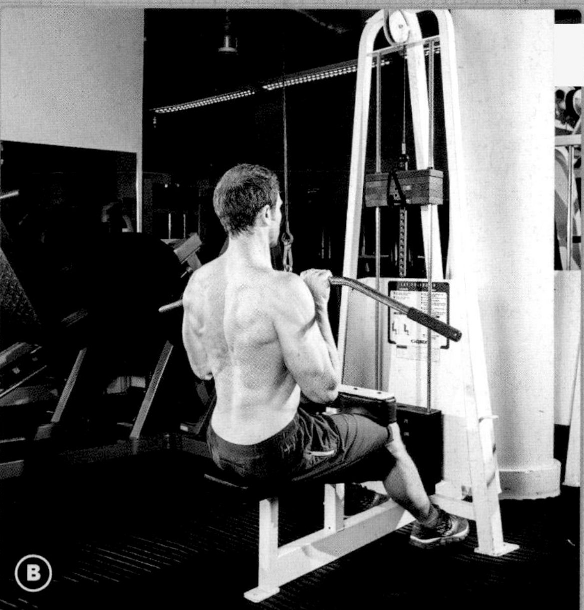

Taking a shoulder-width grip on the bar makes the move easier.

ONE-ARM DUMBBELL ROW

Targets *Traps, lats, rhomboids*

This move allows you to go heavy while working both sides of your back and each arm individually for big muscle benefits

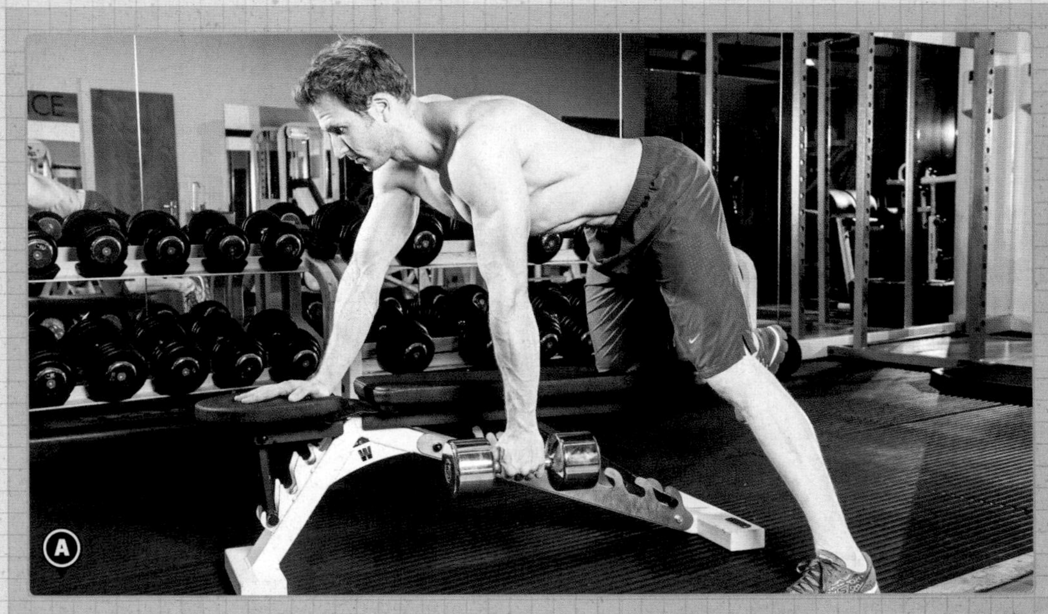

A

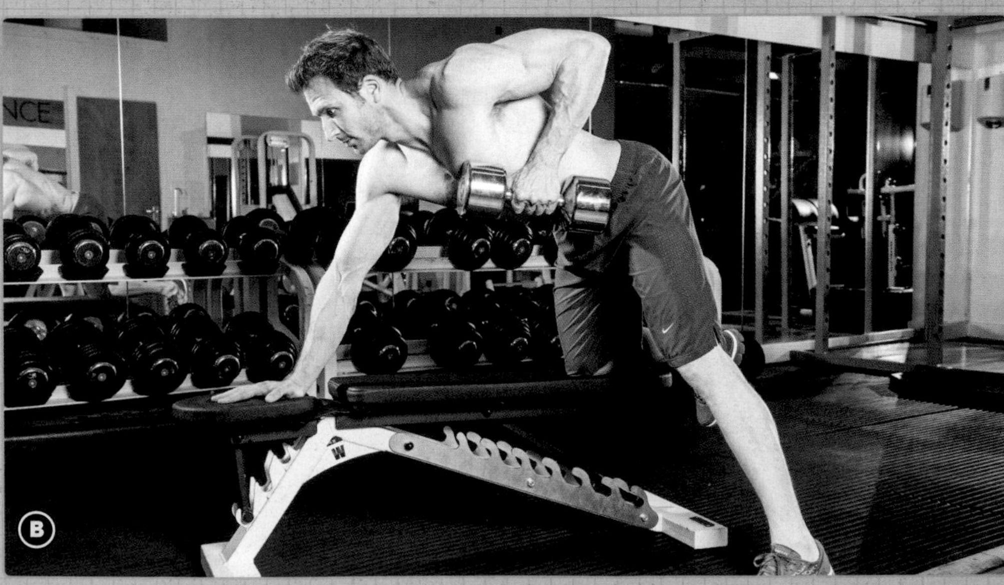

B

- Place your right knee and right hand flat on a bench, with your left leg out to the side. Hold a dumbbell in your left hand with your arm hanging straight down.
- With a natural arch in your back and core braced, lift the weight towards your side, leading with the elbow.
- Pause at the top before returning to the start. Repeat on the other side.

One-arm cable row

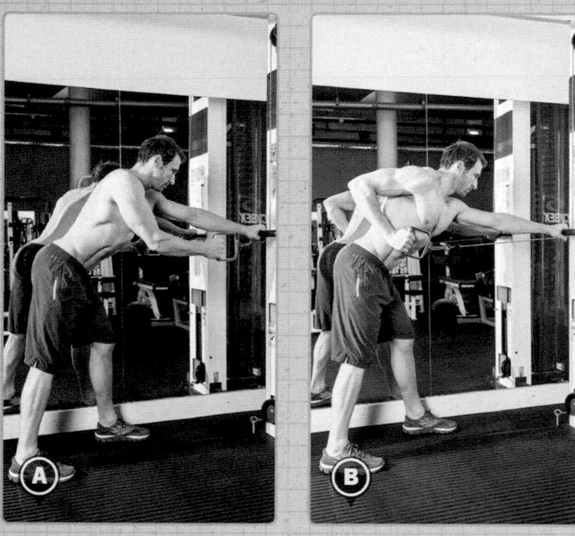

The cable keeps the tension on your target muscles throughout the move and forces your core to engage and stabilise your body.

Split squat to one-arm row

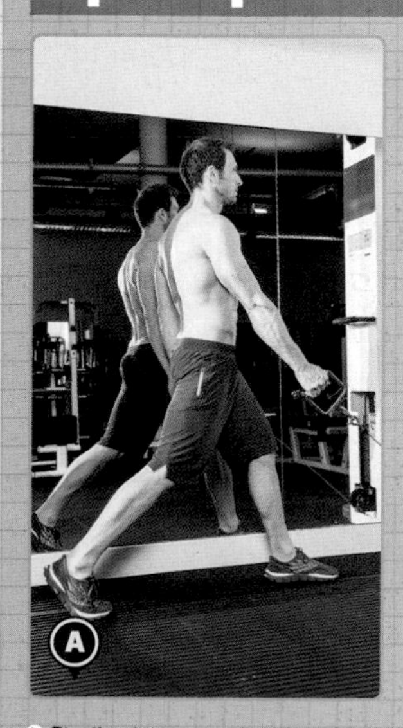

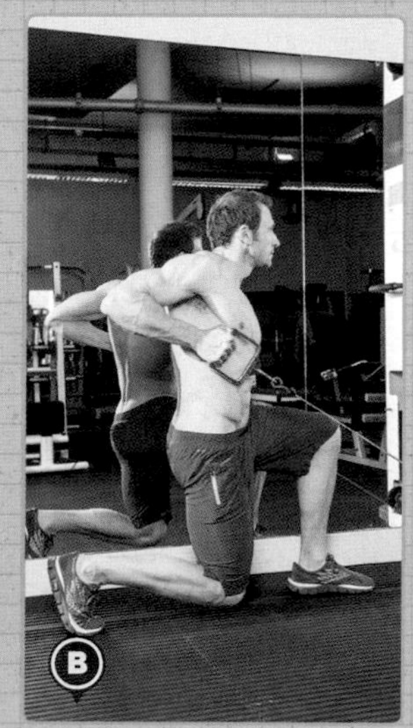

Starting in a squat then standing while rowing makes this a total-body move that targets multiple muscle groups.

One-arm reverse flye

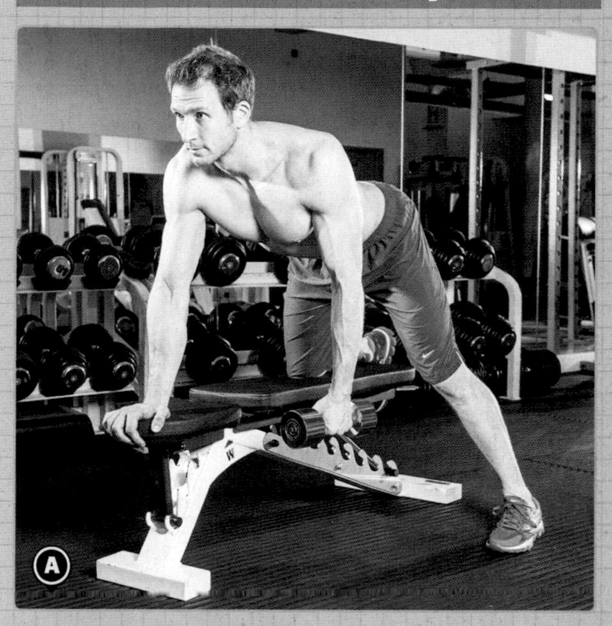

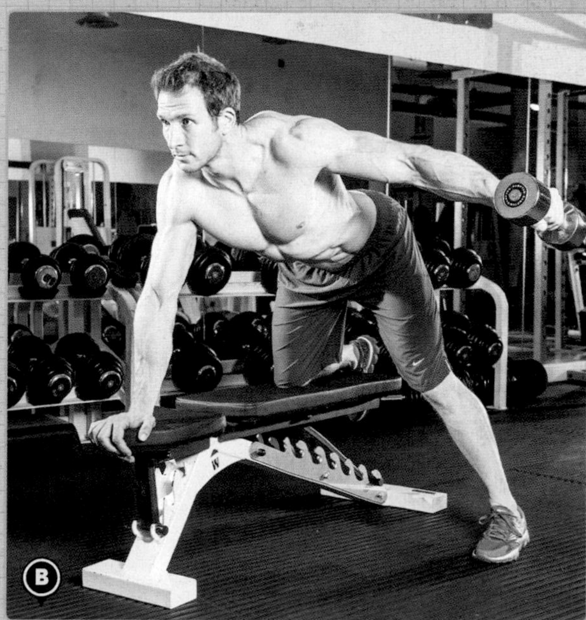

Keeping your arm straight shifts the emphasis of the move to your rear delts and upper back.

SEATED CABLE ROW

***Targets** Lats, traps, rhomboids, biceps*

Effectively target your upper back and biceps with this seated move that allows you to go heavy while maintaining perfect form for maximum muscle gains

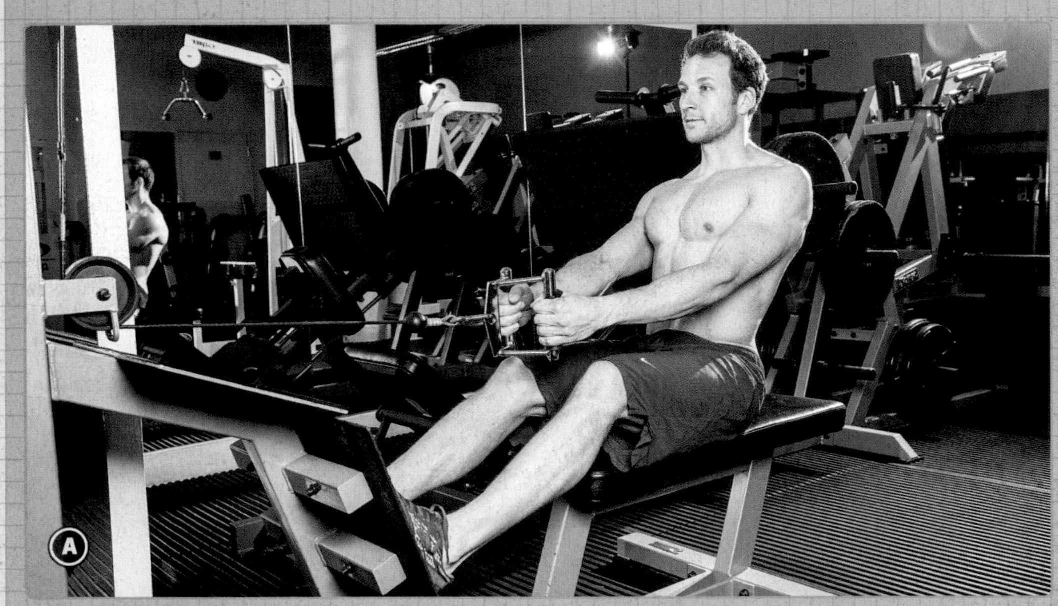

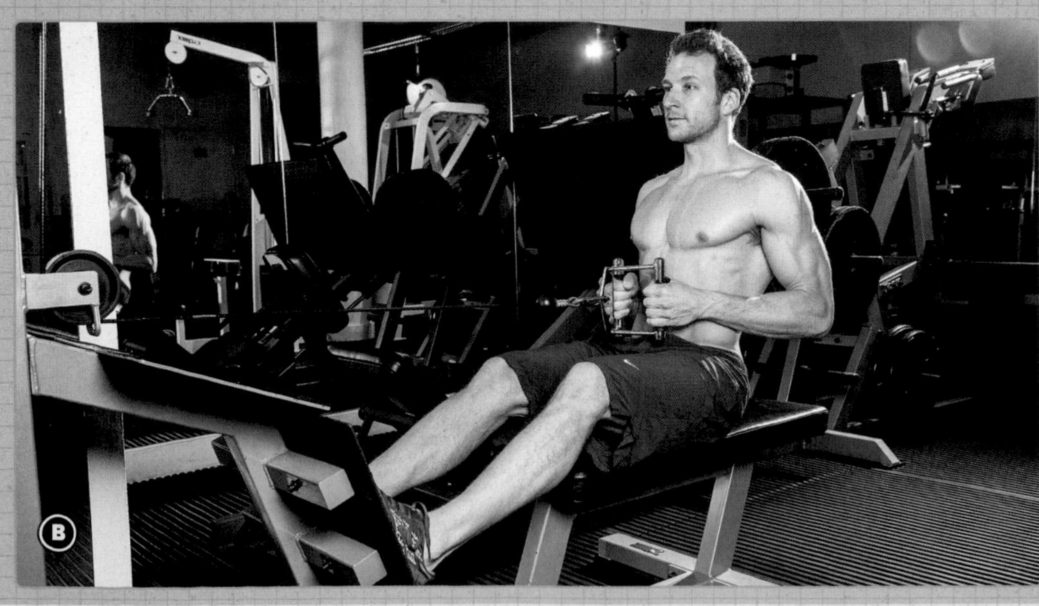

- Sit on the bench with a slight bend in your knees. With a neutral grip, hold a double-D handle attached to the lower pulley of a cable machine.
- Ensure there's tension in the cable before you begin.
- Pull the handle into your sternum, keeping upper-body movement to a minimum, and squeeze your shoulder blades together.
- Return slowly to the start.

Face pull

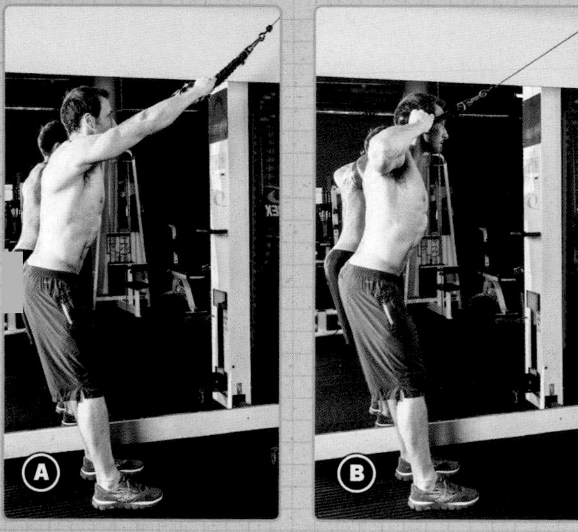

Pulling the double handles to either side of your face hits your traps, rhomboids and rear delts effectively.

Wide-grip cable row

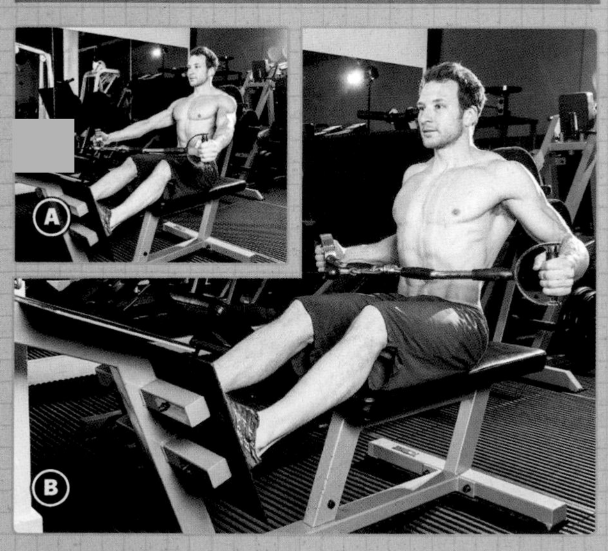

Taking a wide grip on a straight bar removes your biceps from the equation and forces the back and rear shoulders to work harder.

Inverted row

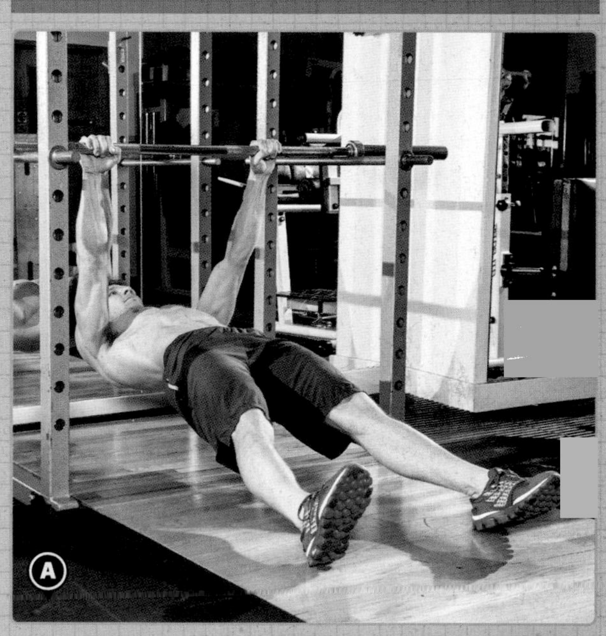

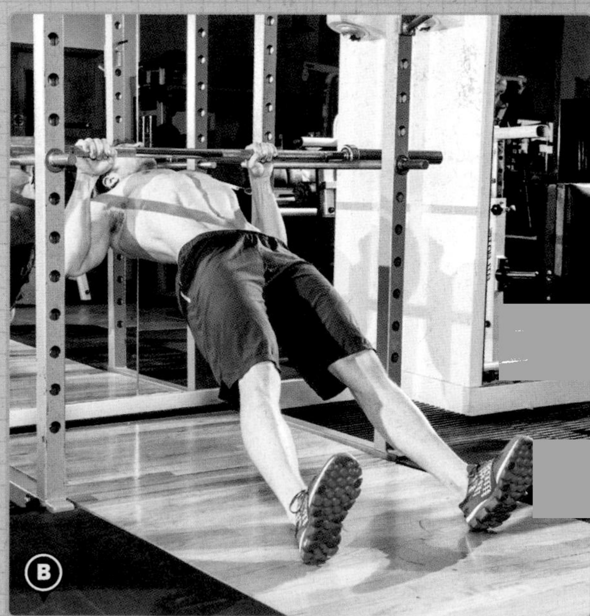

Raise your chest to the bar to use your bodyweight and work your back and biceps.

BARBELL SHRUG

***Targets* Traps**

Build big, strong traps with this move – the limited range of motion means you can lift heavy as long as you keep to strict form

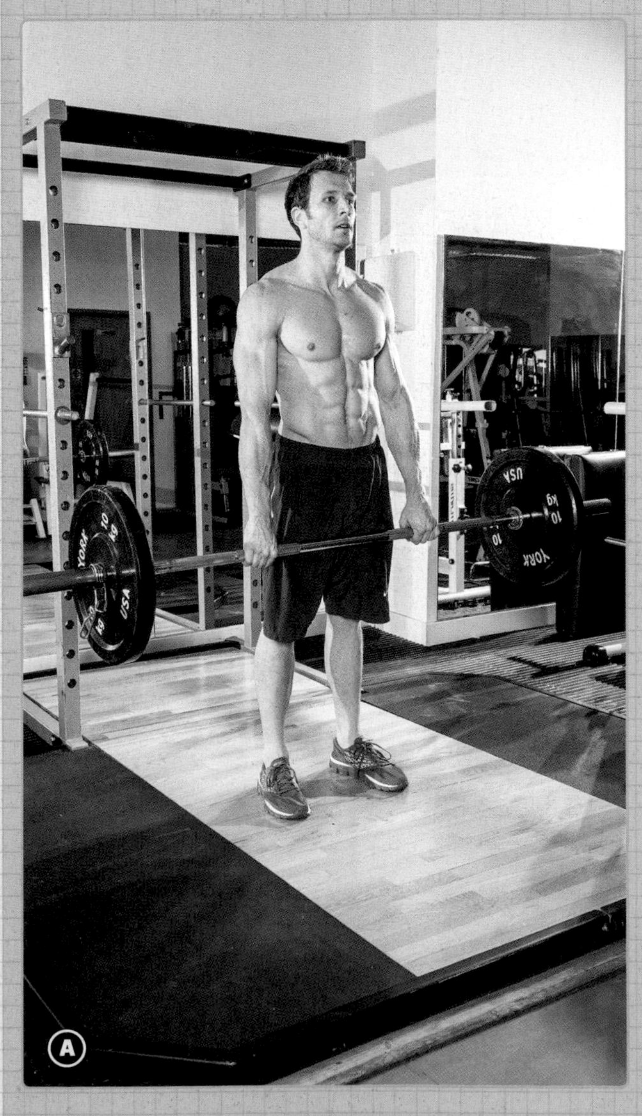

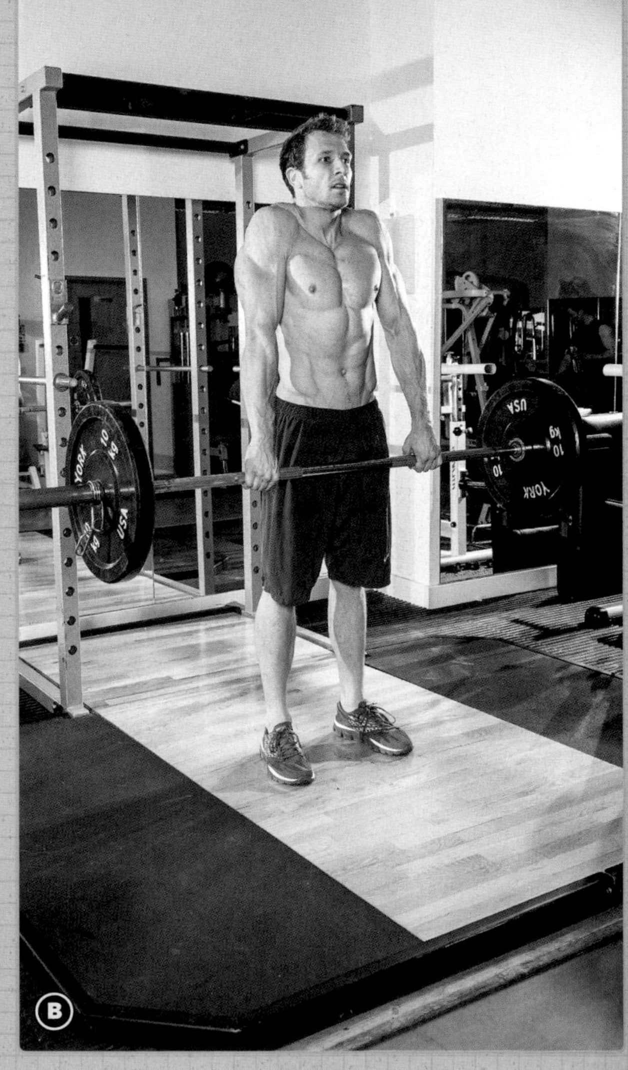

- Hold a bar with an overhand grip with your hands just outside your thighs.
- Keeping your core braced, chest up and a natural arch in your back, shrug your shoulders up towards your ears, keeping your arms straight.
- Hold at the top briefly then lower the bar back to the start position.

Snatch-grip shrug

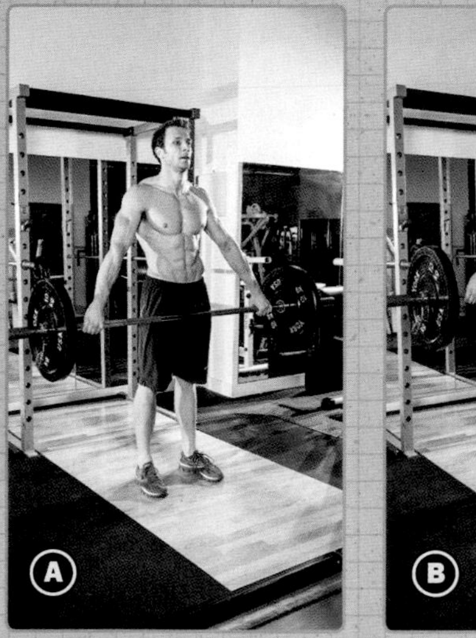

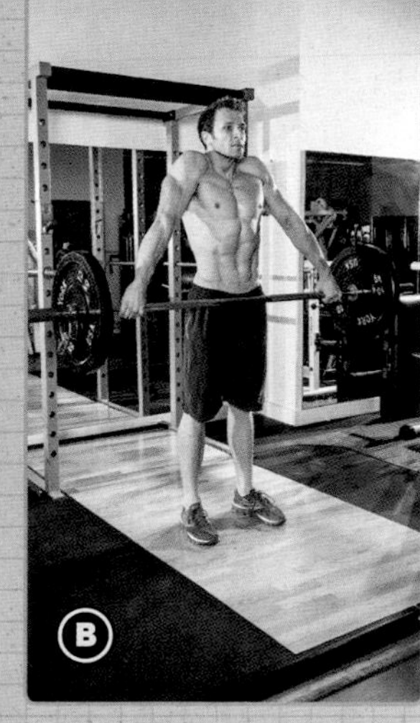

Taking a wider grip on the bar will target different parts of your traps for better muscle growth.

Snatch pull

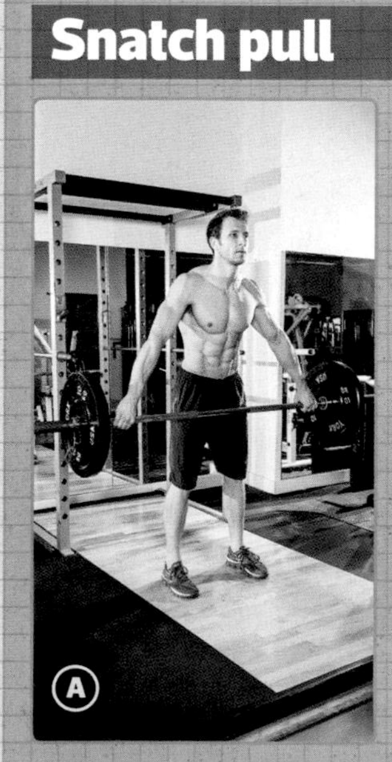

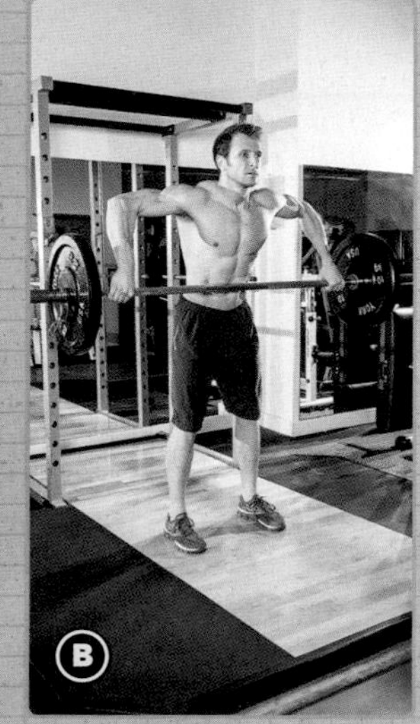

A wide-grip snatch pull will recruit more muscles of your upper back than just your traps for faster muscle gains.

Dumbbell shrug

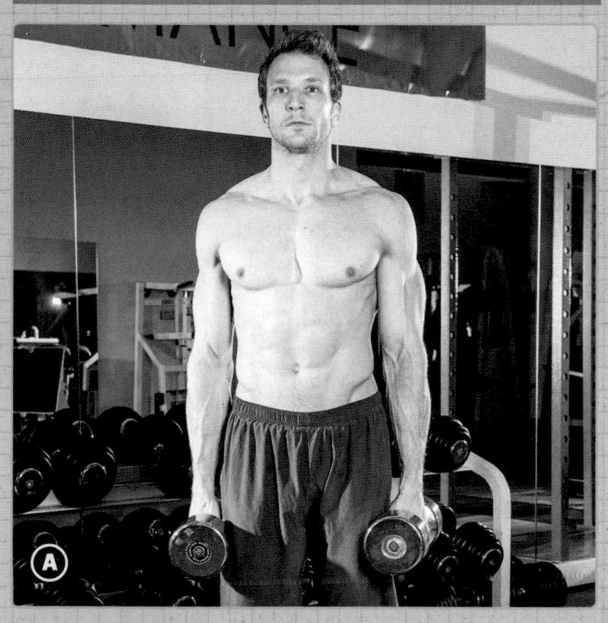

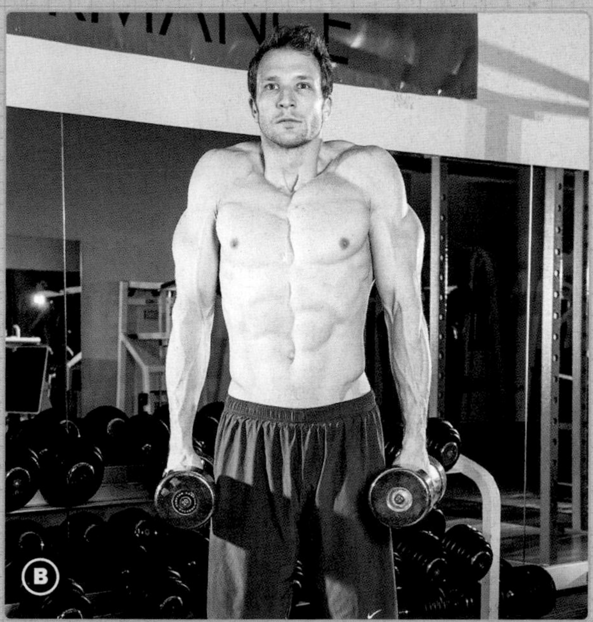

Using dumbbells allows you to keep your hands by your sides for increased comfort, while also working each side of your upper back individually.

GOOD MORNING

Targets *Lower back, hamstrings, glutes*

This move will strengthen the erector spinae muscles of your lower back, which will make your core stronger and assist the transfer of power between your upper and lower body

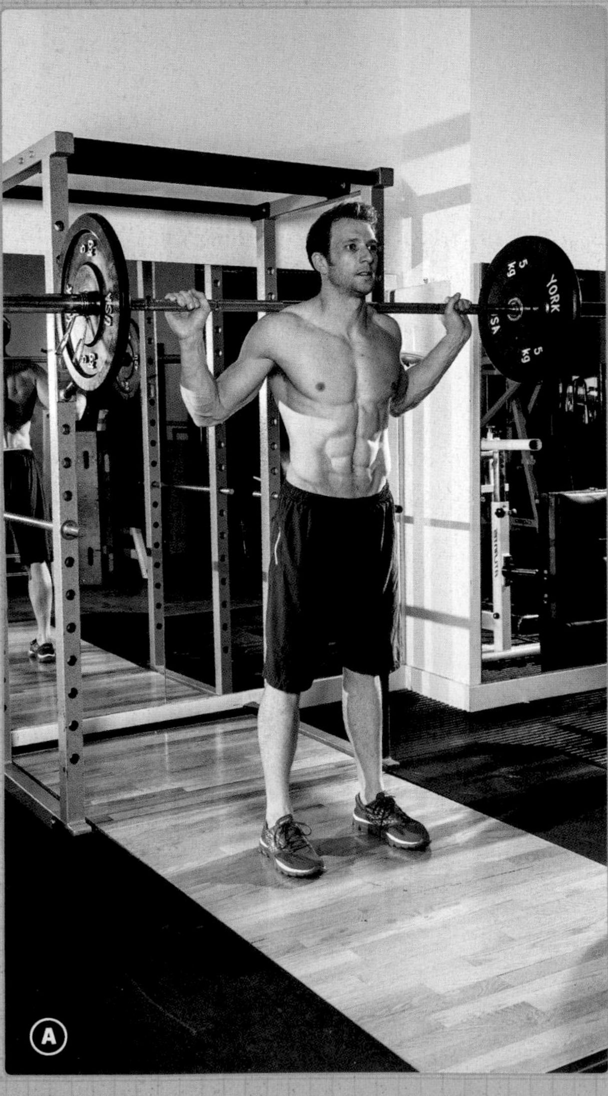

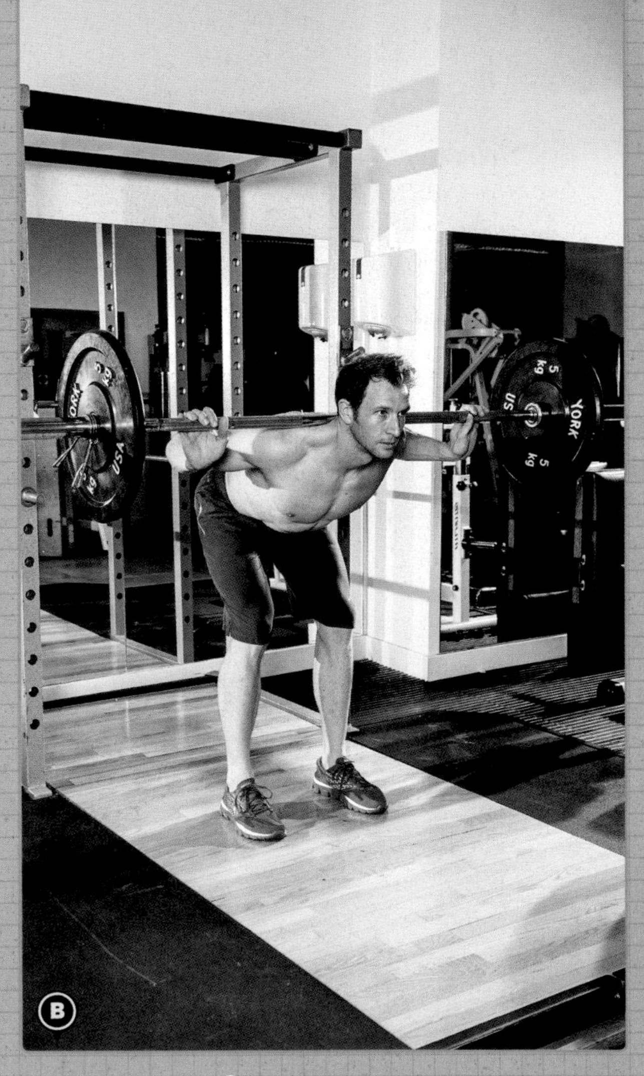

- Stand tall with your feet shoulder-width apart with a light barbell resting across the back of your shoulders.
- Keeping your core braced and a slight bend in your knees, bend forwards from the hips – not the waist – as far as your hamstrings will allow, but not beyond horizontal.
- Return to the start position.

One-leg good morning

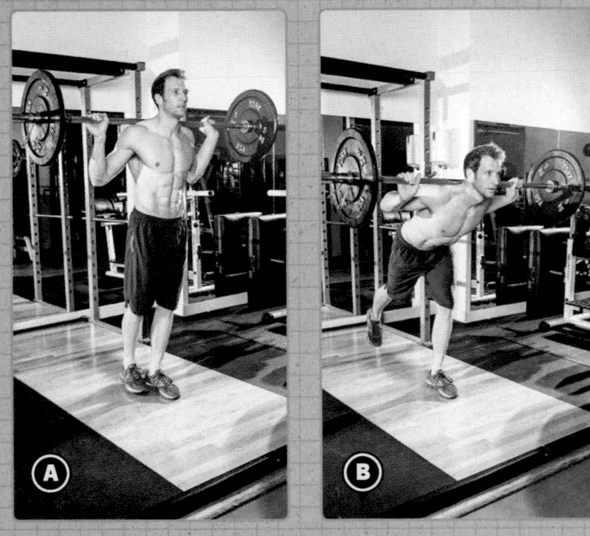

Test your working leg hard by lifting the other off the ground.

Split good morning

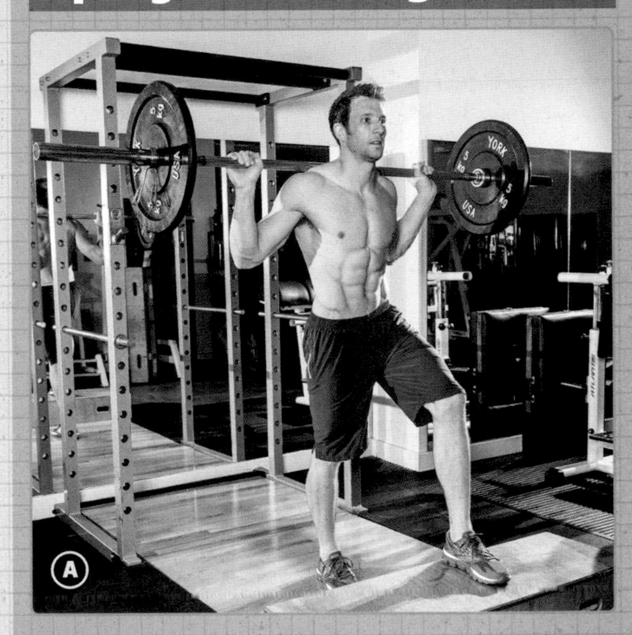

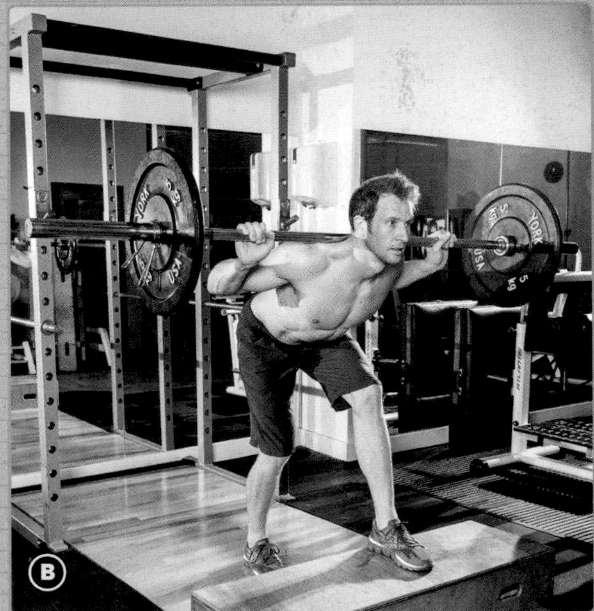

Place greater demands on your lower back and one leg by having one leg forwards or on a raised platform.

Med ball sledgehammer

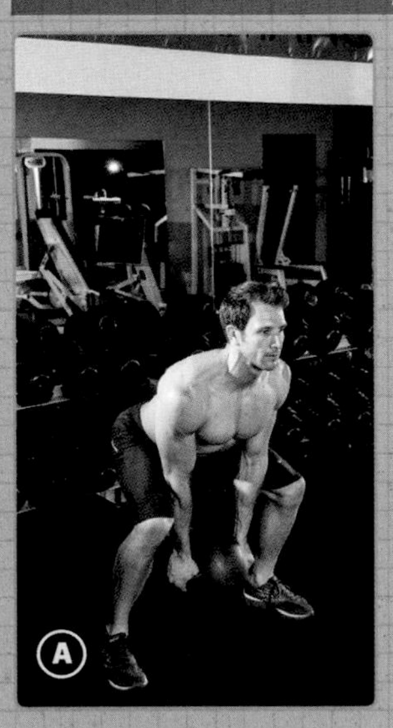

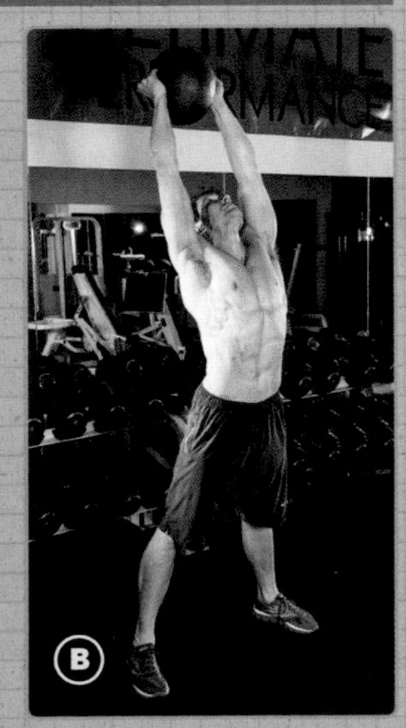

Gripping a medicine ball and explosively moving it up and down will fire up the small stabilising muscles of the lower back and abs.

TWO-POINT BOX

***Targets** Lower back, core*

This simple move will improve the strength and stability of your lower back and core, which will allow you to perform other, more complex moves safely and effectively

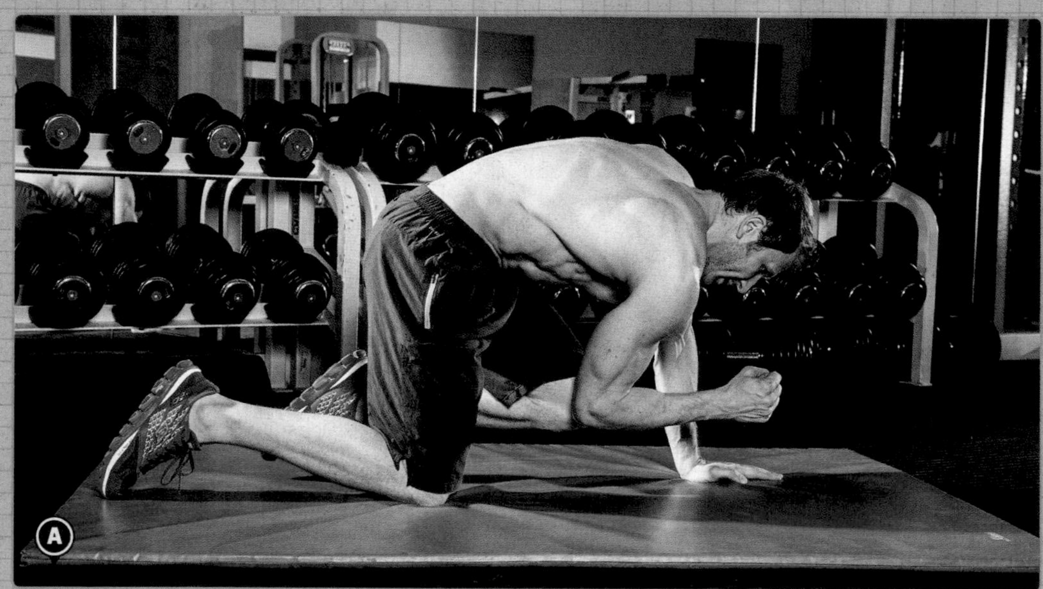

A

- Start with both knees and hands on the floor and your core braced.
- Extend your right arm and left leg until they are fully straight.
- Return to the start position then repeat with the opposite limbs.

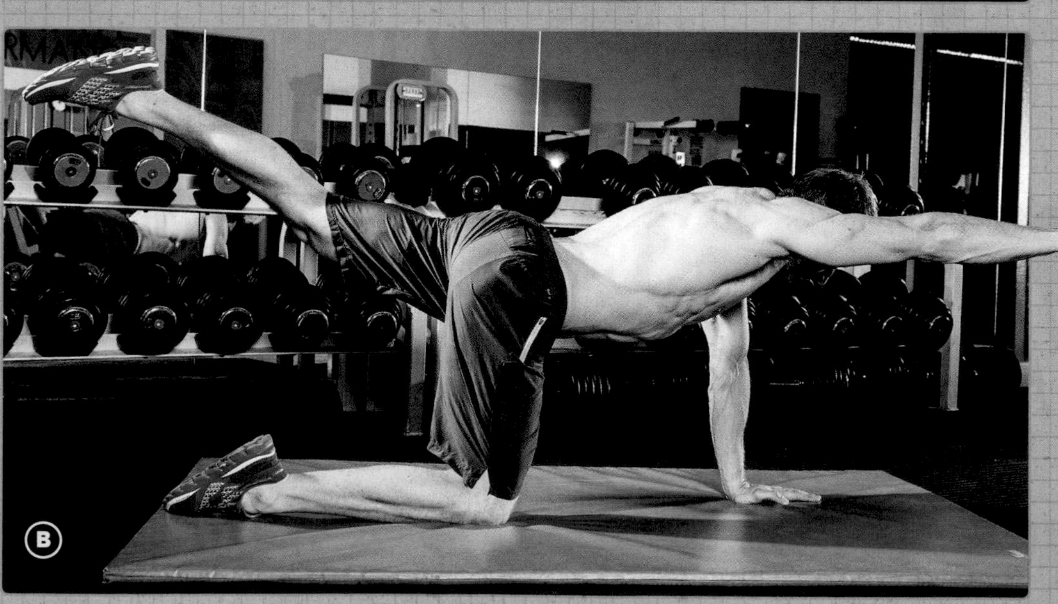

B

Superman raise

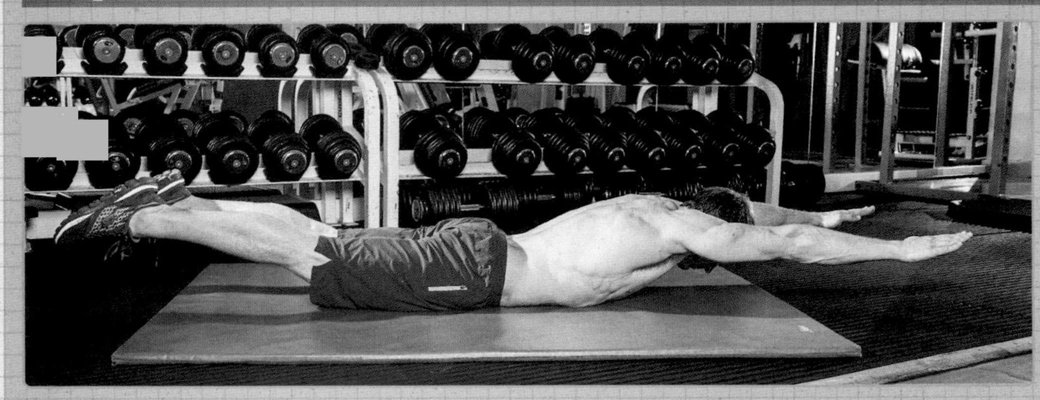

Raising both arms when lying flat on the floor is an easy and simple way to work your lower back.

Aquaman

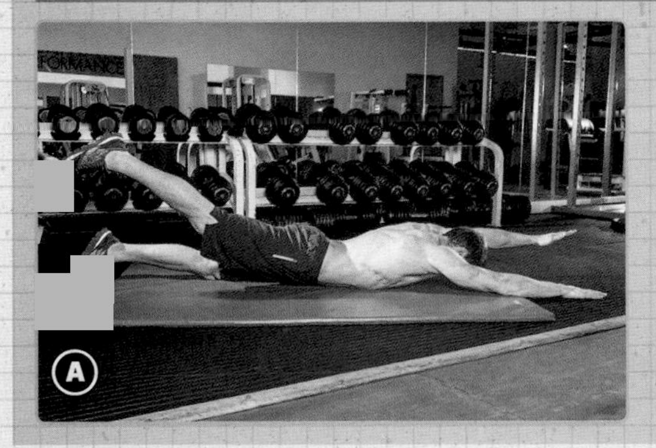

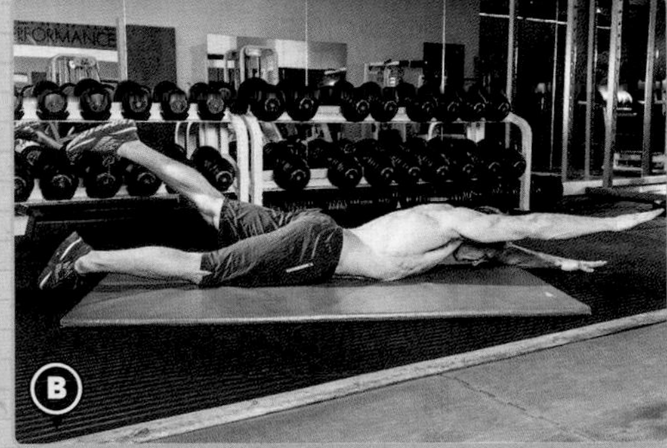

Raising your opposite arm and leg off the floor isn't as easy as it looks and is a great lower-back builder.

Dorsal raise with shoulder rotation

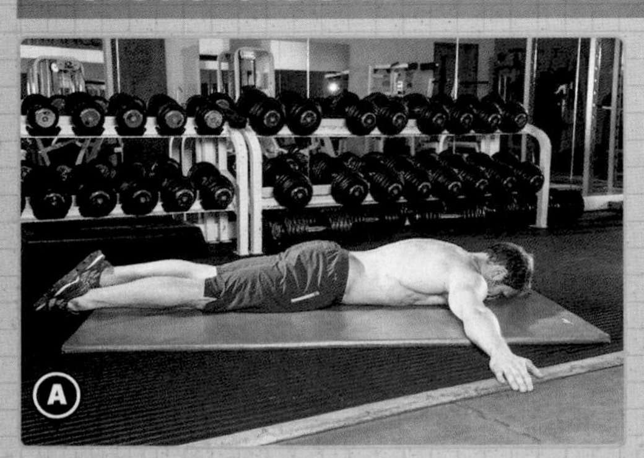

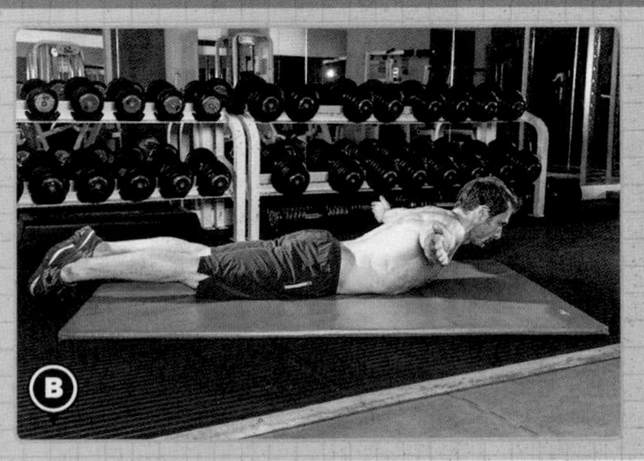

Raising your arms then twisting your hands until your thumbs point towards the ceiling recruits the small but crucial stabilising muscles of the shoulder joint.

INCLINE BACK EXTENSION

***Targets** Lower back*

A surprisingly tough but effective bodyweight move that will strengthen your lower back so you can stay injury free and lift heavier on the big moves

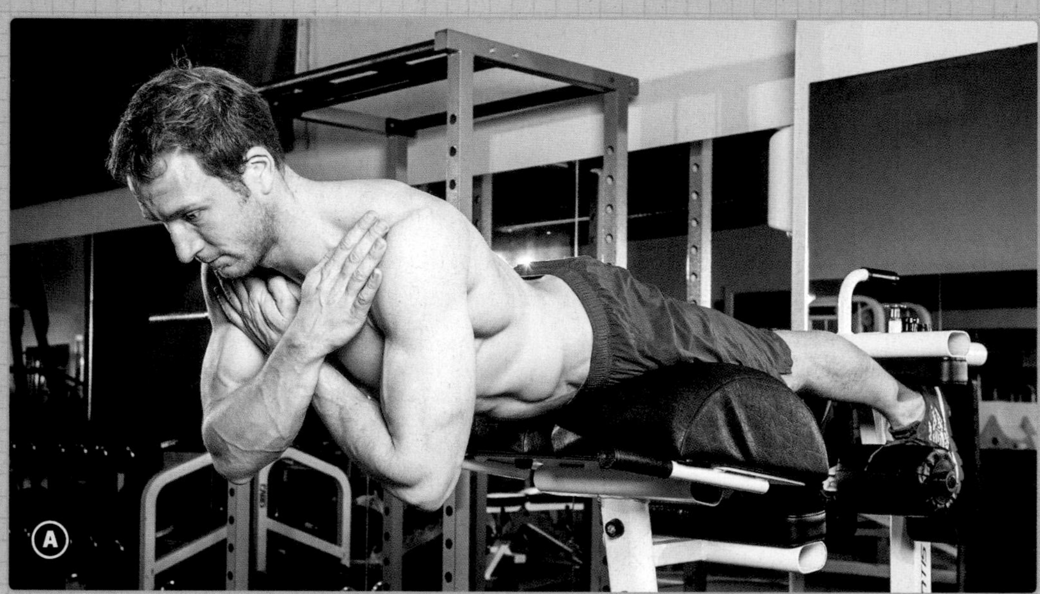

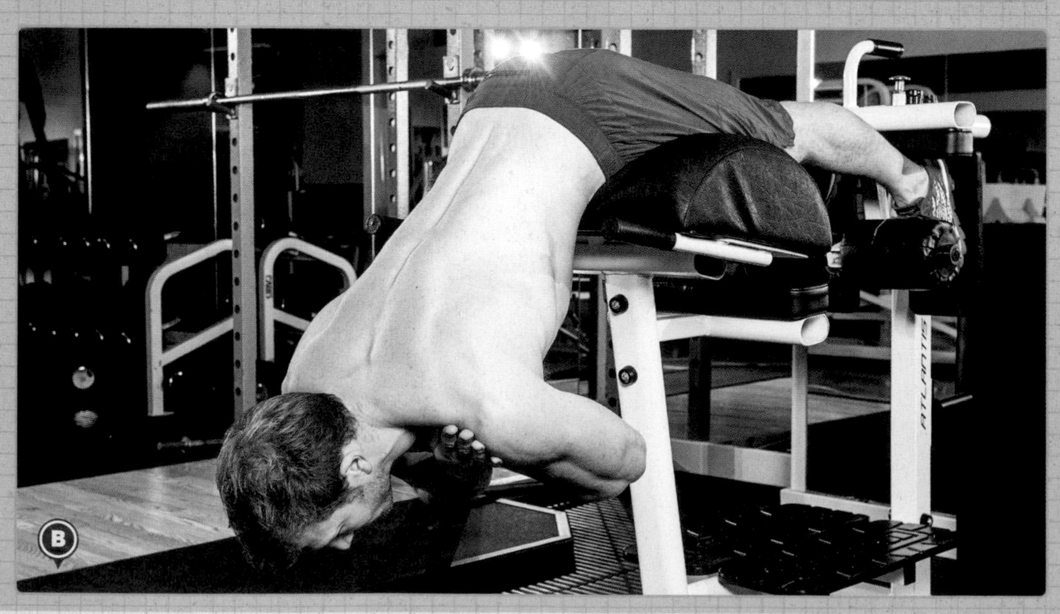

- Position yourself on the bench so your feet and thighs are supported.
- With your hands on your chest and your core braced, lower your torso as far as is comfortable.
- Use your lower back muscles to return to the start.

Decline back extension

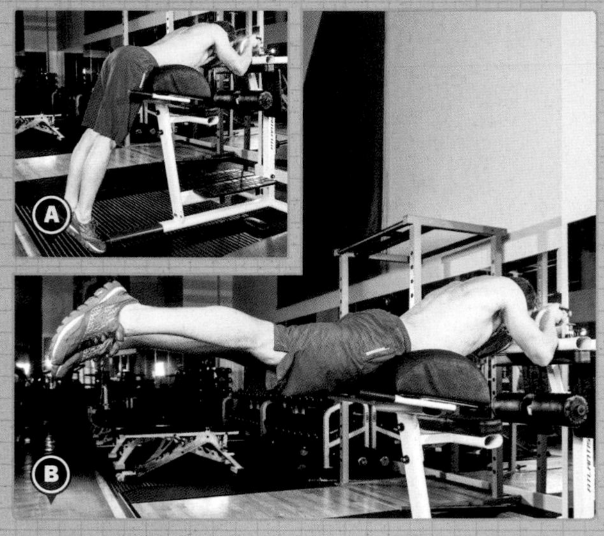

Raising your legs works the muscles from a different angle to keep them growing.

Gym ball back extension

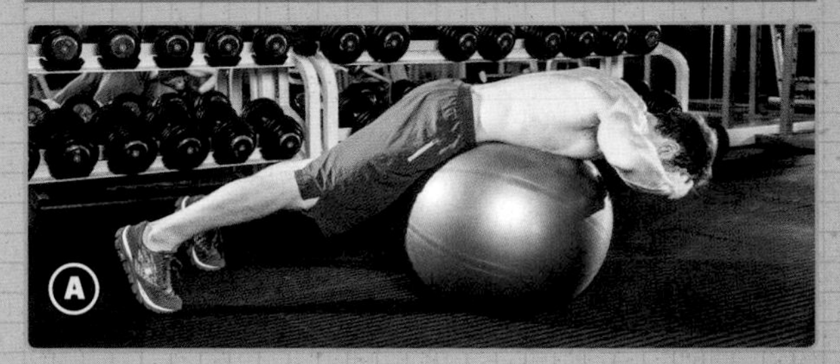

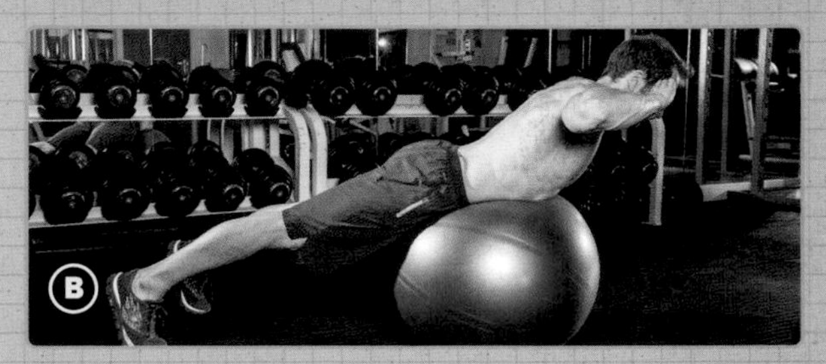

Using a gym ball makes the move easier by decreasing the range of motion, but you must still use your core to stay balanced.

Weighted back extension

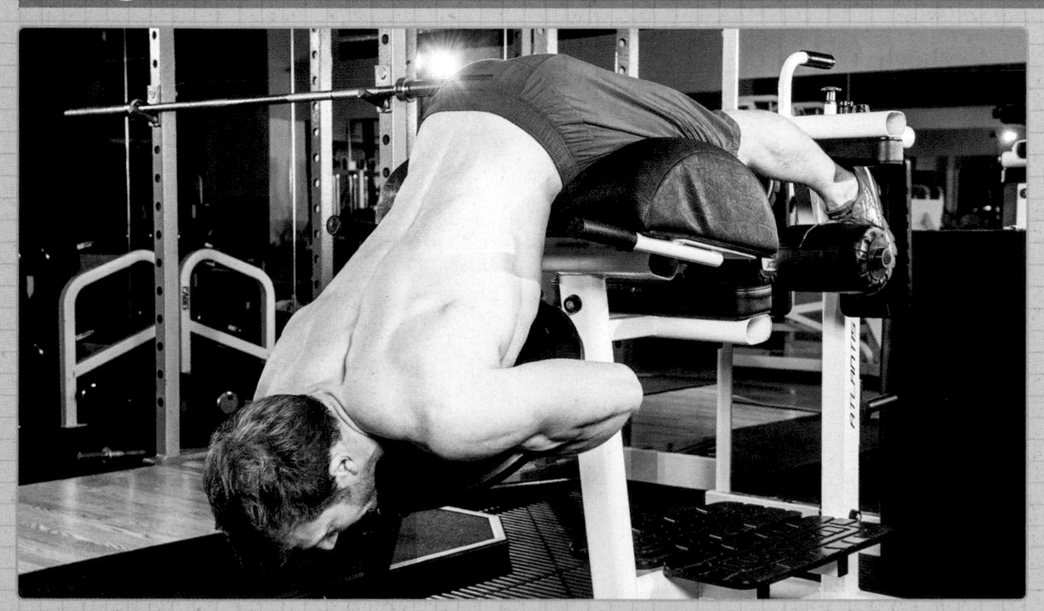

Holding additional weight across your chest makes this move even harder and more effective.

CHEST

Build a strong and broad chest by hitting these muscles from multiple angles

Getting a big, strong chest is a primary objective for many gym-goers, which is why the bench press is the one move most men perform regularly. The chest muscles consist of the pectoralis major and minor – commonly referred to as the pecs – and the serratus anterior.

These muscles are primarily responsible for pushing objects away from you, which is why the bench press is so popular and the main test of upper-body strength. However, it is important to work this significant muscle group in a variety of ways and from multiple angles to target the upper, middle and lower parts of the pectorals to elicit maximum muscle strength and size.

> **"It's important to work the chest muscles in a variety of ways to elicit growth"**

This chapter details all the moves that will work each part of your chest effectively for rapid results.

Chest explained

Here's how your chest muscles work

- The pectoralis major is a thick, fan-shaped muscle that makes up the bulk of the muscles on your chest and is responsible for the movement of your shoulder joint, specifically when pushing objects away from you.

- The pectoralis minor is a thin, triangular muscle that sits underneath the pectoralis major and draws the shoulder blades down and forwards.

- The serratus anterior are thin, finger-like muscles on each side of your body that allow the upward rotation of the shoulder blades. These are important when lifting weights overhead.

The chest muscles

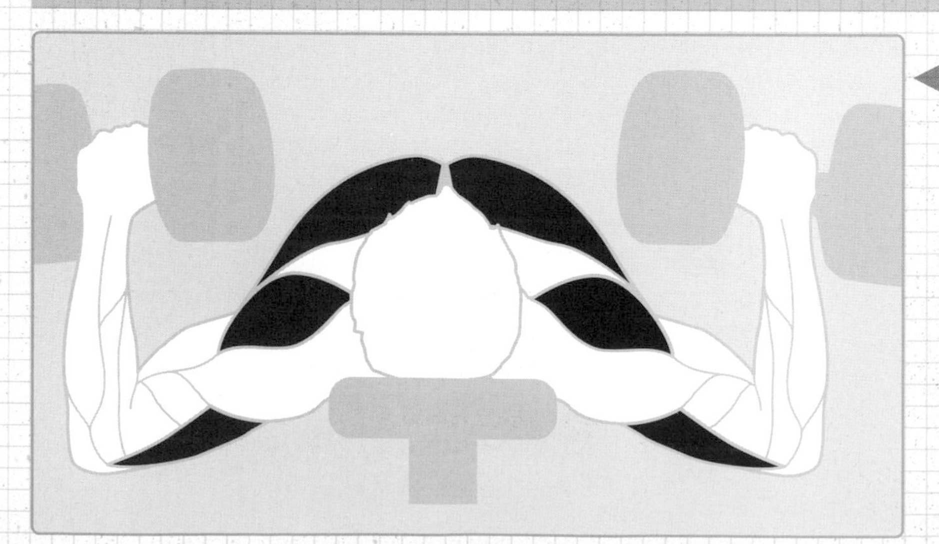

The chest muscles work closely with the anterior deltoids and triceps when pushing an object away from you, whether that's dumbbells on a bench press or the floor when doing press-ups.

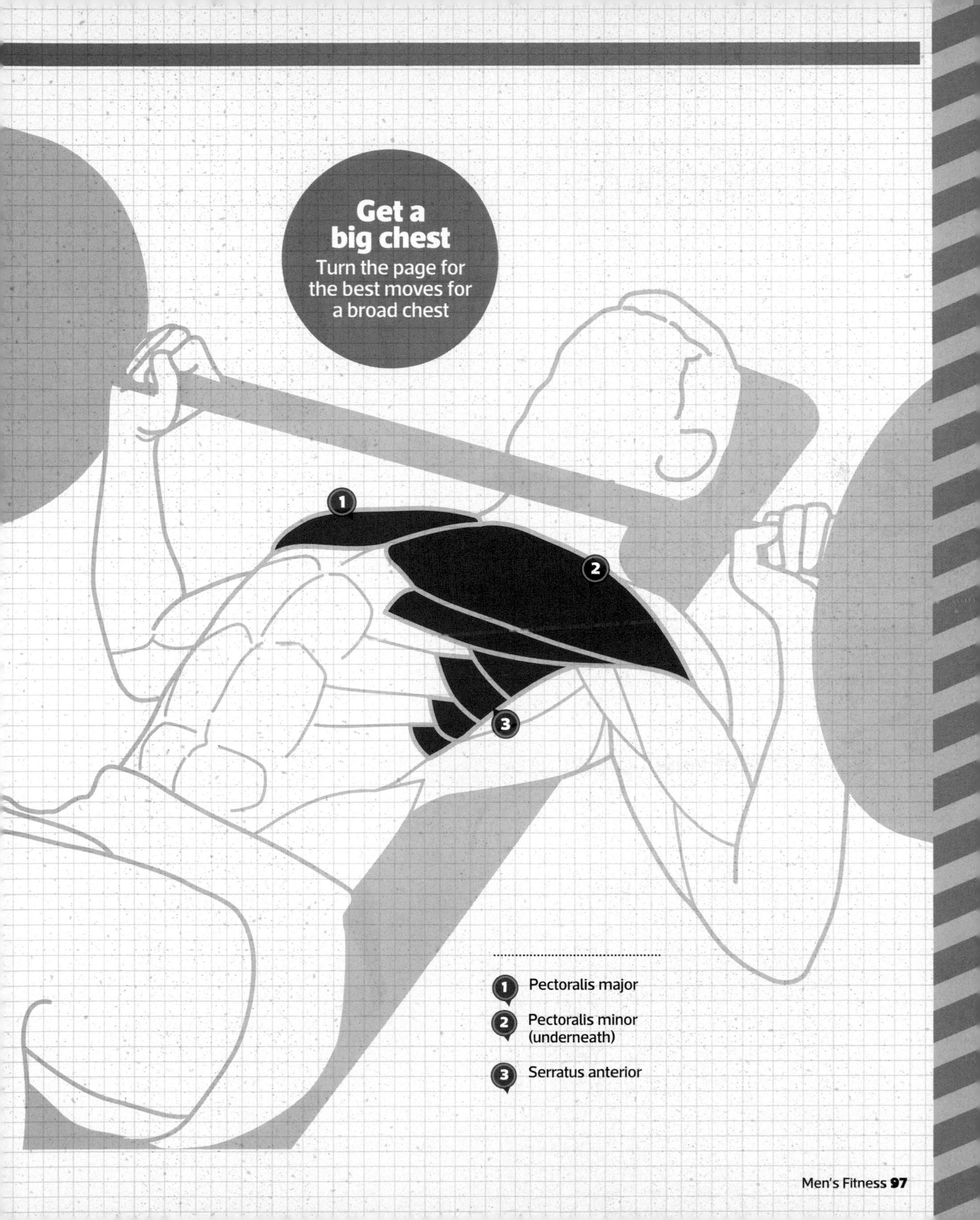
Get a big chest
Turn the page for the best moves for a broad chest
1
2
3
1 Pectoralis major
2 Pectoralis minor (underneath)
3 Serratus anterior

BENCH PRESS

***Targets** Pecs, triceps, shoulders*

The classic big lift is still one of the best ways to build a bigger, stronger chest

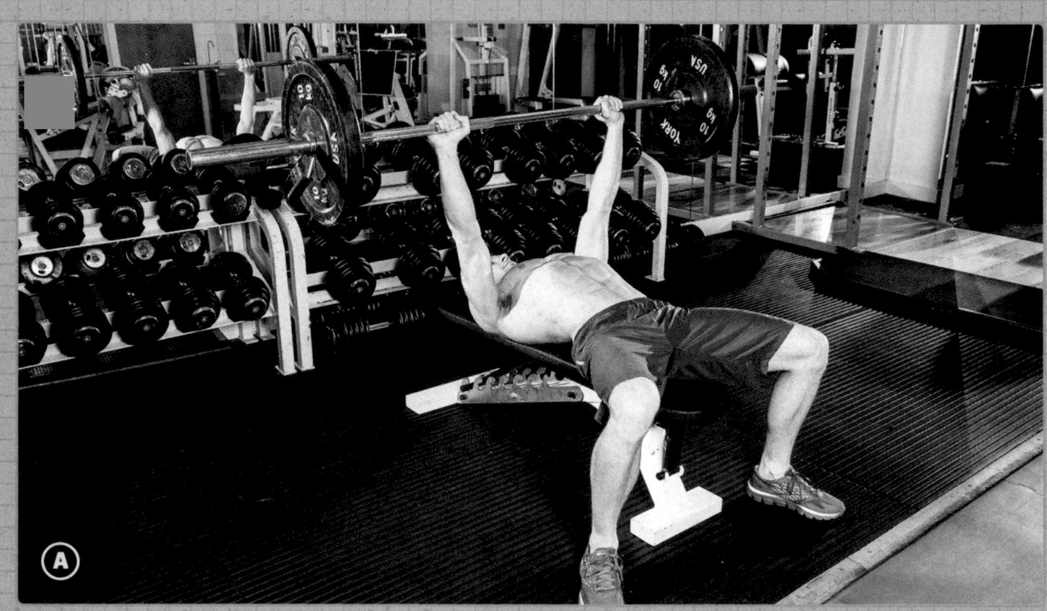

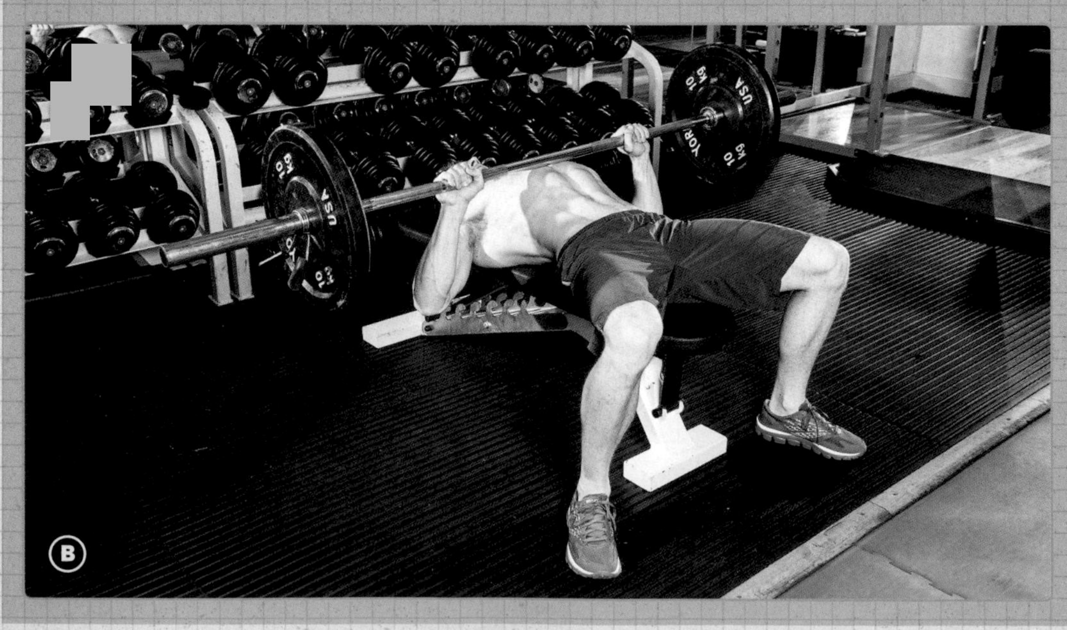

- Lie on the bench with your feet on the floor, directly underneath your knees.
- Hold the bar with an overhand grip with your hands shoulder-width apart.
- Slowly lower the bar to your chest, taking your elbows out to 90°, until the bar is almost touching the middle of chest or just over your nipples.
- Drive your feet hard into the floor and push the bar back strongly to the start position.

Ballistic bench press

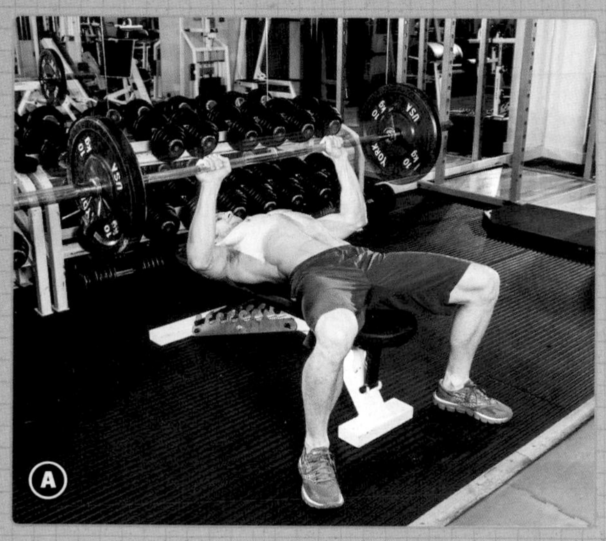

Pressing the bar up explosively will fire up your fast-twitch muscle fibres and lead to greater power gains. Just make sure you don't let go.

Press-up

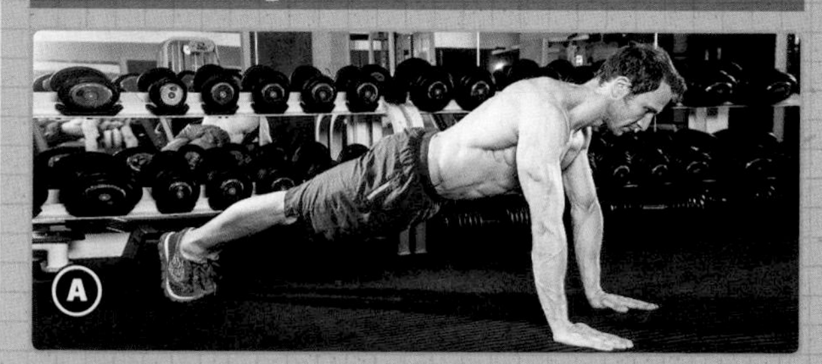

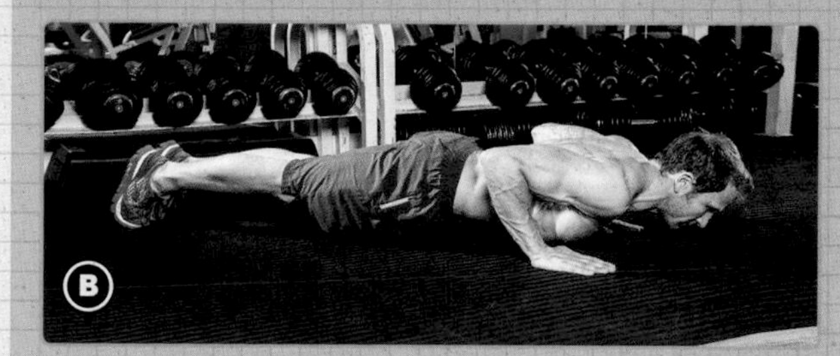

This simple and safe move allows you to work the target muscles any time and any place.

Dumbbell bench press

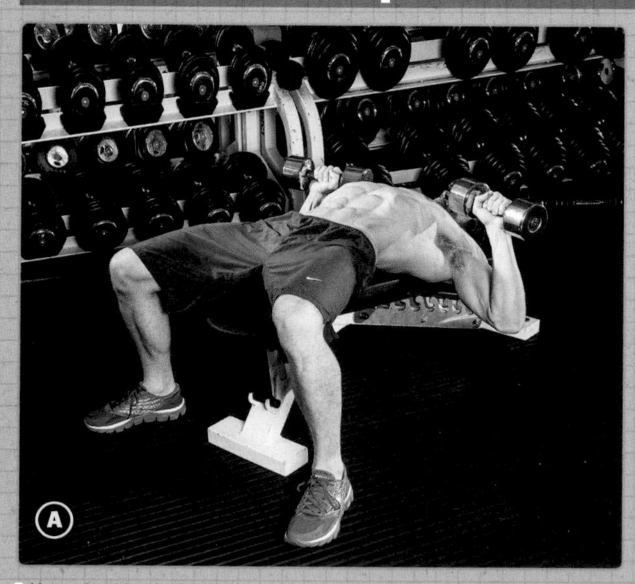

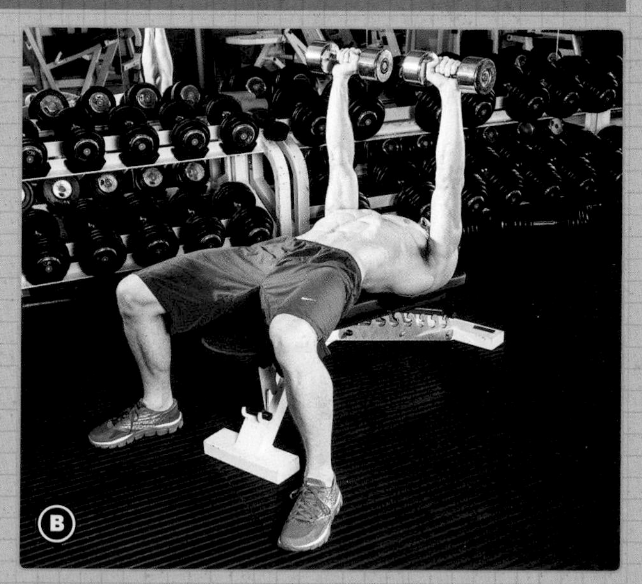

Using dumbbells allows a greater range of motion and requires more effort to stabilise your body.

INCLINE BENCH PRESS

***Targets** Upper pecs, triceps, shoulders*

Lying on an incline bench shifts the focus towards the muscle fibres of your upper chest and front of your shoulders

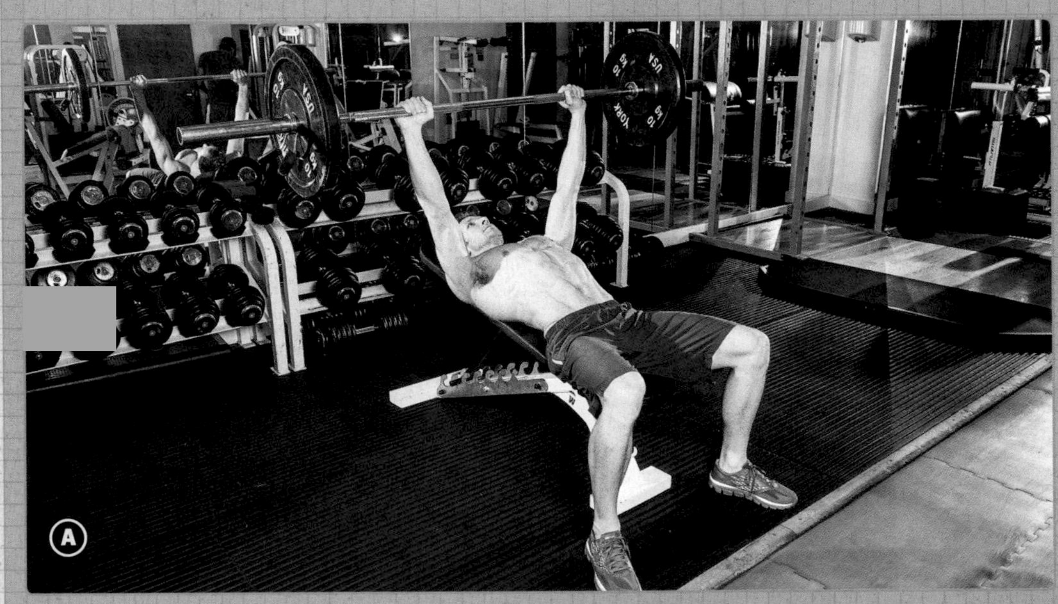

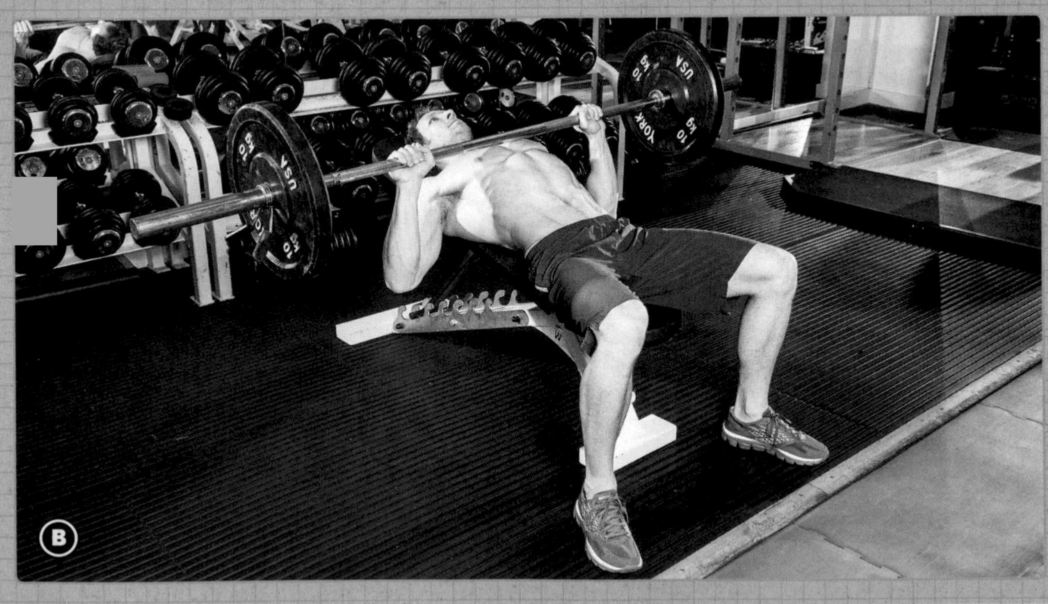

- Lie on an incline bench with your feet on the floor, directly underneath your knees.
- Hold the bar with an overhand grip with your hands shoulder-width apart.
- Slowly lower the bar to your chest, taking your elbows out to 90°, until the bar is almost touching the middle of chest or just over your nipples.
- Drive your feet hard into the floor and push the bar back strongly to the start position.

Incline dumbbell press

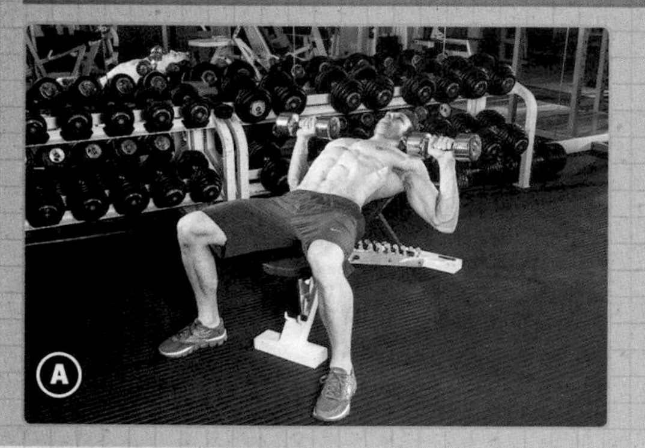

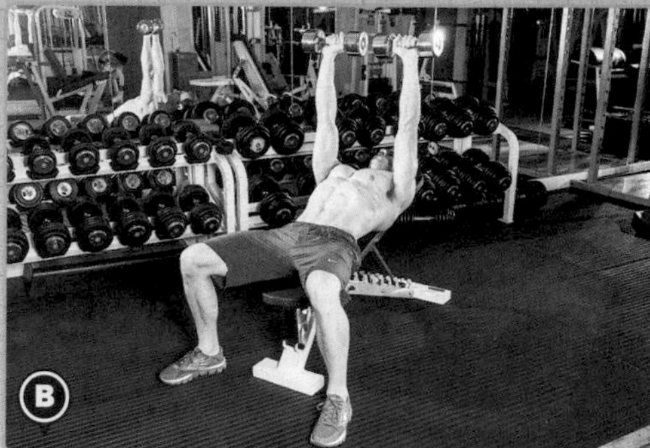

- Using dumbbells allows a greater range of motion and ensures you work both sides of your chest evenly.

Incline alternating dumbbell press

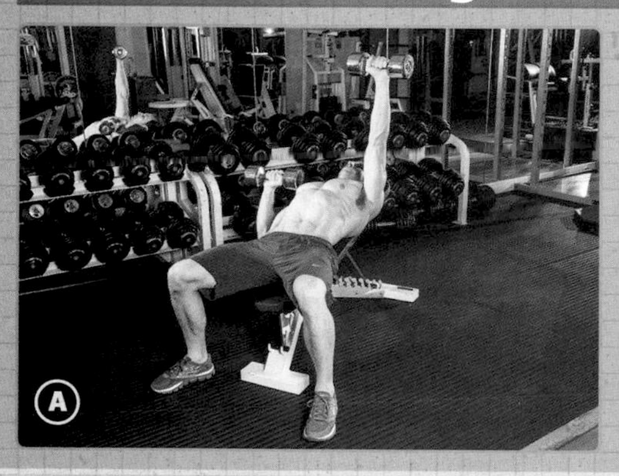

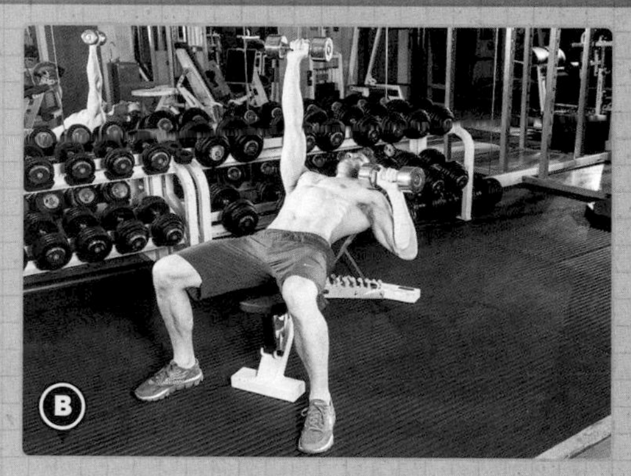

- Lifting one weight at a time requires greater core control and recruits more of the small but important stabilising muscles of your torso.

Decline press-up

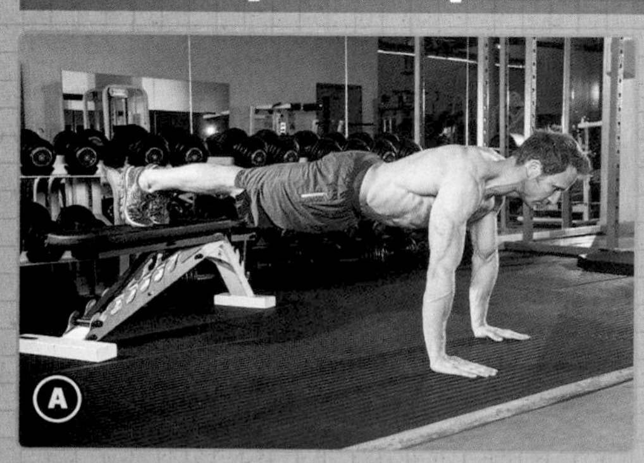

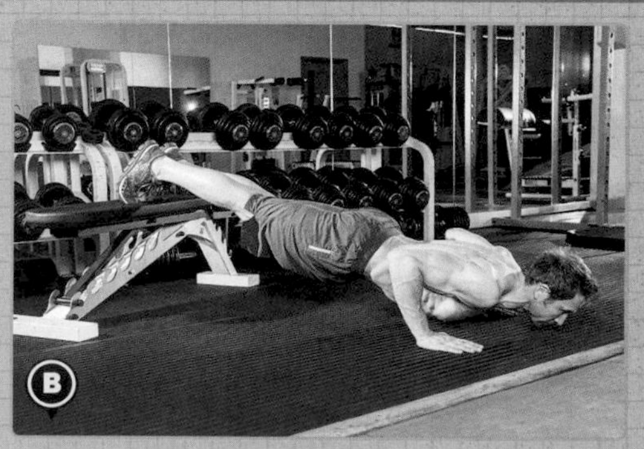

- Raising your feet off the ground places more of your bodyweight on the target muscles, making this a harder variation that also targets your upper chest.

DECLINE BENCH PRESS

***Targets** Lower pecs, triceps, shoulders*

Lying on a decline bench moves the focus of the move to the lower part of the chest while still working your triceps and the front of your shoulders

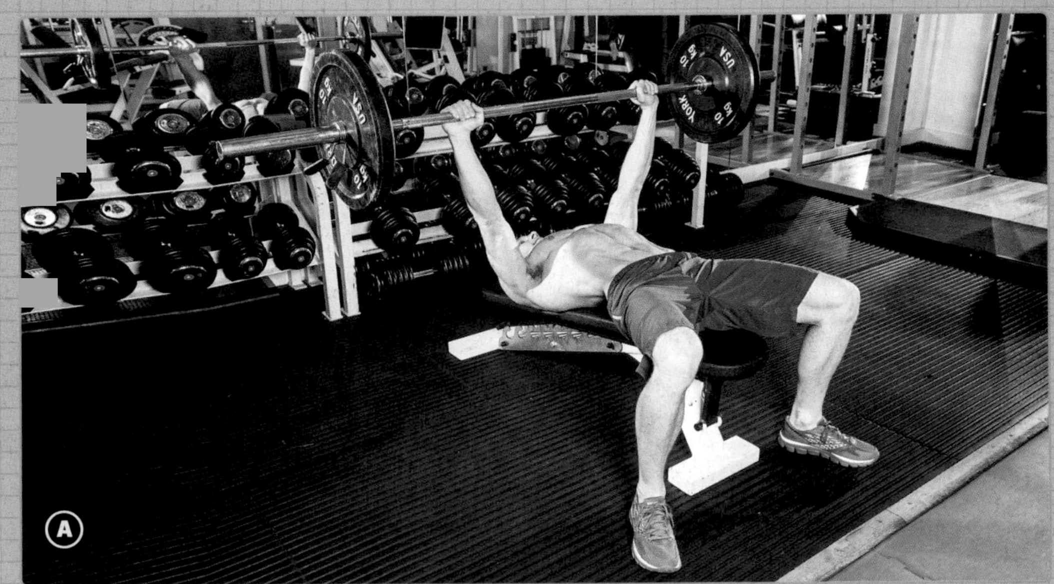

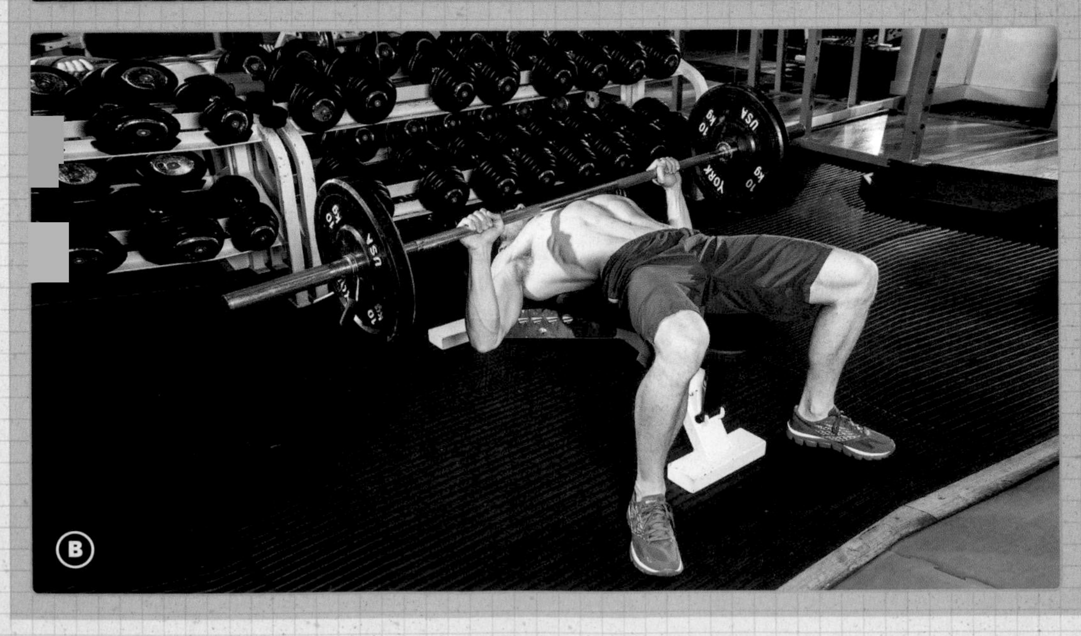

- Lie on a decline bench with your feet on the floor, directly underneath your knees.
- Hold the bar with an overhand grip with your hands shoulder-width apart.
- Slowly lower the bar to your chest, taking your elbows out to 90°, until the bar is almost touching the middle of chest or just over your nipples.
- Drive your feet hard into the floor and push the bar back strongly to the start position.

Decline dumbbell press

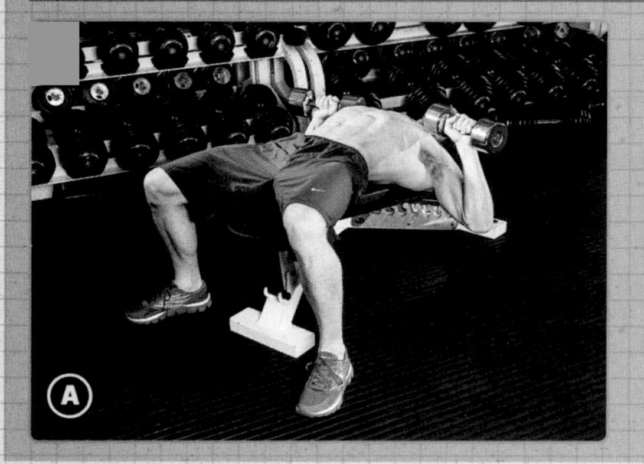

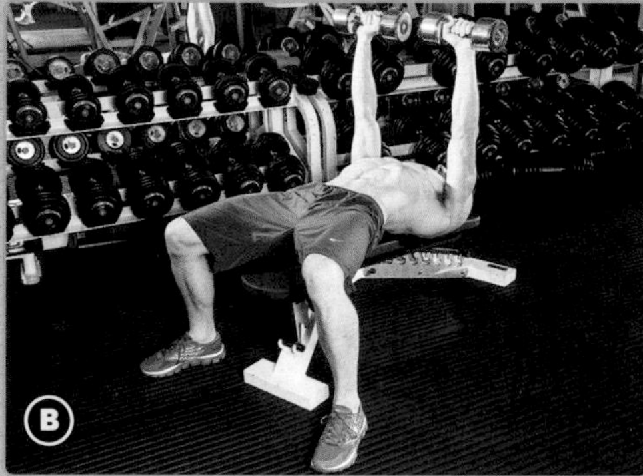

Using dumbbells works both sides of your chest independently and through a greater range of motion.

Decline alternating dumbbell press

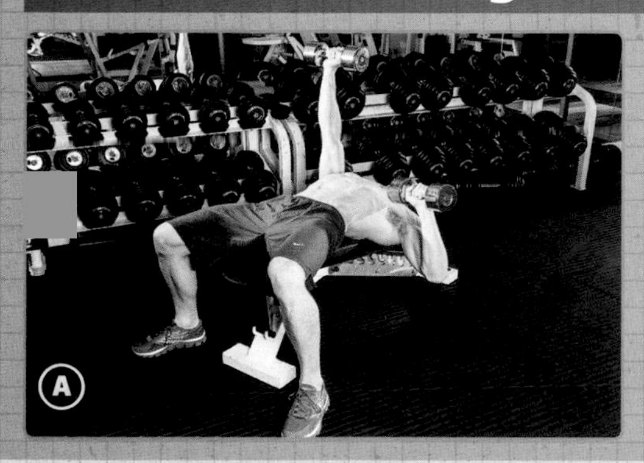

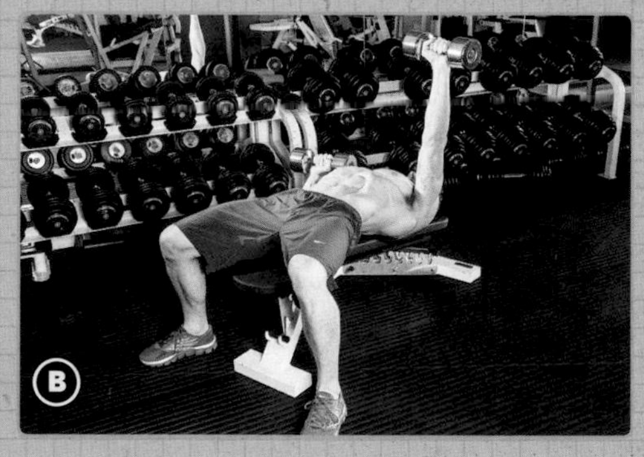

Lifting one weight at a time requires greater core control and recruits more of the small but important stabilising muscles of your torso, while also hitting your lower chest.

Incline press-up

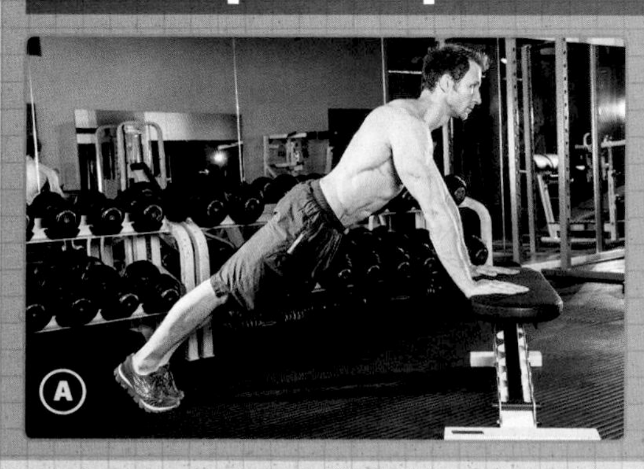

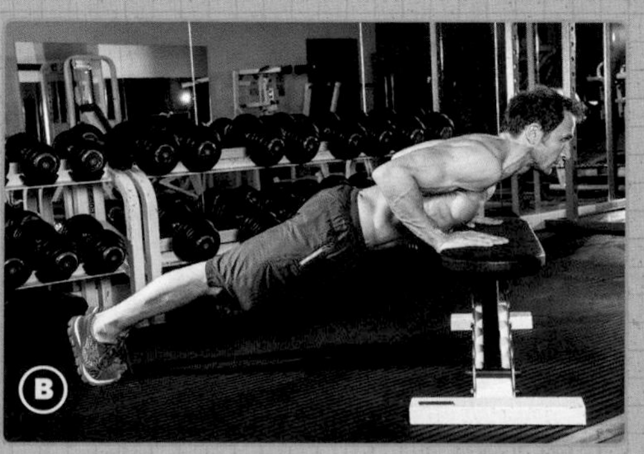

Starting with your hands higher than your feet reduces the amount of bodyweight the target muscles must manage, making this an easier version of a standard press-up.

DUMBBELL FLYE

Targets *Pecs*

This more advanced move places the emphasis squarely on your chest muscles, but use lighter dumbbells to protect your shoulder joints

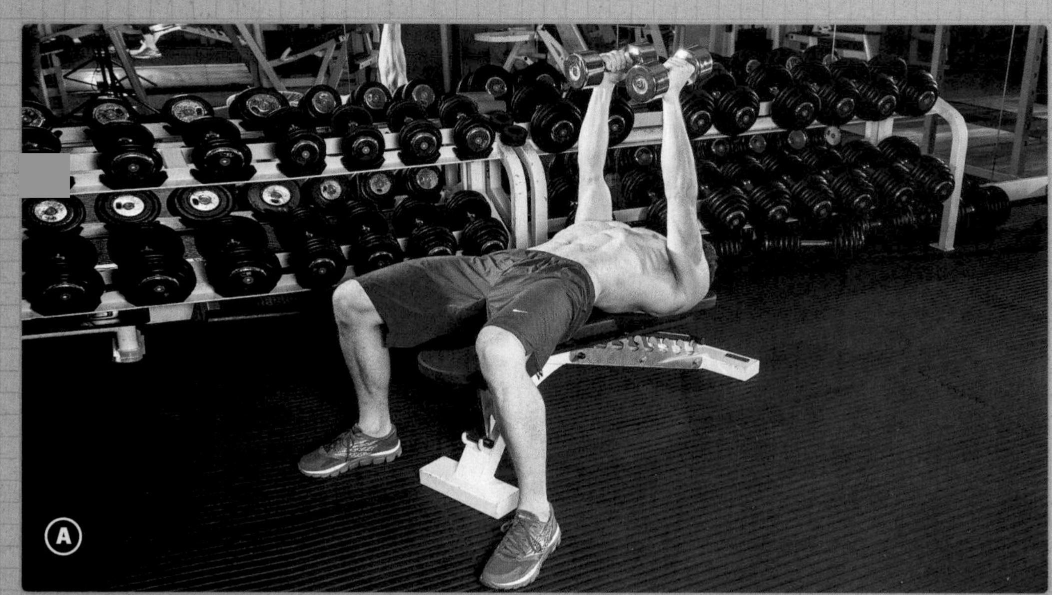

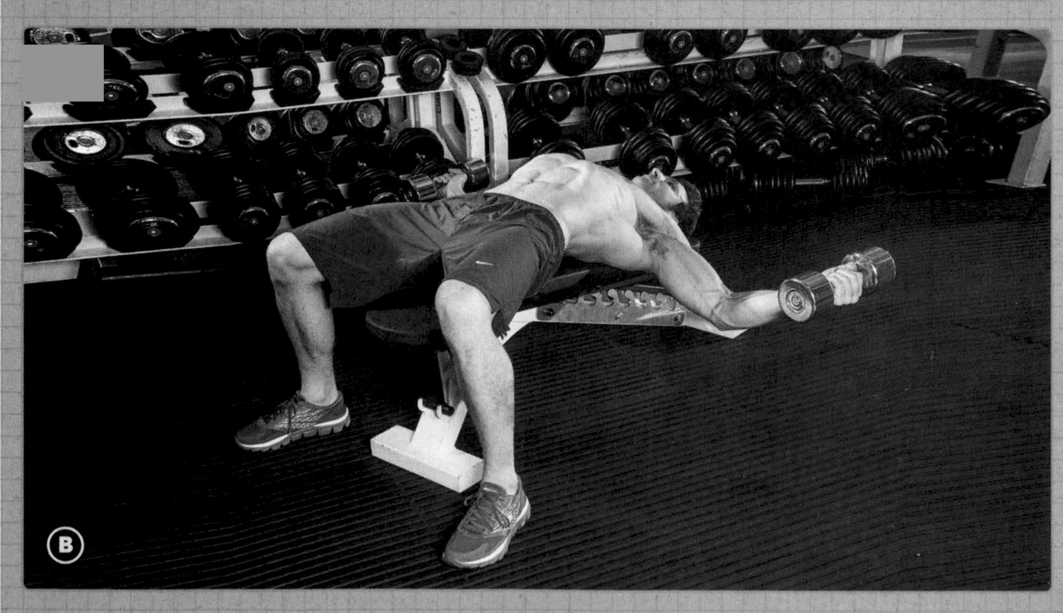

- Lie on a flat bench holding a dumbbell in each hand directly above your chest with your palms facing.
- Make sure your head and upper back are supported on the bench and your feet are flat on the floor.
- Keeping a slight bend in your elbows, slowly lower the weights out to the side as far as is comfortable.
- Squeeze your chest to reverse the movement and raise the weights back to the top.

Cable flye

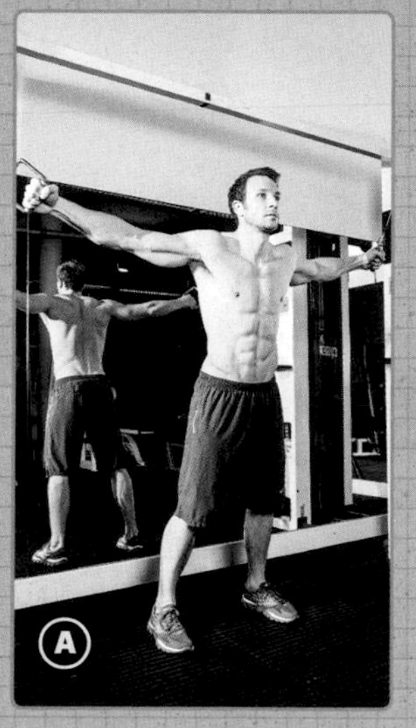

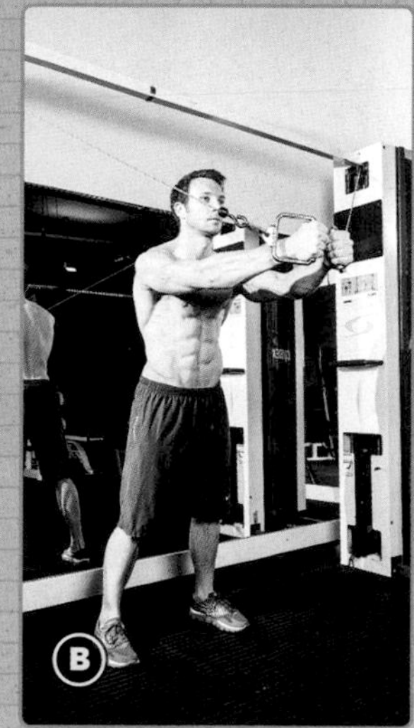

The resistance of the cable makes your muscles work throughout each rep, while standing up recruits your core stabilising muscles.

Cable crossover

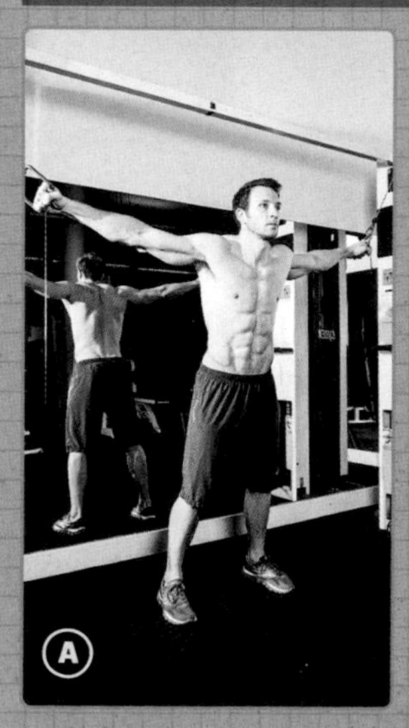

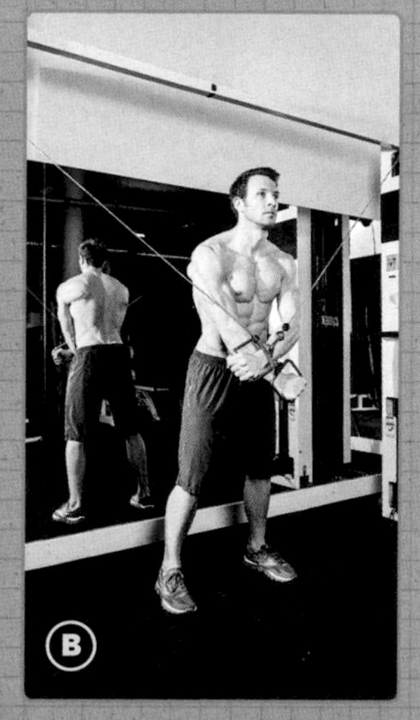

Bringing your hands down in a wide arc so they meet in front of you hits the target muscles from a different angle and forces a powerful contraction in your chest muscles.

Incline dumbbell flye

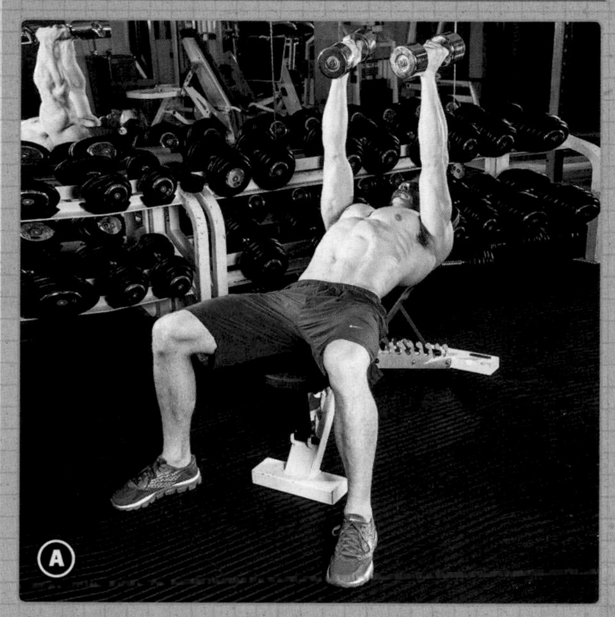

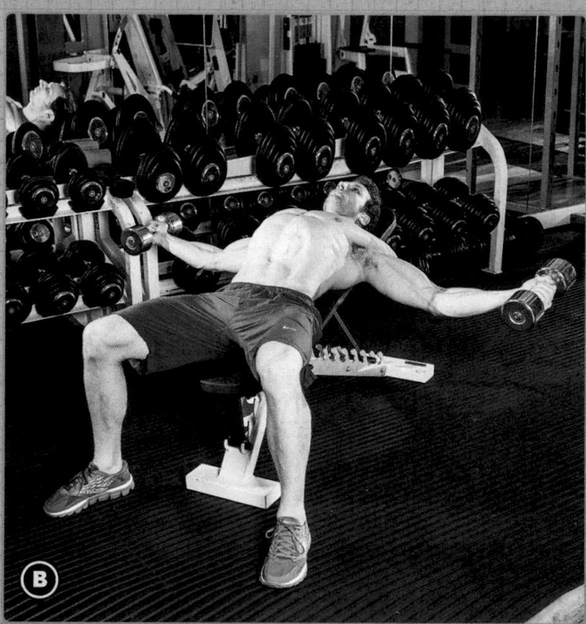

Performing the move on an incline hits your chest from a different angle and works the upper-chest muscles harder.

T PRESS-UP

Targets *Pecs, triceps, core*

Make the humble press-up harder and work the shoulders, arms and core with this dynamic move

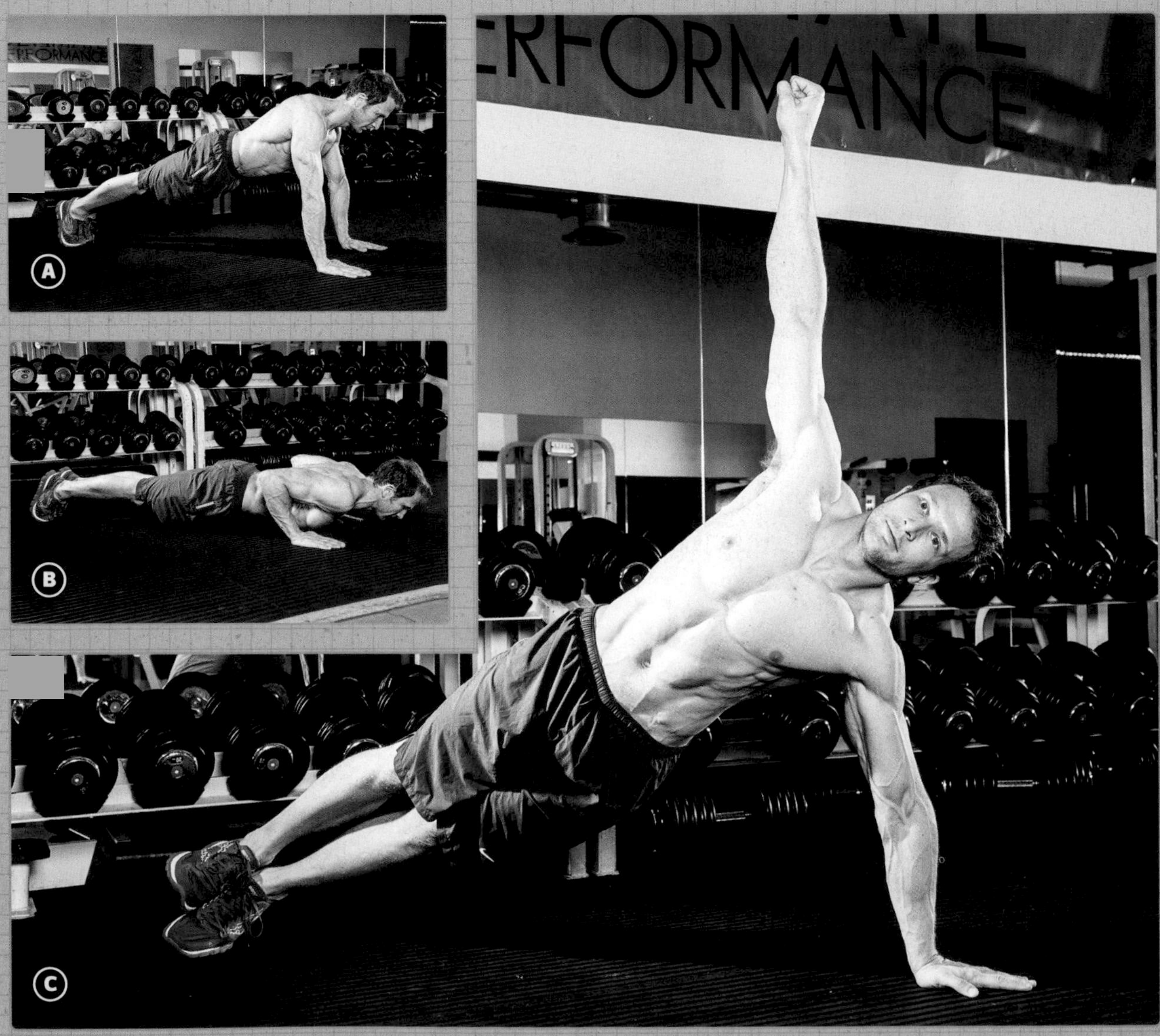

- Start in a press-up position and lower your chest to the floor, keeping your elbows close to your side.
- Press back up powerfully. At the top of the move lift one arm off the ground and twist your torso until that arm is pointing towards the ceiling.
- Lower back down before repeating on the other side.

Dumbbell floor press

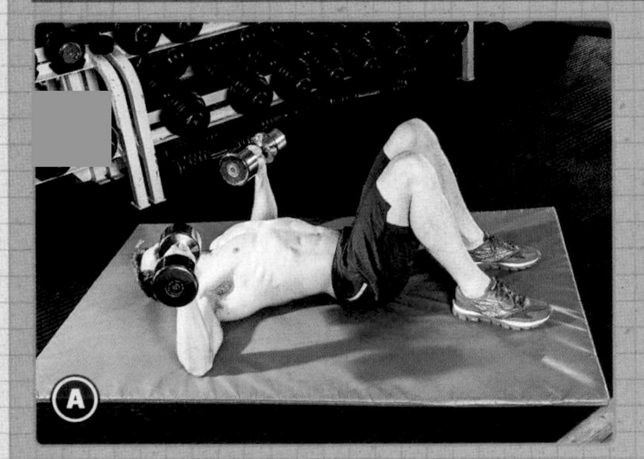

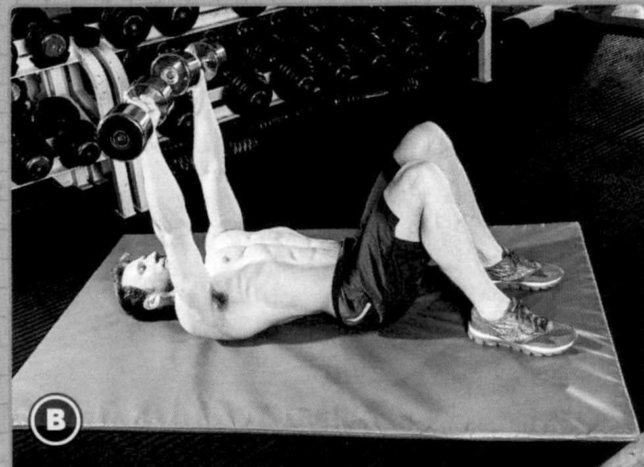

Pressing the dumbbells from the floor provides a more stable base but limits the range of motion.

Clap press-up

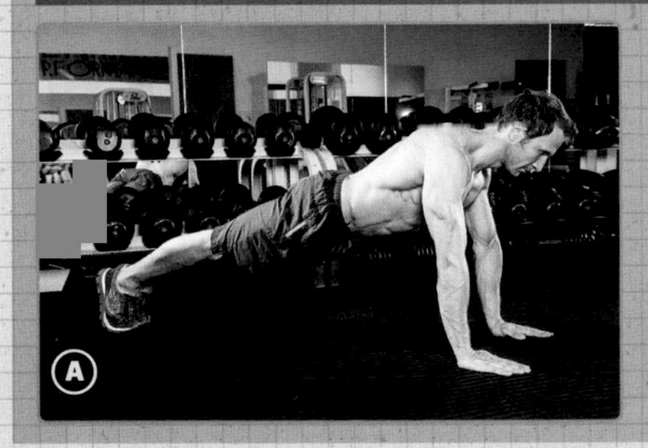

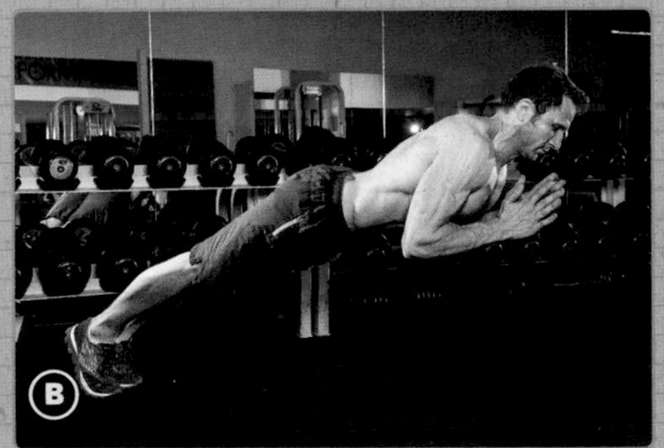

Pressing up powerfully so your hands leave the floor and clapping them together fires up your fast-twitch muscle fibres.

Offset press-up

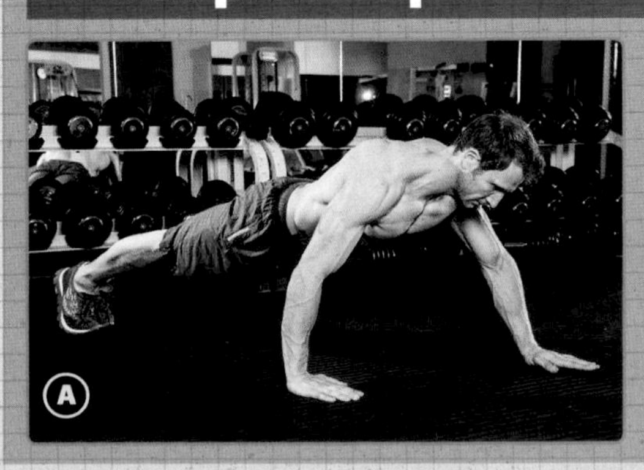

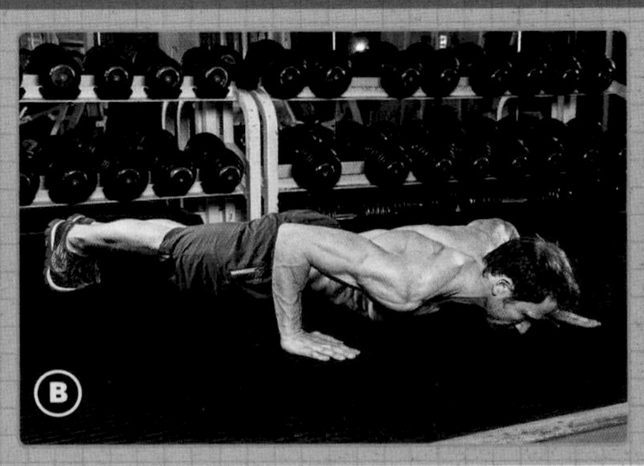

Having one hand in front of the other changes the angle of the press-up so your muscles must work in a different way to lower and raise your body.

DUMBBELL PULL-OVER

***Targets** Pecs, lats*

One of the few exercises to work your chest and back at once, this works your chest through a wide range of motion for impressive results

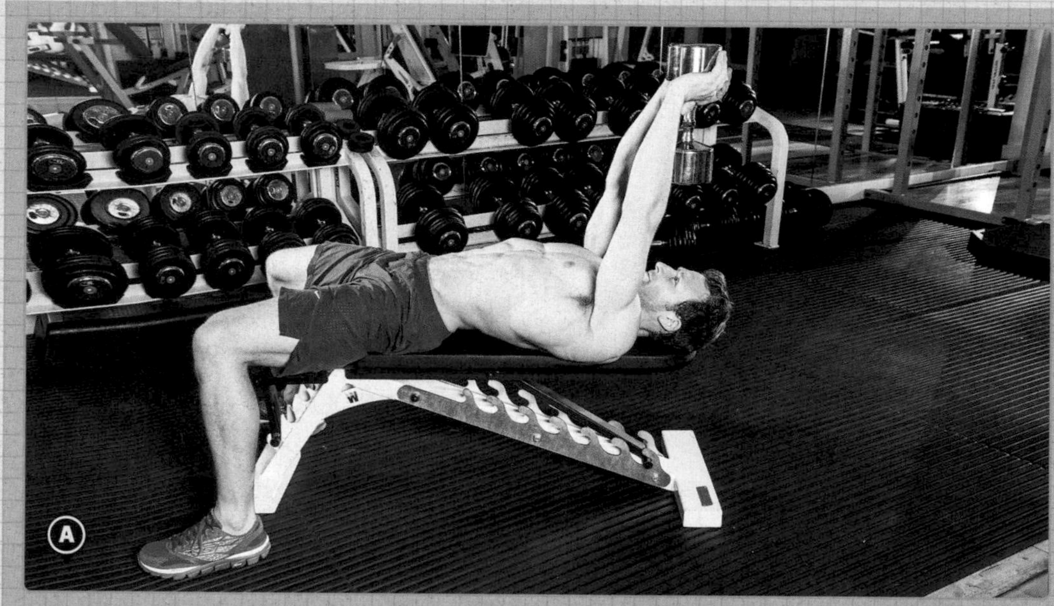

A

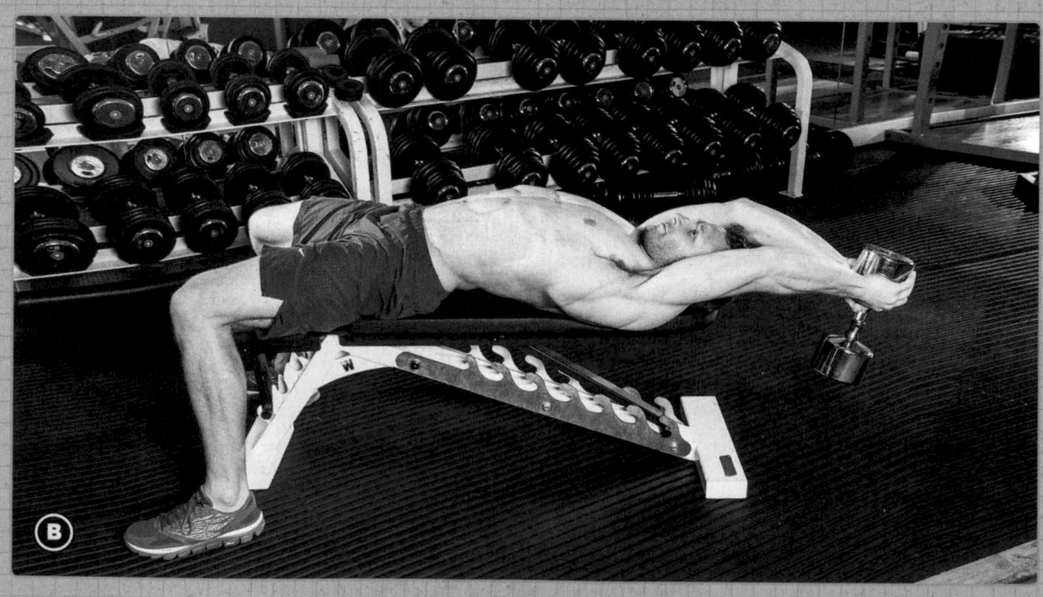

B

- Lie flat on a bench with your head and shoulders supported and your feet flat on the floor.
- Hold a single dumbbell with both hands over your chest and engage your core.
- Slowly lower the weight behind your head, keeping a slight bend in your elbows.
- Raise the weight back over your head to return to the start position.

Cable pull-over

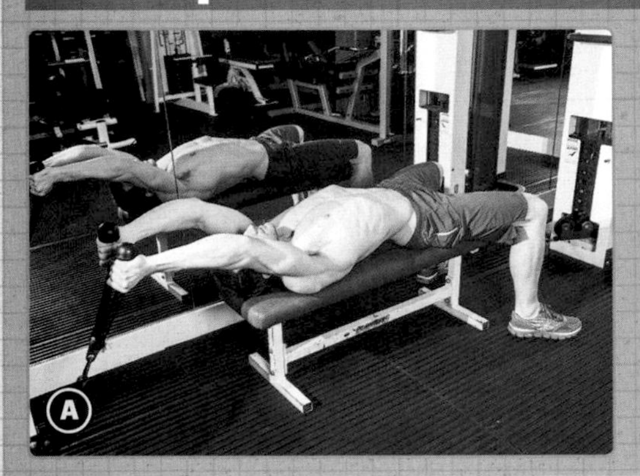

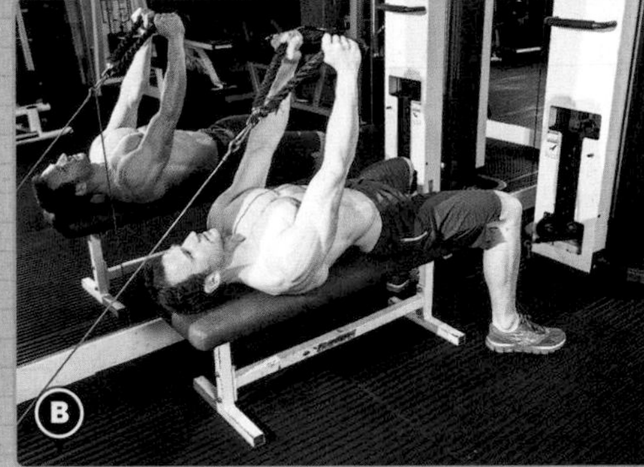

The cable provides a safer version of the move while also working your muscles through a greater range of motion under constant tension.

Gym ball dumbbell pull-over

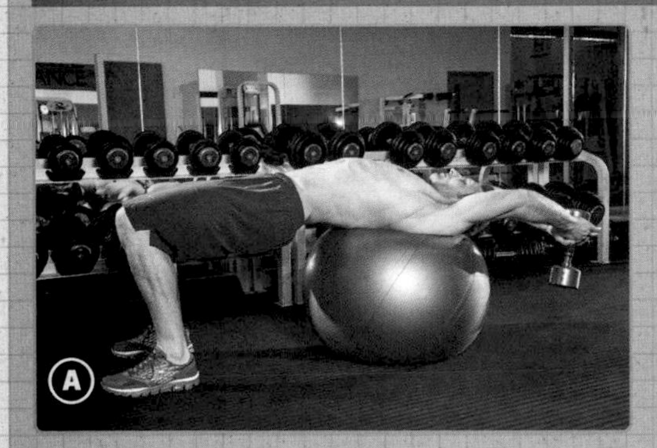

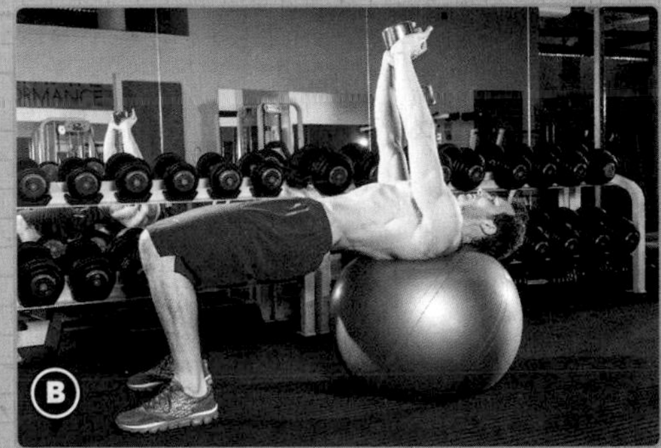

The instability of the ball forces your core into action to keep your body balanced.

Dumbbell pull-over press

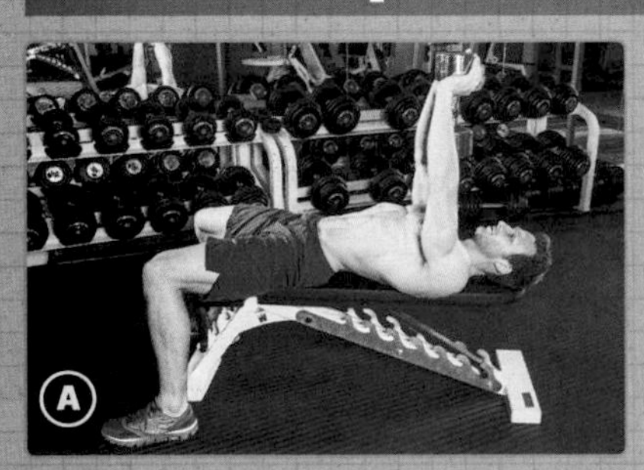

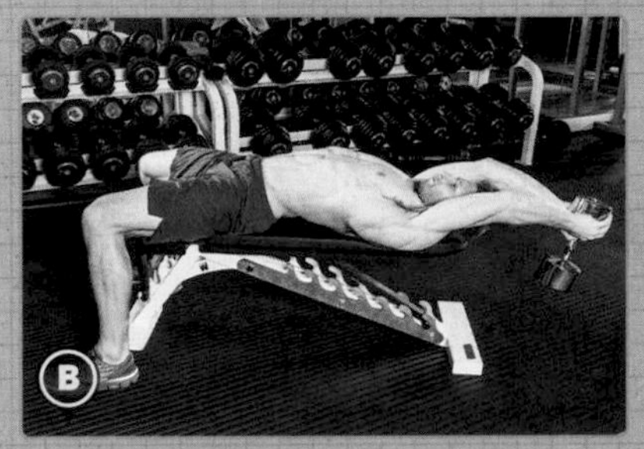

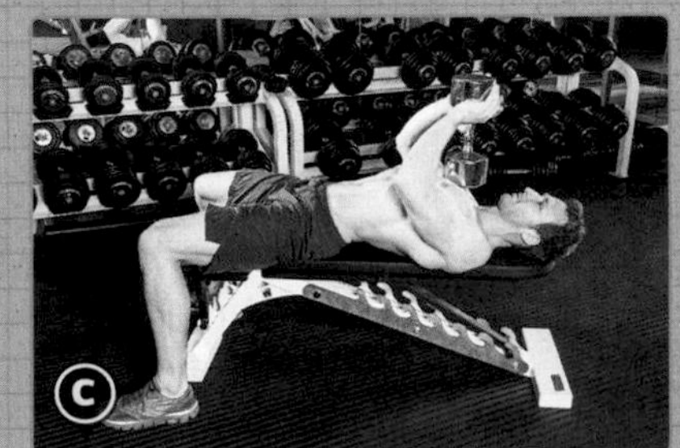

Bending your elbows as you lower the weight behind your head and then straightening them as you return it to the start position brings your triceps into play.

LEGS

Hit your legs hard to build lean muscle mass all over your body

The muscles of your legs and buttocks are the biggest in your body. Training them effectively means they will look impressive, but in addition to that is has more significant benefits for the rest of your body.

Because these muscles are so large, they can lift a lot of weight, so working these major muscles groups hard creates a post-workout surge in testosterone and other growth hormones. These hormones not only build bigger, stronger legs, but also create an overall anabolic, or muscle-building, environment that helps add lean muscle mass all over your body. They also instruct your body to burn body fat, so training your lower body will build bigger arms and reveal your six-pack.

Most lower-body lifts are far more complex than upper-body moves, so it can be tempting to skip them in favour of easier exercises. But learning the correct movement patterns and maintaining perfect form will allow you to increase rapidly the amount of weight you lift, which in turn will make you stronger and have a huge positive impact on your physique. This chapter explains all you need to know.

The leg muscles

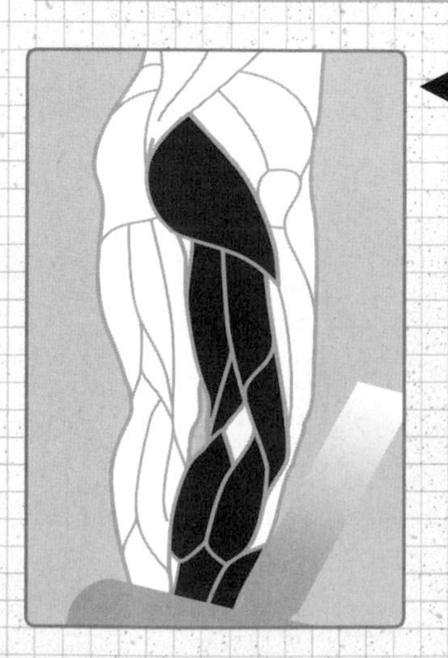

◀ The quadriceps and hamstrings are antagonist muscles, which mean they work together to straighten or bend the knee joint. The glutes work to move the hips and stabilise your pelvis, while your calves move your ankle joint.

Legs explained

Here's how your leg muscles work

- The quadriceps femoris, or quads, is a powerful extensor, or straightener, of the knee joint. It is made up of four heads: the rectus femoris, which is the middle of the thigh and covers the other three; the vastus intermedius, which lies directly beneath the rectus femoris; the vastus lateralis, on the outer thigh; and the vastus medialis, on the inner thigh.

- The hamstring crosses the hip and knee joint and is responsible for extending the hip and flexing the knee. It is the antagonist muscle to the quads and is made up of three parts: the semitendinosus, the semimembranosus and the biceps femoris, which has a long and short head.

- The gluteal muscles, or glutes, are four muscles, of which the gluteus maximus is the largest. The other three are called the gluteus medius, gluteus minimus and tensor fasciae latae. Their main responsibilities include extending the femur, or thigh bone, supporting and stabilising the pelvis and drawing the pelvis backwards to return your body to an upright position. The lower parts are also involved in abducting and externally rotating the legs.

- The gastrocnemius is the major muscle at the back of your lower leg that, along with the soleus, makes up the calf. It's job is plantar flexing at the ankle, the action of going on to tiptoes and flexing the leg at the knee joint.

- The powerful soleus muscle sits beneath the gastrocnemius, with which is shares responsibilities.

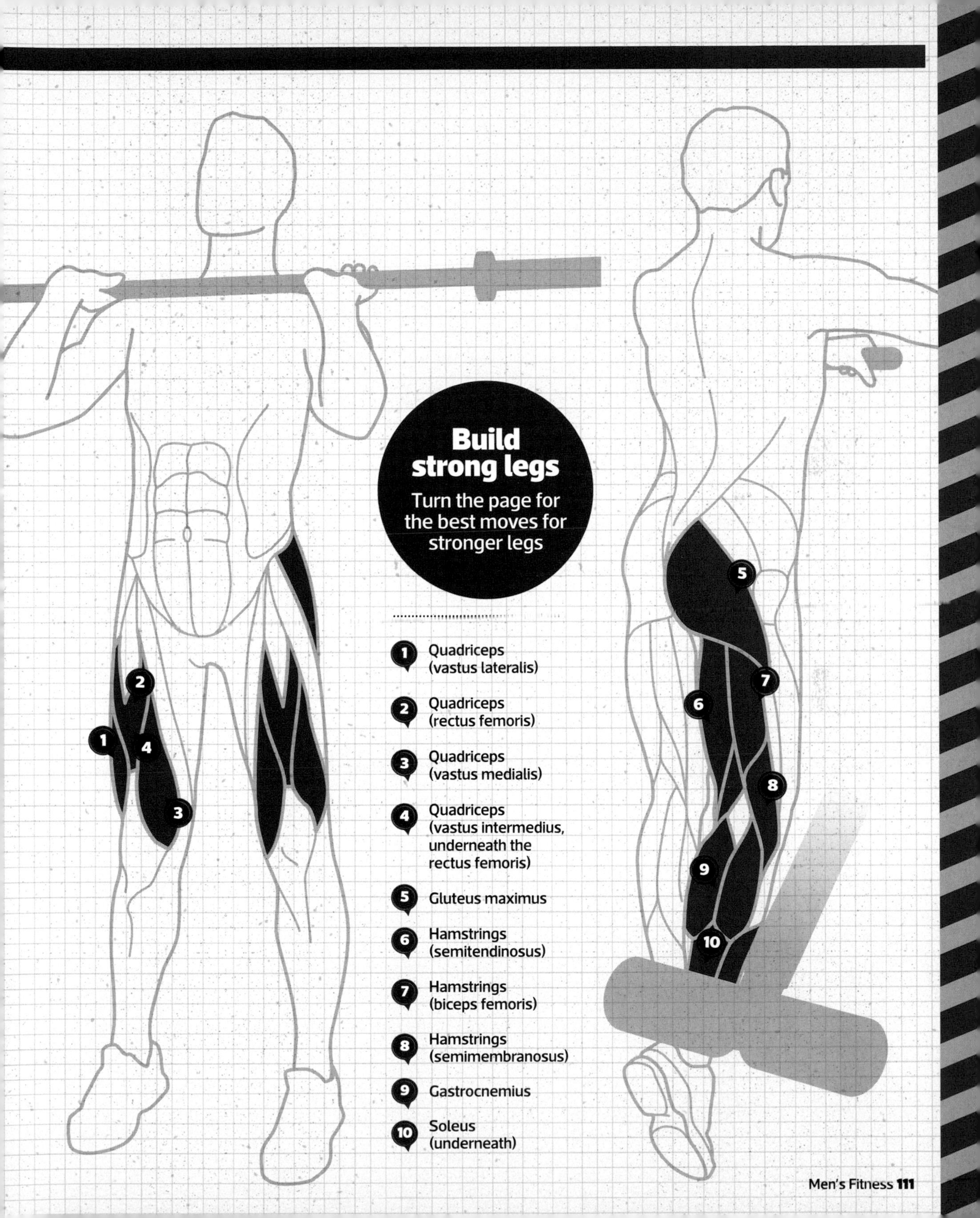

Build strong legs
Turn the page for the best moves for stronger legs
1 Quadriceps (vastus lateralis)
2 Quadriceps (rectus femoris)
3 Quadriceps (vastus medialis)
4 Quadriceps (vastus intermedius, underneath the rectus femoris)
5 Gluteus maximus
6 Hamstrings (semitendinosus)
7 Hamstrings (biceps femoris)
8 Hamstrings (semimembranosus)
9 Gastrocnemius
10 Soleus (underneath)

BODYWEIGHT SQUAT

***Targets** Quads, glutes, hamstrings*

Master this basic movement and start to add serious muscle mass across your body

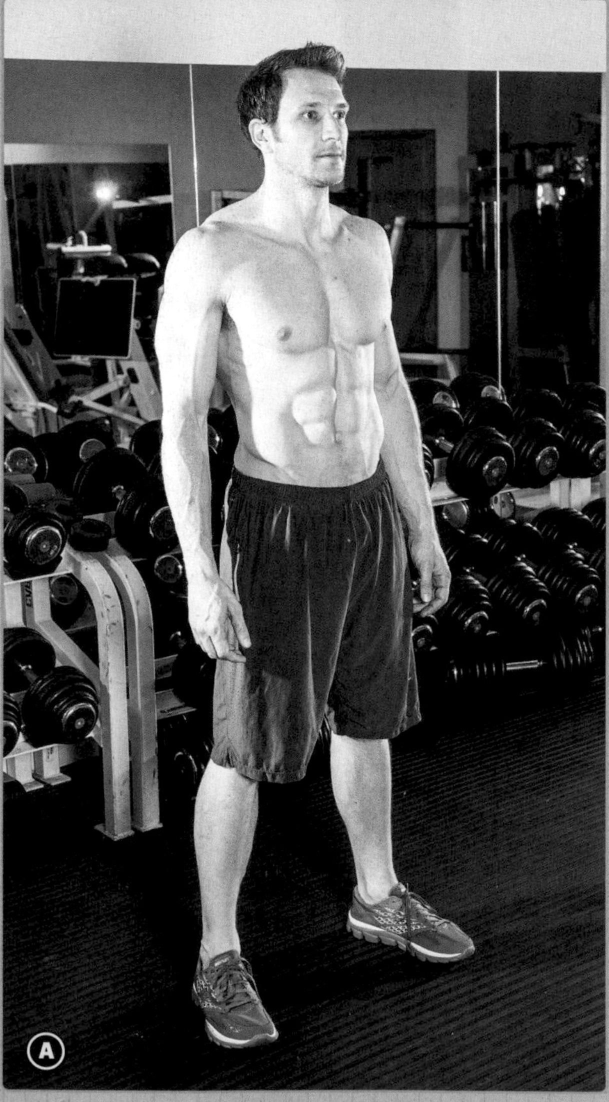

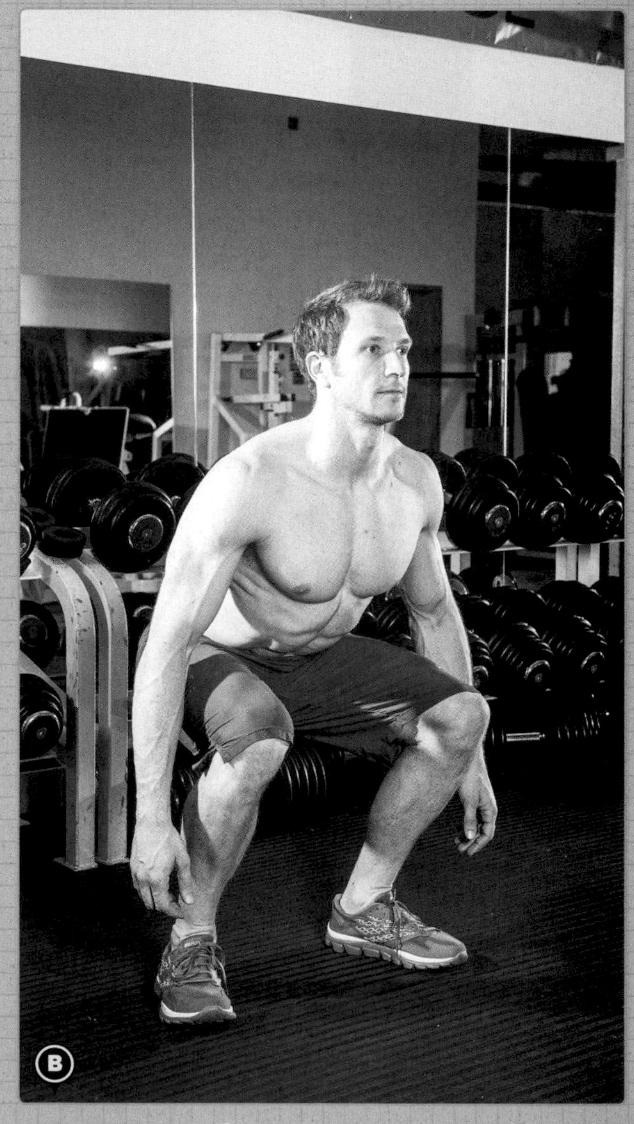

- Stand with your feet slightly wider than shoulder-width apart with your toes pointing outwards slightly.
- Squat until your thighs are at least parallel to the floor. The deeper you can squat, the better.
- Drive back up through your heels to return to the start position.

Jump squat

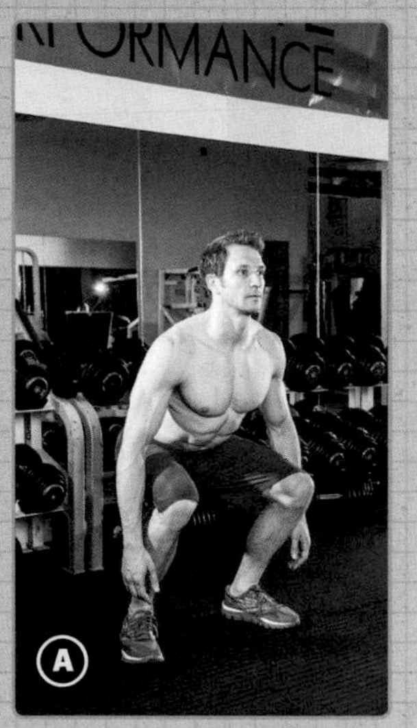

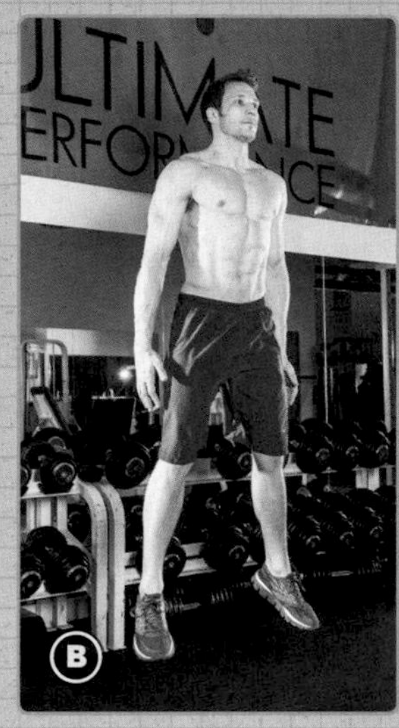

Squatting then jumping powerfully into the air fires your fast-twitch muscle fibres, which are responsible for explosive power and strength

Bodyweight lunge

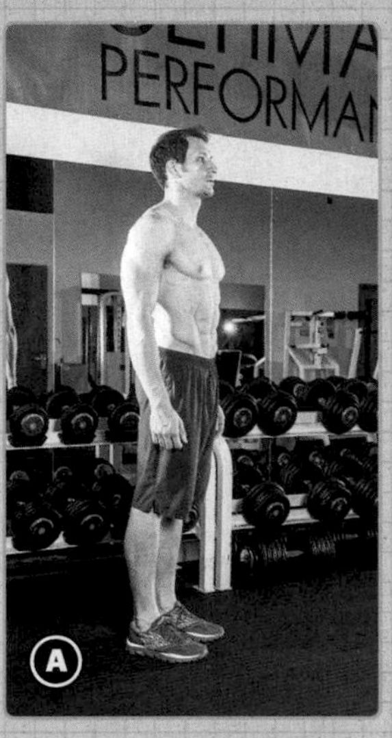

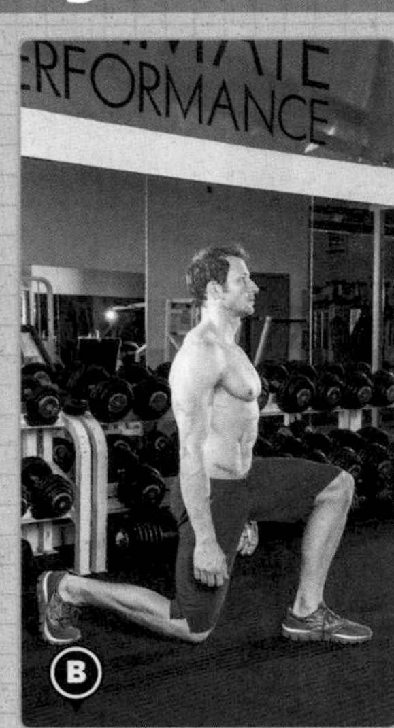

Taking one step forwards and lowering your body until both knees are bent at right angles will work your hamstrings harder.

Jump lunge

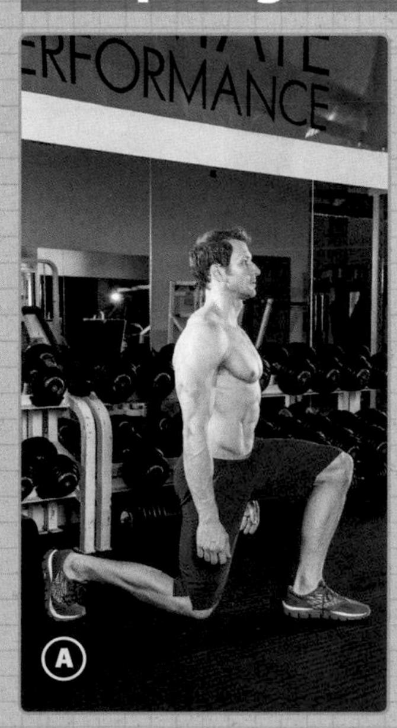

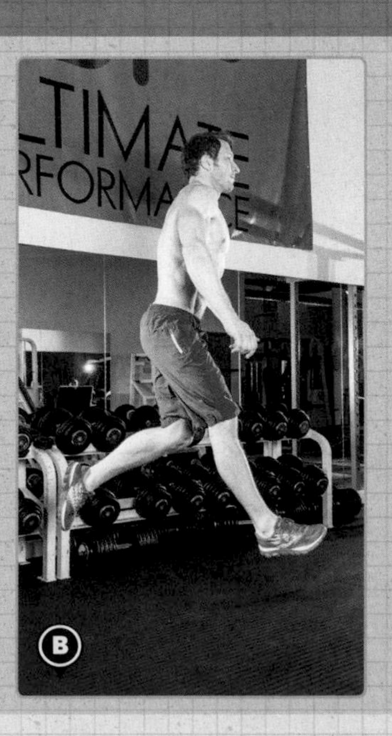

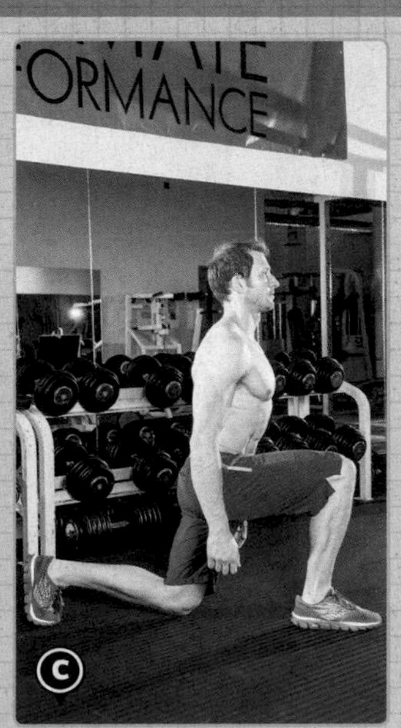

Lungeing then launching yourself and swapping legs in mid-air to land and lunge on your other leg is a great way to hit your hamstrings.

SQUAT

***Targets** Quads, glutes, hamstrings, core*

A key exercise for building bigger and stronger legs, the squat also works many other muscle groups and should be a staple in everyone's training programme

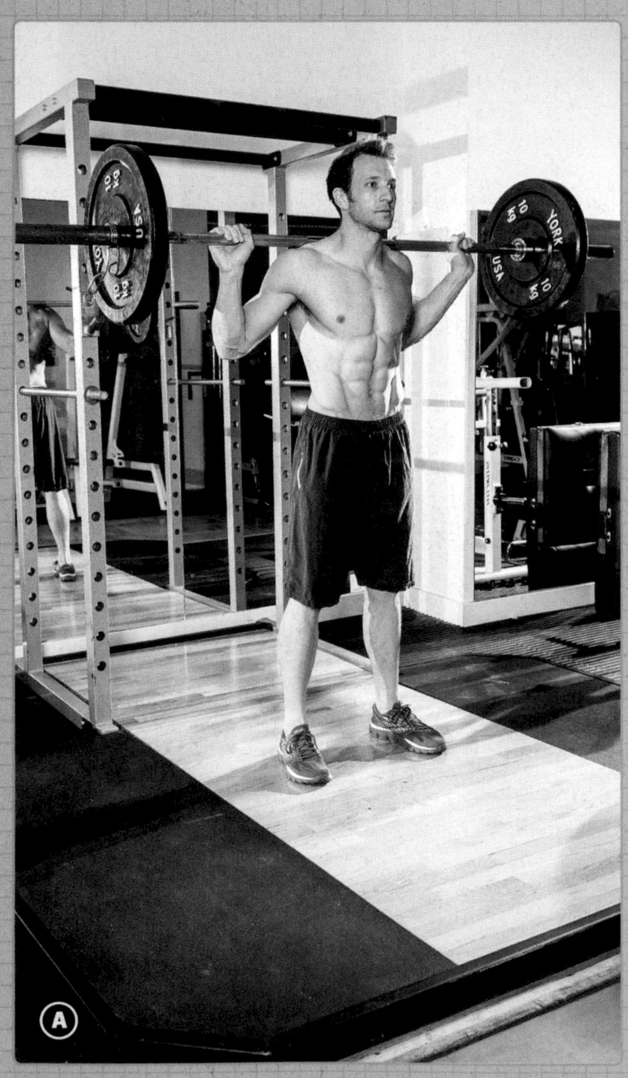

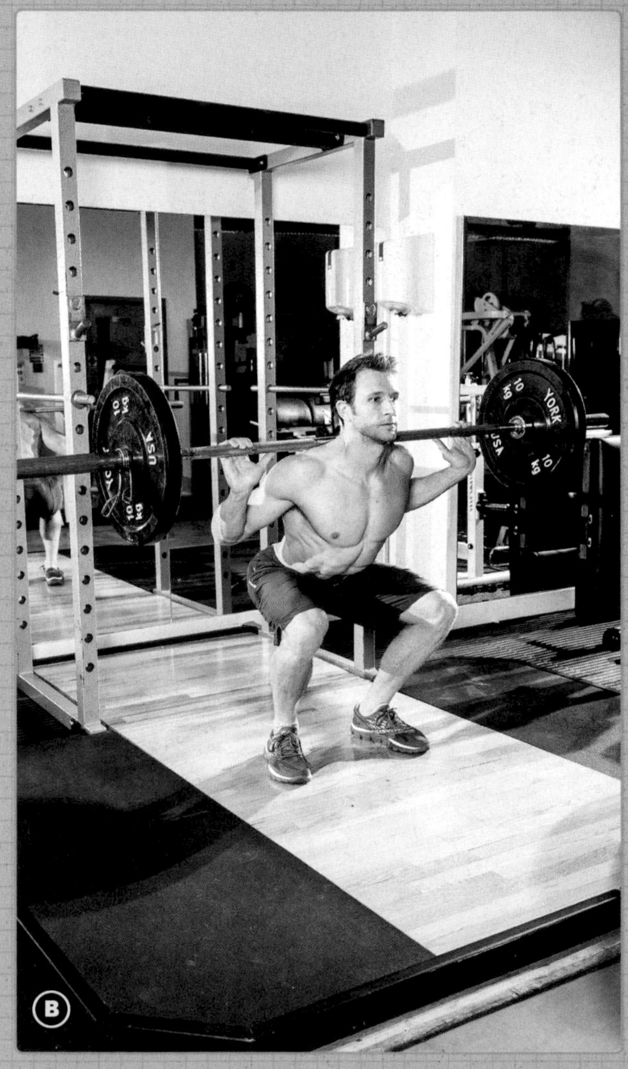

- Rest the bar against the back of your shoulders – not on your neck – and hold the bar with an overhand grip slightly wider than your shoulders. Keep your elbows pointing down.
- Your feet should be a little more than shoulder-width apart with your toes pointing outwards slightly.
- Squat until your thighs are at least parallel to the floor. The deeper you can squat, the better.
- Drive back up through your heels to return to the start position.

Dumbbell squat

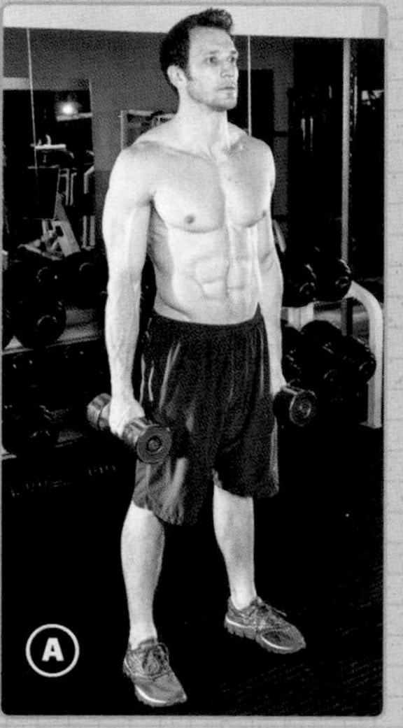

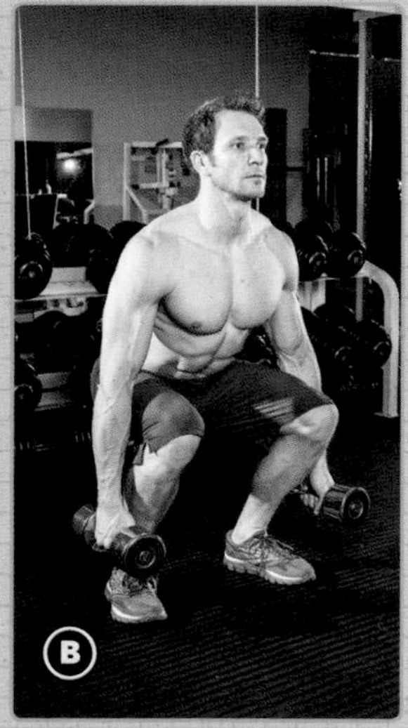

Using dumbbells allows you to maintain better form than with a barbell so it's a good starting point that still works the target muscles hard.

One-leg squat

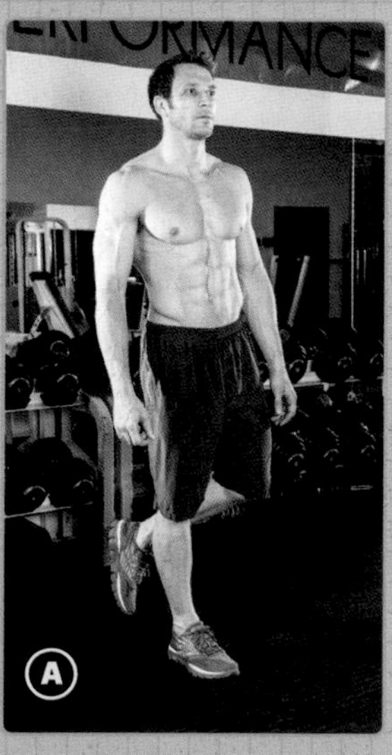

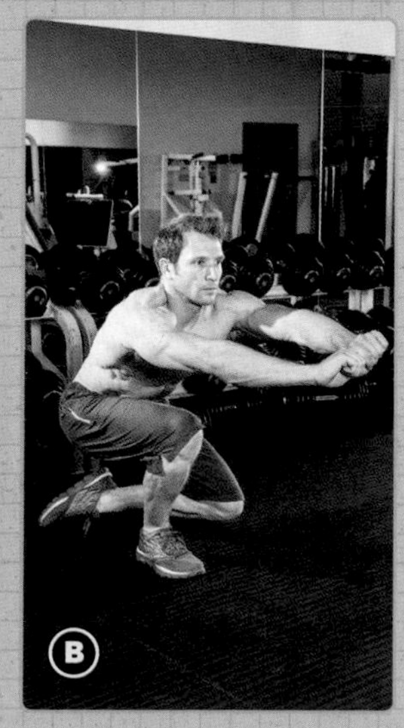

Squatting one leg at a time works the muscles independently, improves balance, co-ordination and core strength, and also improves knee and ankle joint stability.

Pistol squat

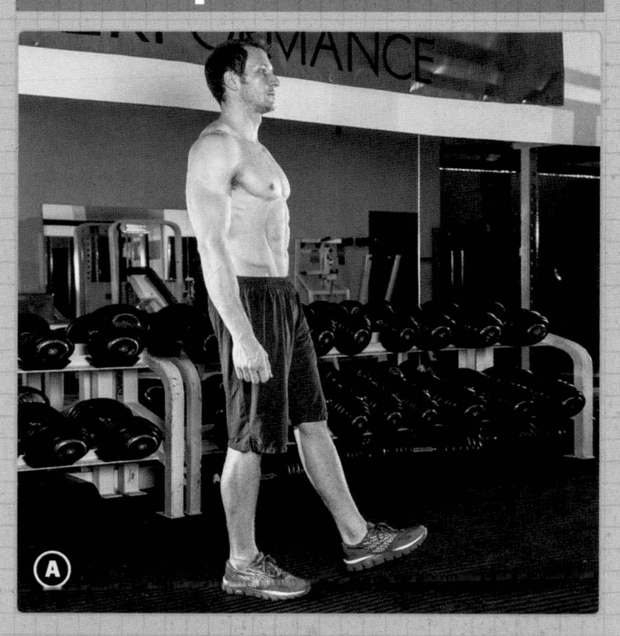

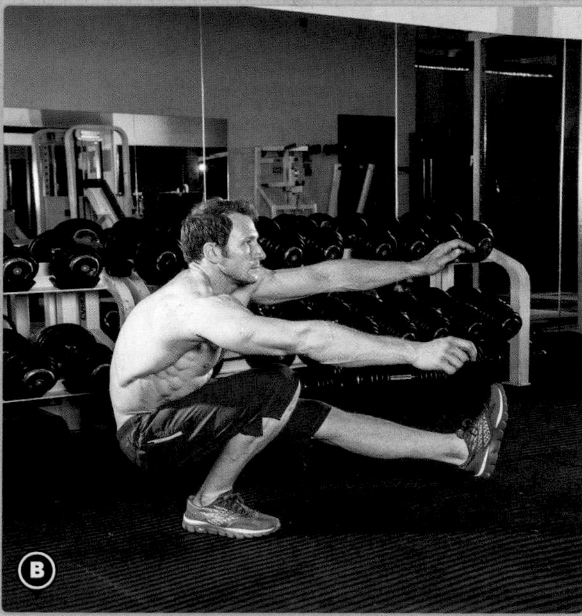

One of the toughest bodyweight moves, this requires balance, co-ordination, flexibility and strong leg muscles.

FRONT SQUAT

***Targets** Quads, glutes, hamstrings*

Holding the bar across the front of your shoulders shifts more of the load on to your quads and eases the pressure on your lower back

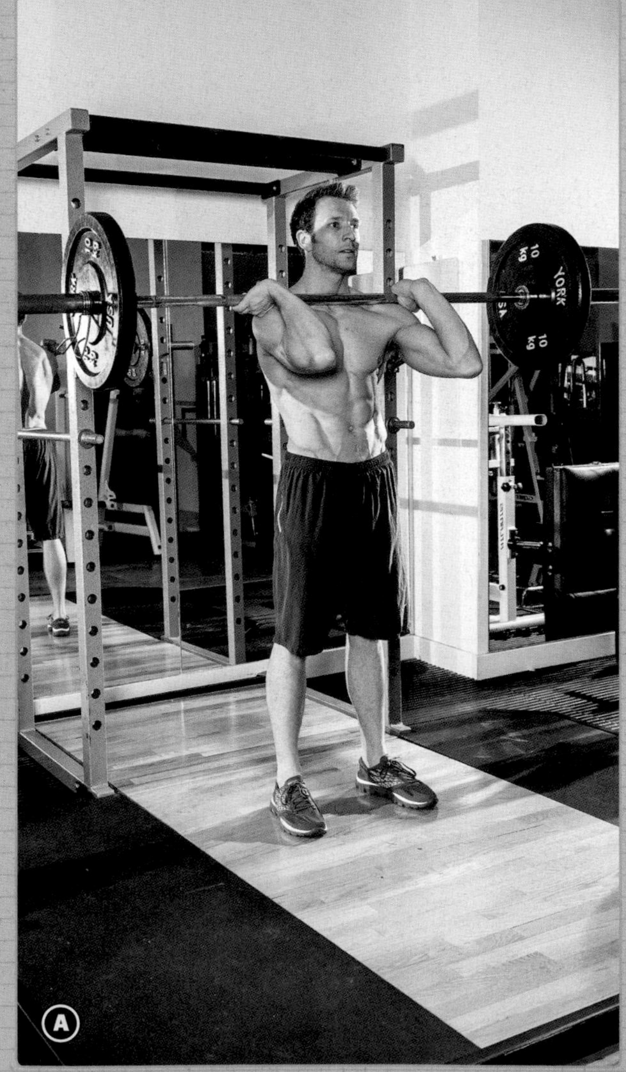

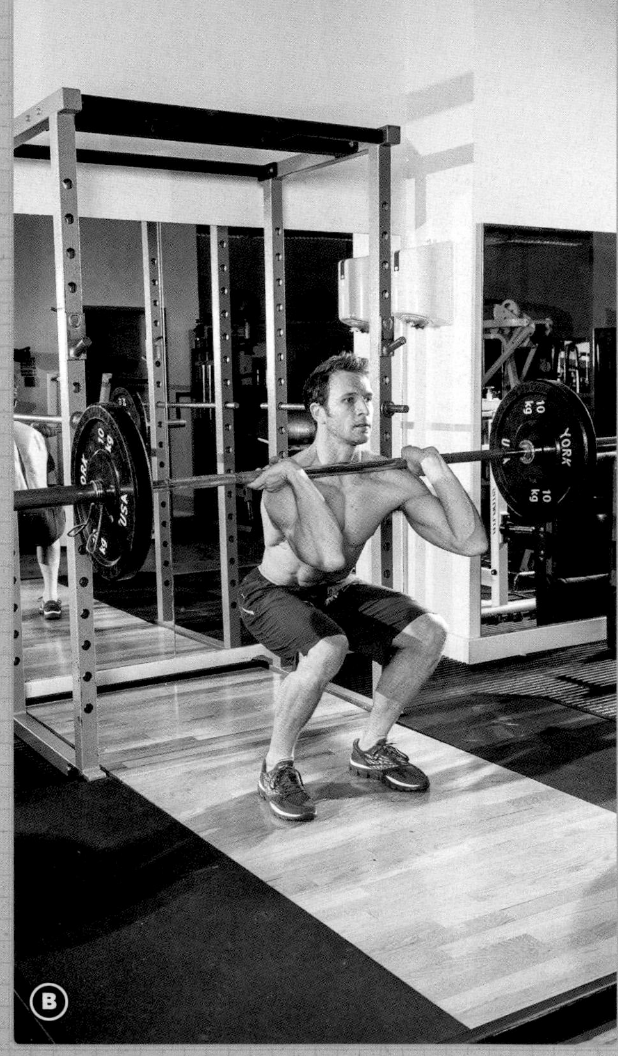

- Stand with your feet shoulder-width apart and rest the bar on the front of your shoulders, gripping it with your hands by your shoulders, your elbows pointing forwards.
- Maintain a natural arch in your back and your core braced throughout the move.
- Squat until your thighs are at least parallel to the floor. The deeper you can squat, the better.
- Drive back up through your heels to return to the start position.

Sumo squat

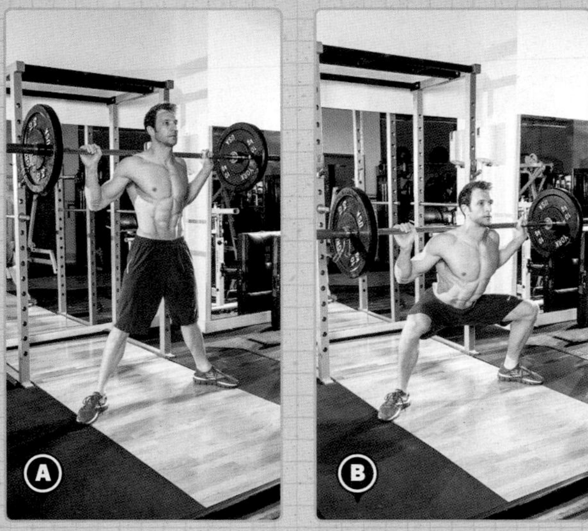

A wide stance works your adductors, or inner thighs, and your glutes harder as you squat and stand back up.

Hack squat

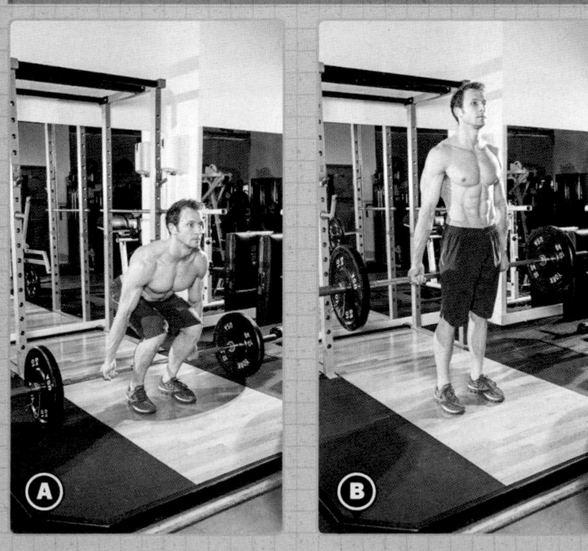

Holding the bar behind your back reduces pressure on your lower back and forces your quads to work harder.

Overhead squat

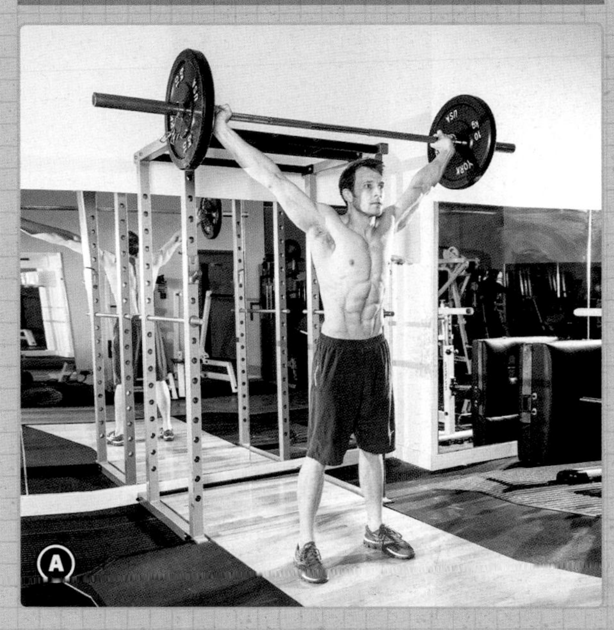

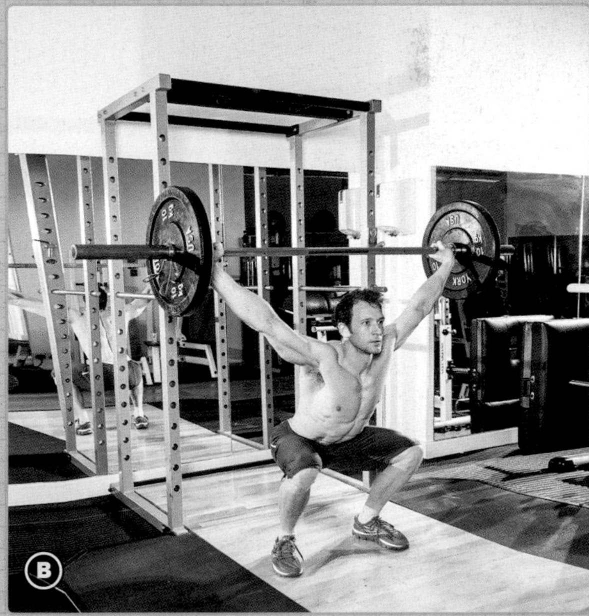

Squatting while holding the bar above your head with your arms fully extended is a major test of leg and core strength, as well as balance, co-ordination and joint stability and flexibility.

BARBELL LUNGE

***Targets** Hamstrings, quads, glutes, core*

Power and co-ordination are crucial for managing the weight as you lunge forwards

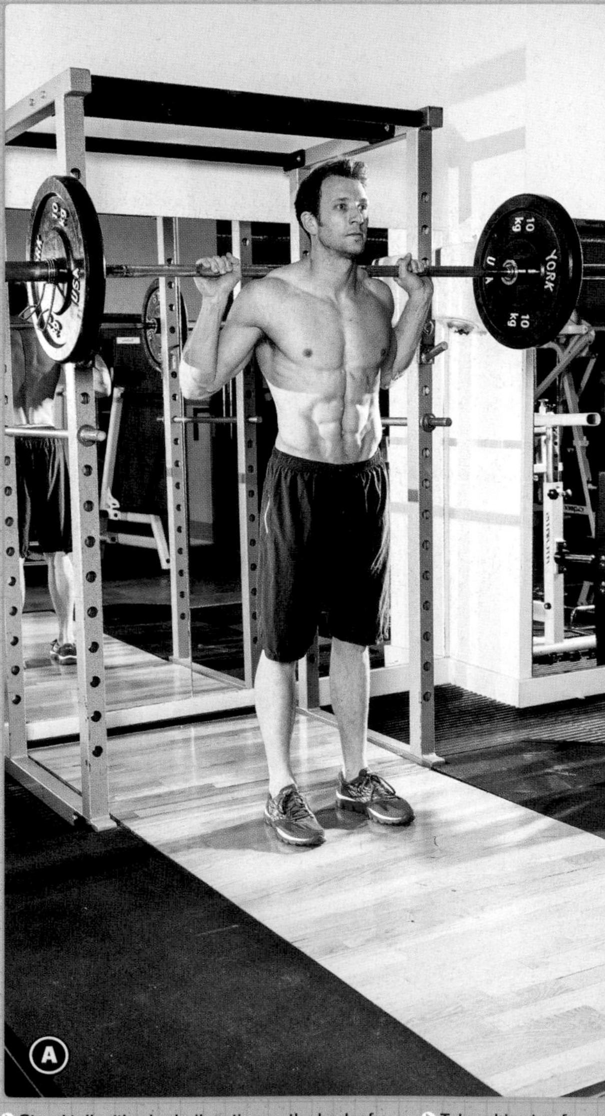

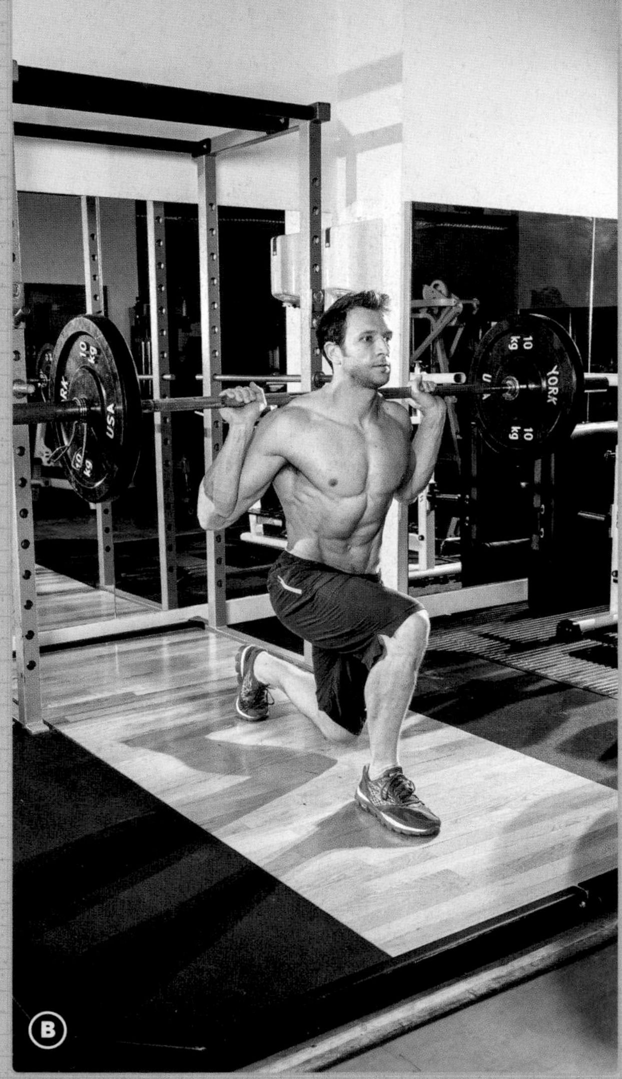

- Stand tall with a barbell resting on the back of your shoulders. Point your elbows behind you to retract your shoulder blades and keep your back upright and core braced throughout.
- Take a big step forwards, taking care to keep your knee over your front foot, not beyond it.
- Lower your body until both knees are bent at 90° before pushing back off your front foot to return to the start position.

Split squat

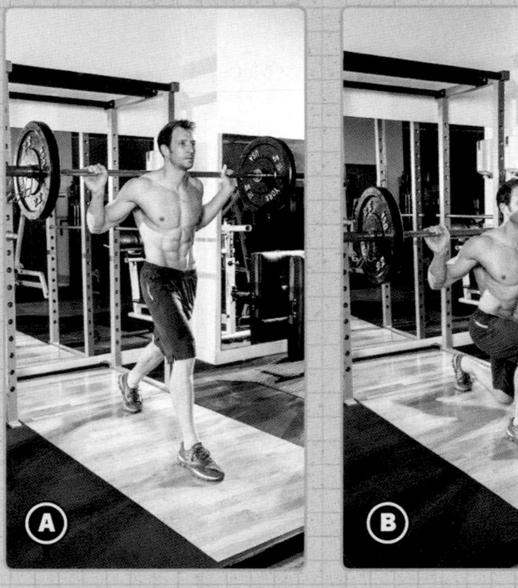

Keeping one foot forwards and squatting works the target muscles but places less pressure on the knee and ankle.

Dumbbell lunge

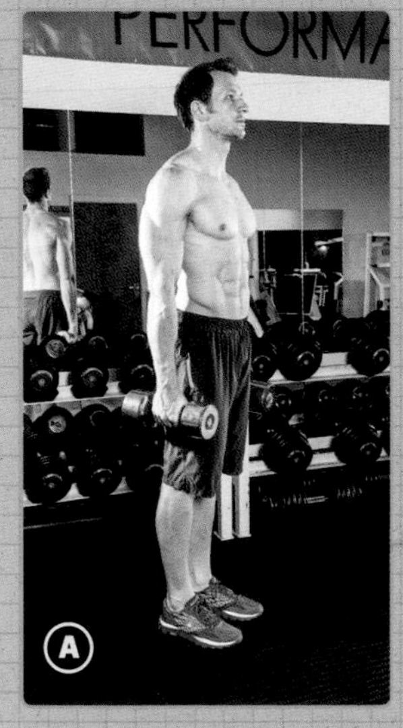

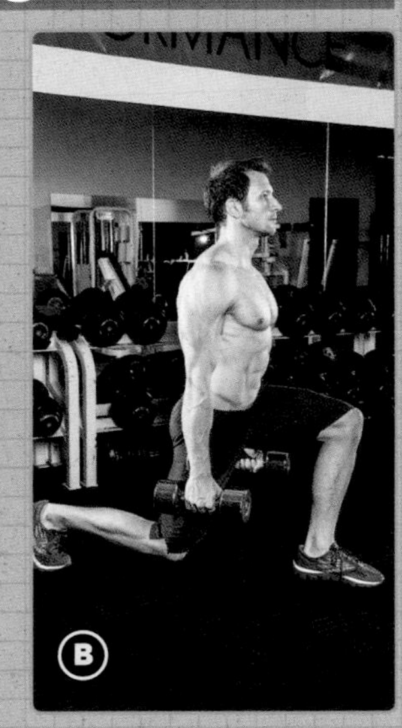

Using dumbbells reduces the stress on your lower back and so makes it a beginner-friendly alternative.

Elevated front foot split squat

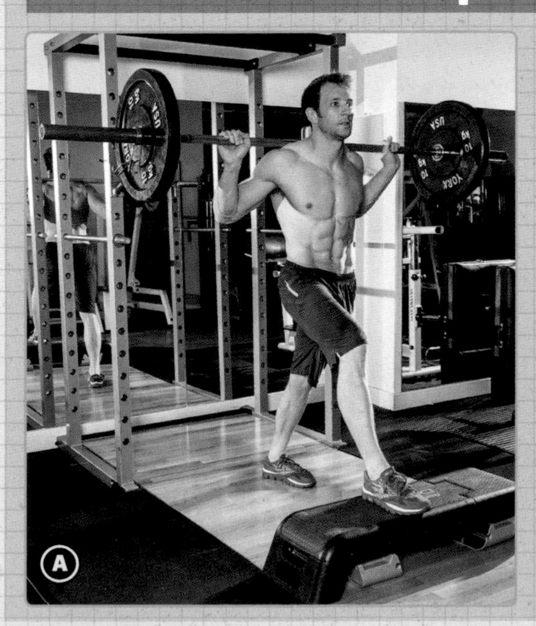

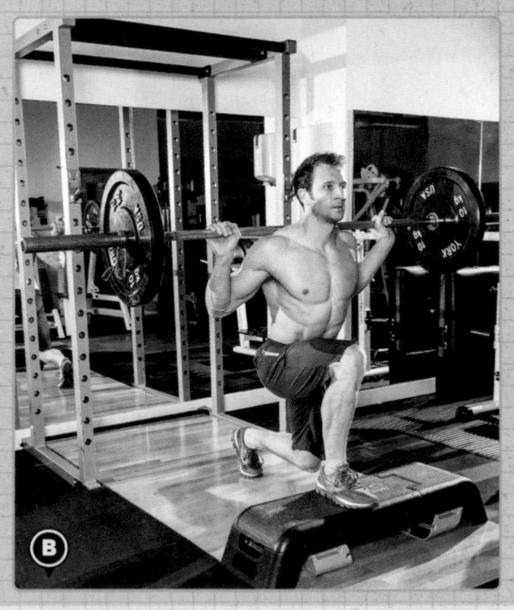

Elevating your front foot limits the range of motion, making it a good progression move to harder variants.

LATERAL LUNGE

Targets *Adductors*

Your inner thighs are crucial to stabilising the legs as well having a huge role in sudden, turning movements crucial in all sports

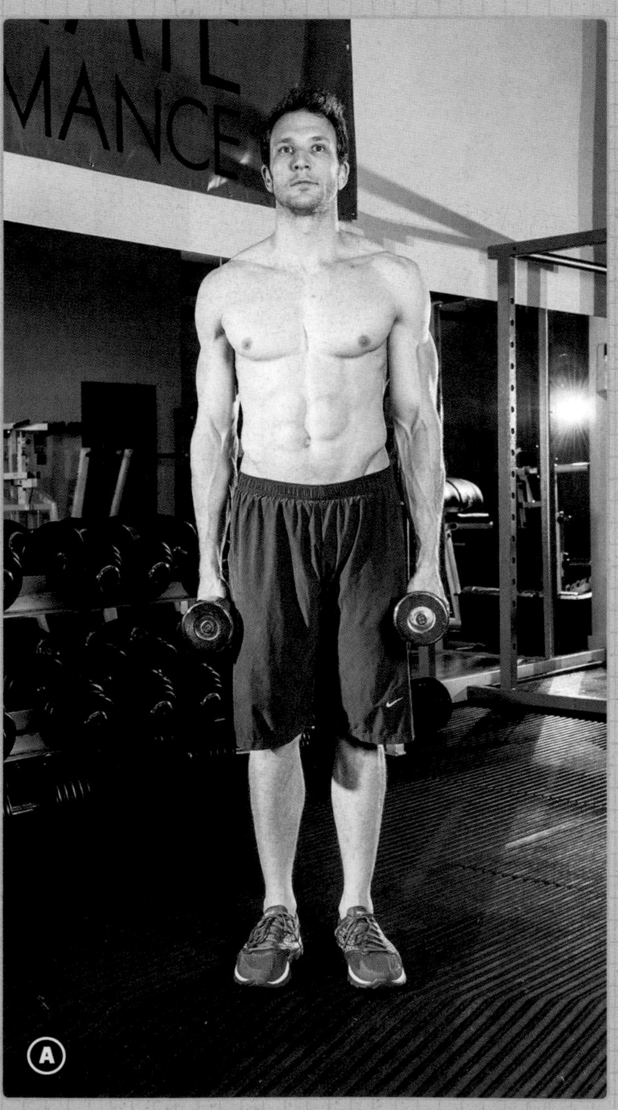

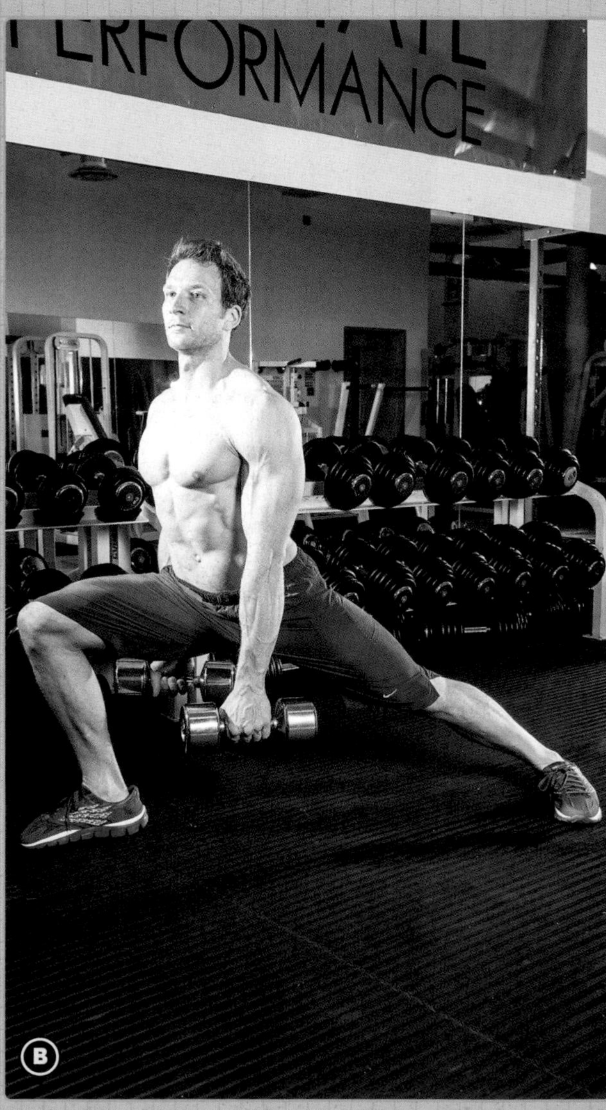

- Stand tall with your feet close together, holding a dumbbell in each hand.
- Keeping your core braced, take a big step to one side and lower your body towards the leading leg, keeping with your knee in line with your toes.
- Push back off the leading leg to return to the start position, then repeat the other side.

Reverse lunge

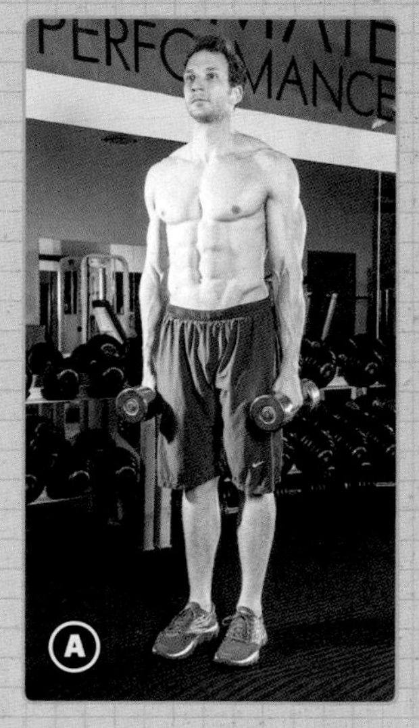

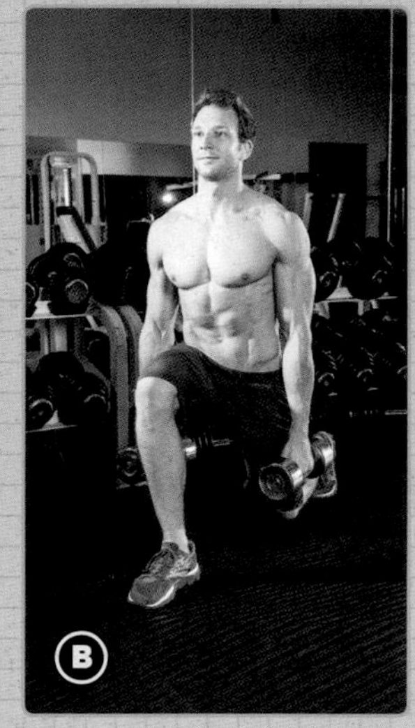

Stepping backwards hits the target muscles differently and improves balance and co-ordination.

Transverse lunge

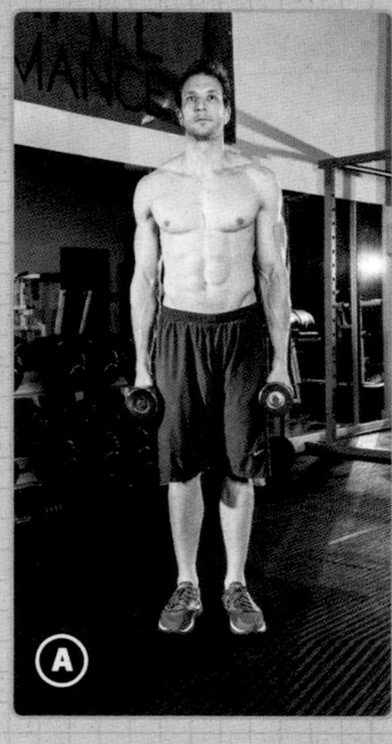

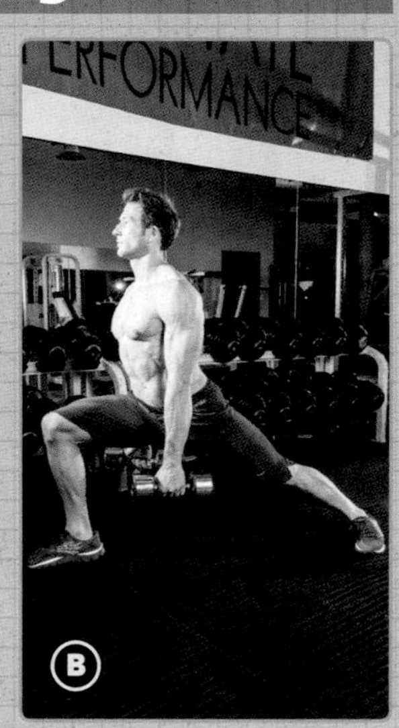

Stepping out and opening your hips will target those small but vital muscles responsible for efficient sudden turning movements.

Lateral lunge and touch

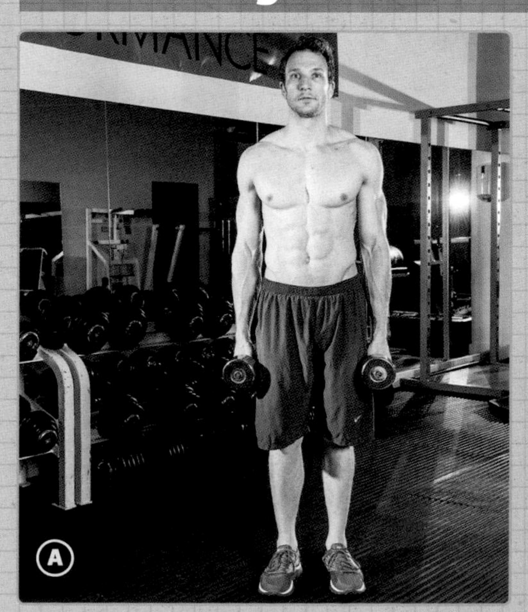

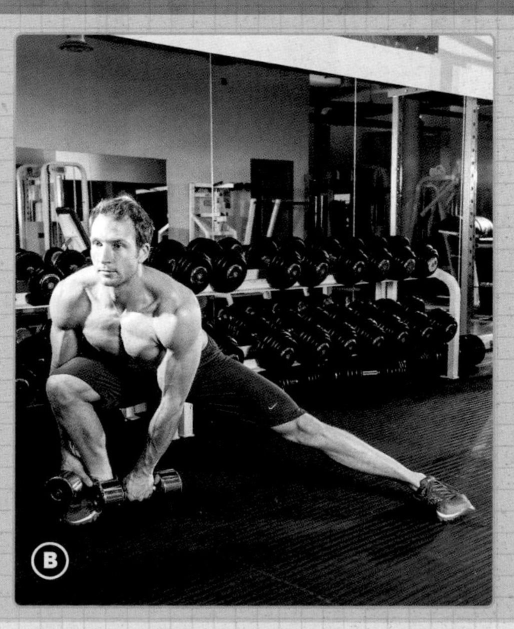

Bending down to touch the weights to the floor works your hamstrings harder.

BULGARIAN SPLIT SQUAT

***Targets** Quads, glutes, hamstrings*

Placing one foot on a raised surface behind you forces the standing leg to do all the work to ensure balanced gains

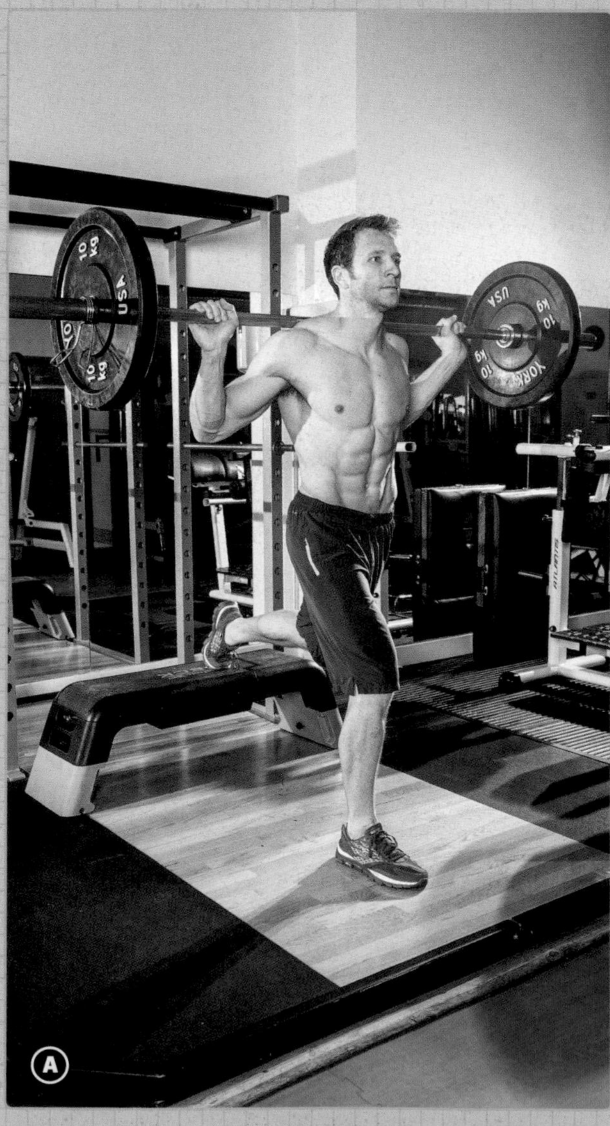

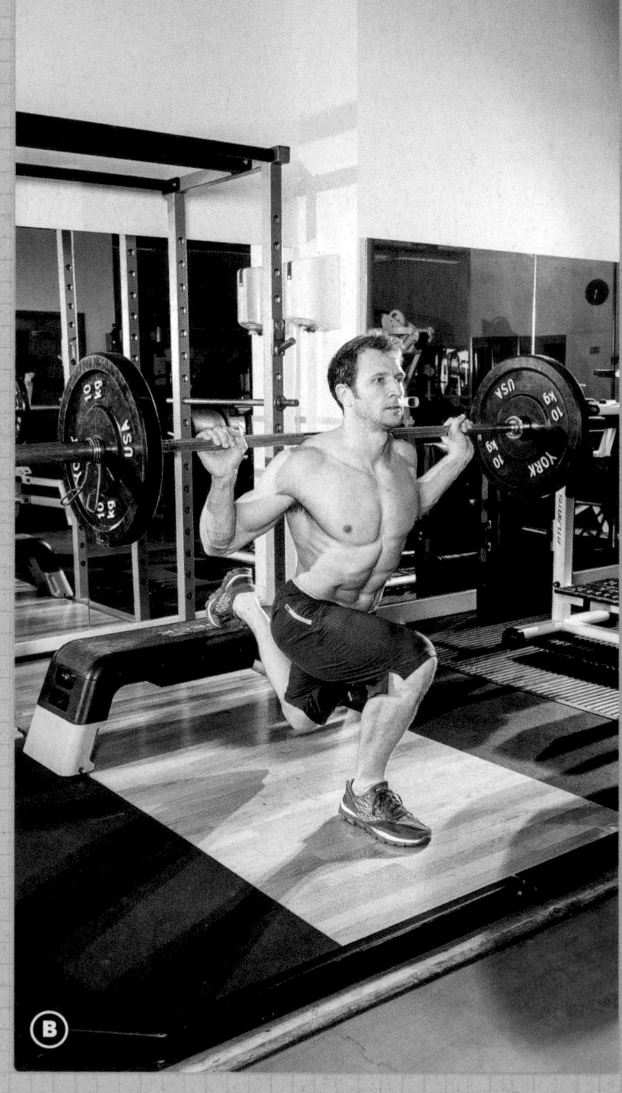

- Stand tall and place one foot behind you on a bench or raised platform. Hold the bar across the back of your shoulders.
- Bend your standing leg until your thigh is parallel to the floor, keeping your core braced and your knee in line with your foot.
- Push into the floor to return to the start.

Gym ball Bulgarian split squat with twist

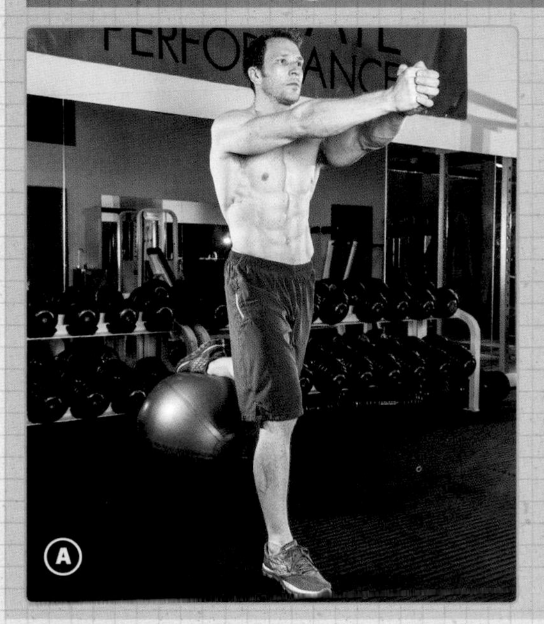

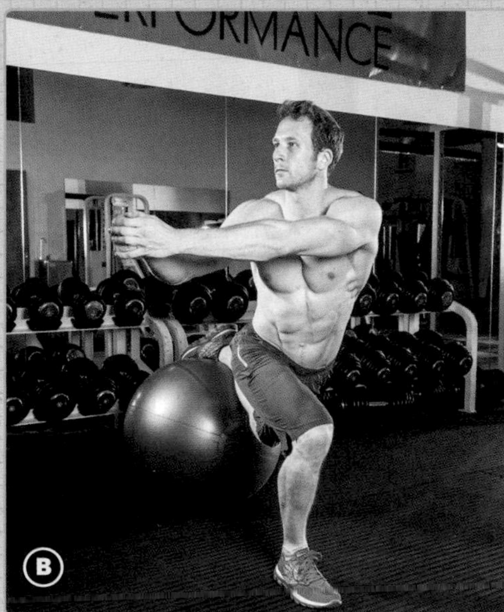

Twisting to the sides while lungeing improves balance, co-ordination and leg and core strength.

Gym ball dumbbell Bulgarian split squat

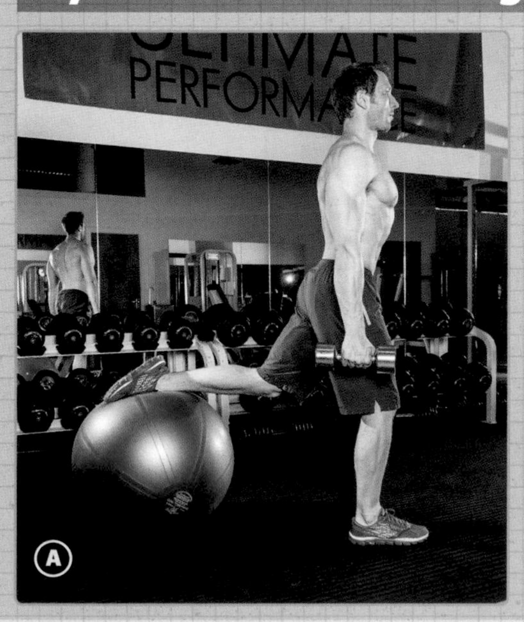

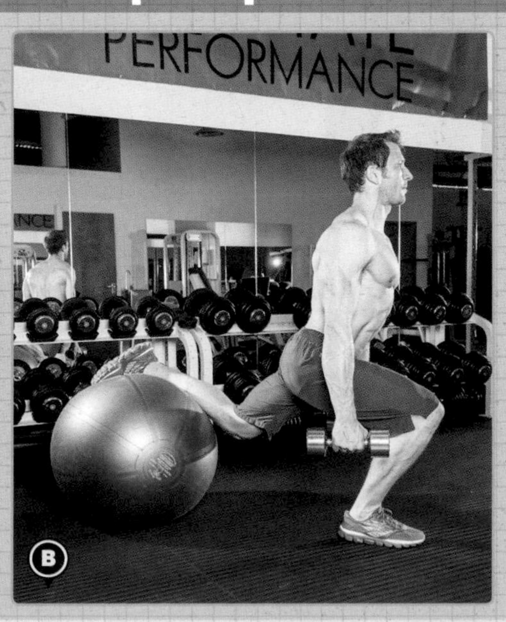

The instability of the gym ball under your back foot forces your core and front leg to work even harder.

DUMBBELL STEP-UP

Targets *Quads, glutes*

Build strength in the target muscles by making this everyday move – you do it every time you walk up steps – harder with weights

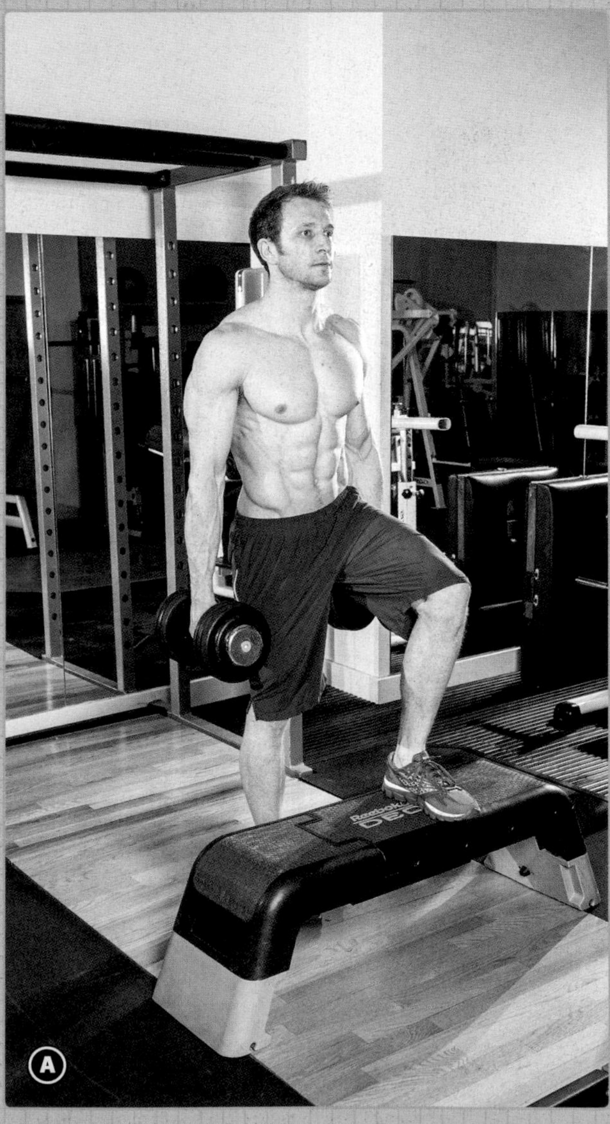

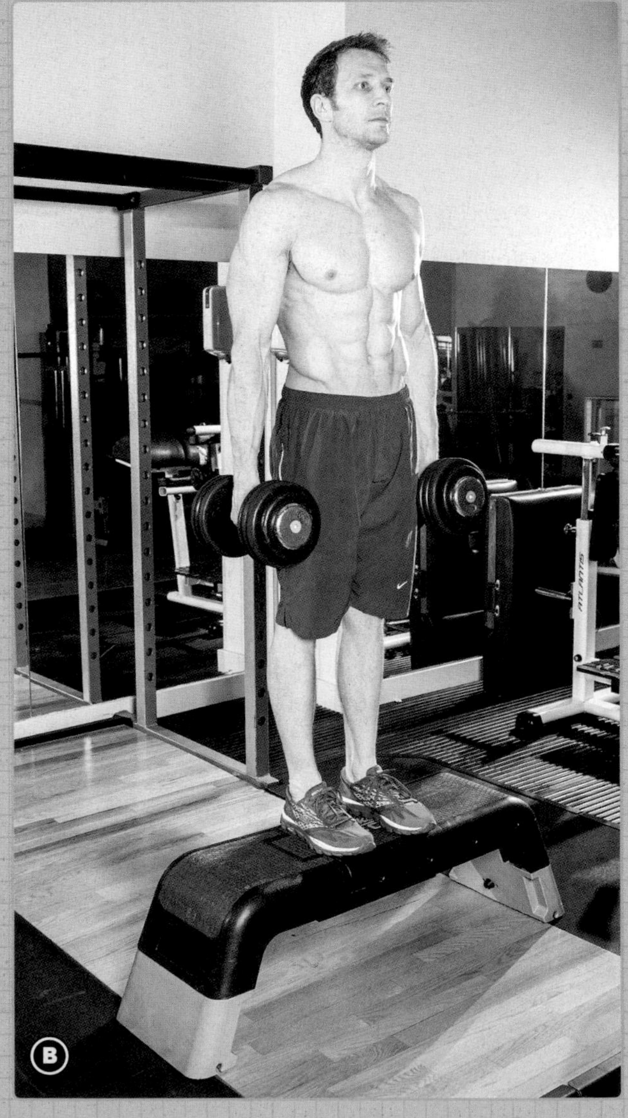

- Stand in front of a platform set at knee height holding a dumbbell in each hand.
- Keep one foot on the platform and step up with the other foot.
- Step back down and repeat with the other leg.

Dumbbell side step-up

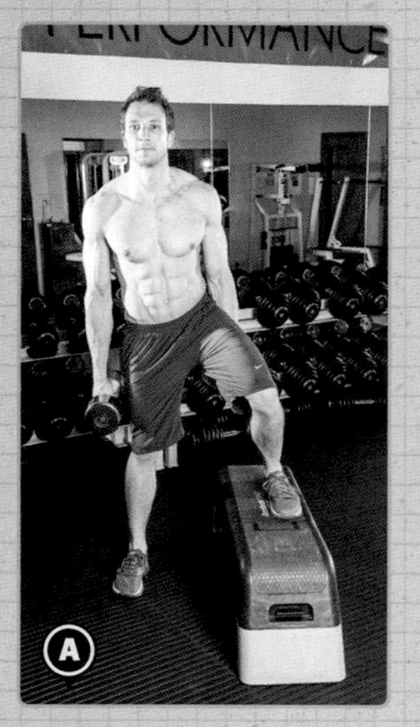

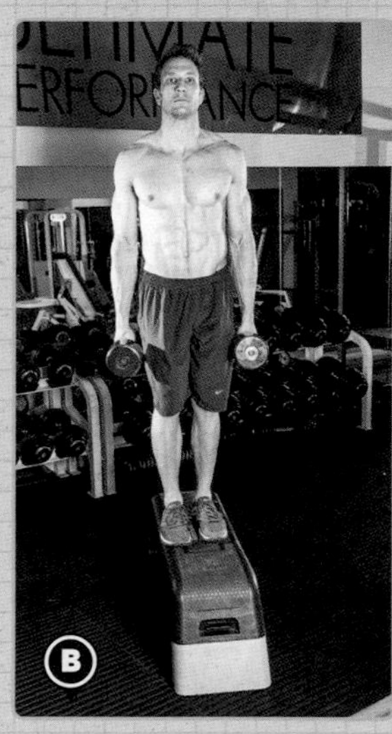

Hit your quads and glutes from a different angle by stepping up sideways on to the bench.

Alternating box jumps

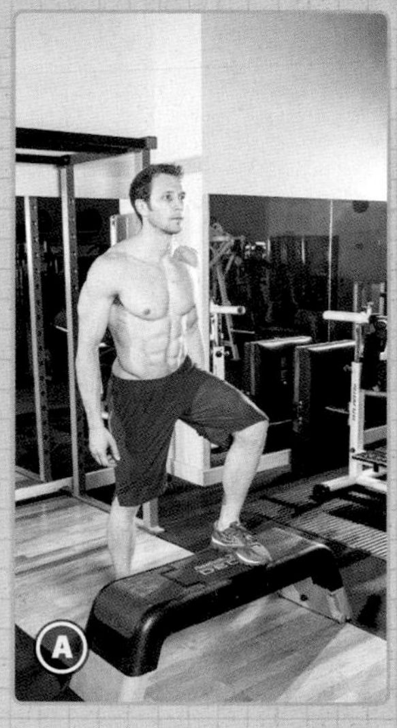

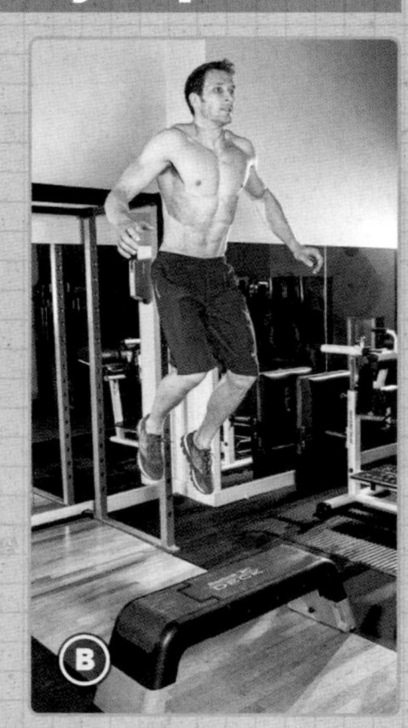

Step up on to the bench with one foot and jump into the air, and then repeat with the opposite leg to work each limb independently.

Box jumps

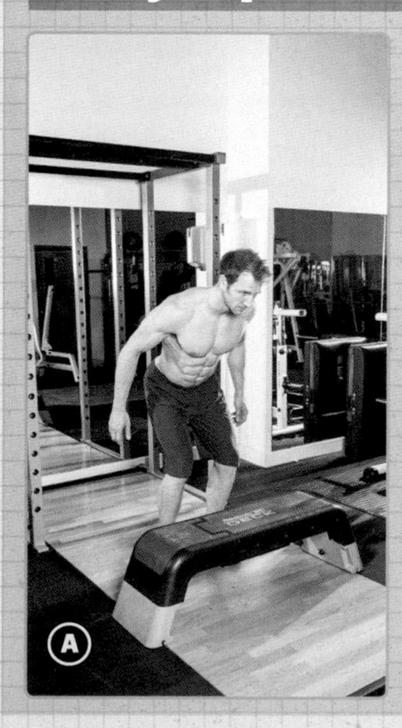

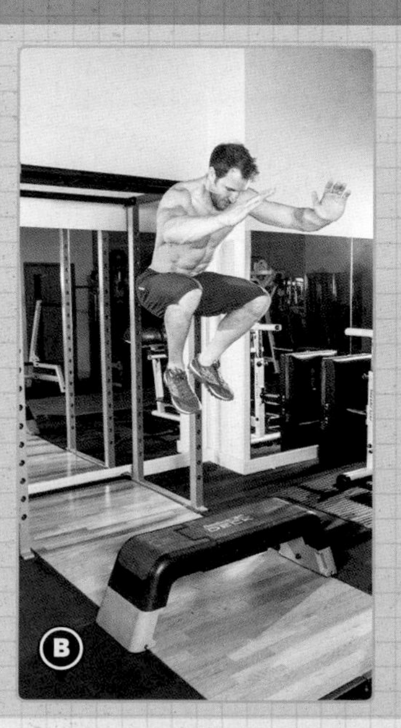

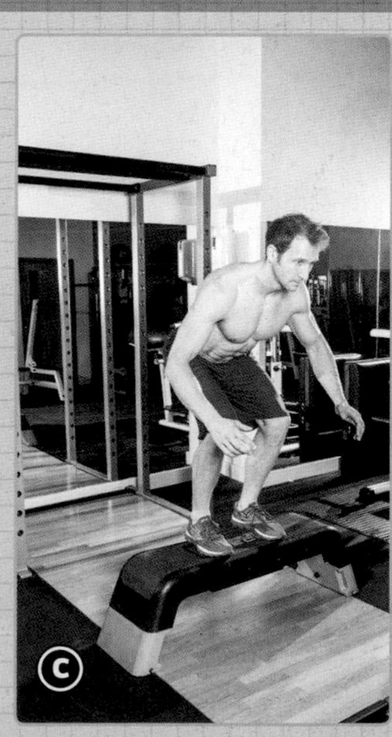

Build explosive power by jumping on to the box to land with both feet, then stepping back down again.

ROMANIAN DEADLIFT

Targets *Hamstrings*

This is one of the best moves to add muscle size and strength on the back of your thighs, but always maintain perfect form to protect your lower back

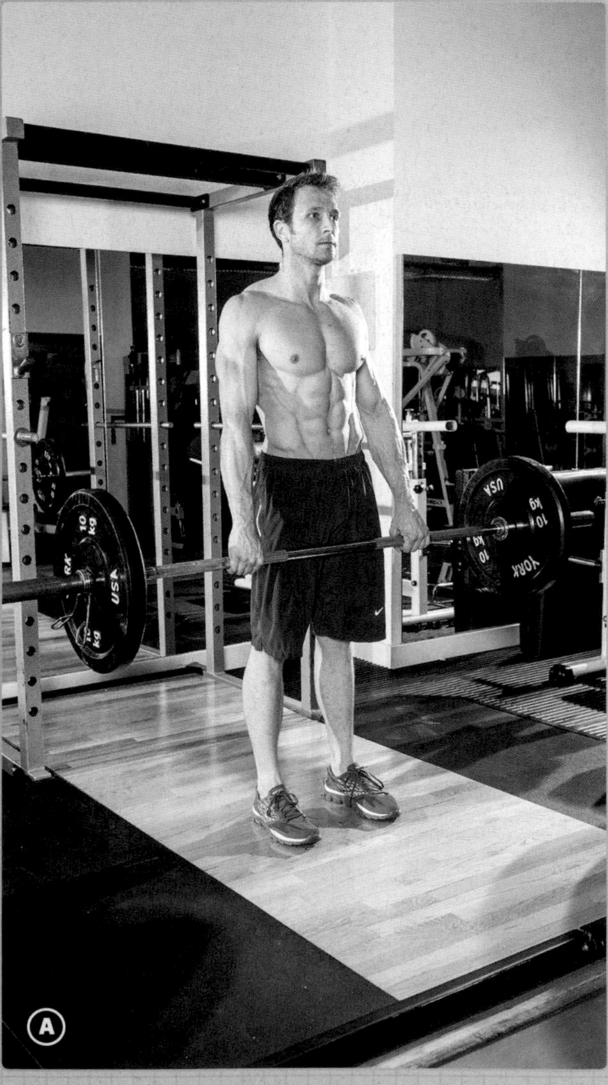

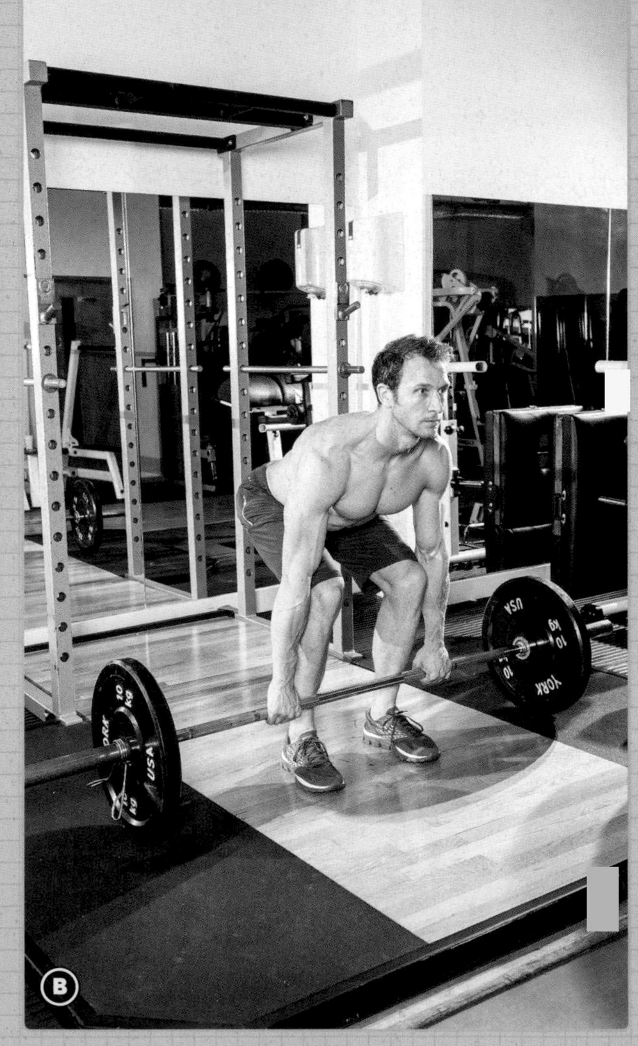

- Stand tall with your feet shoulder-width apart holding a barbell with an overhand grip just outside your thighs.
- Keeping a slight bend in your knees, bend forwards from the hips – not the waist – and lower the bar down the front of your shins until you feel a good stretch in your hamstrings.
- Reverse the move back to the start and push your hips forwards.

Stiff-leg Romanian deadlift

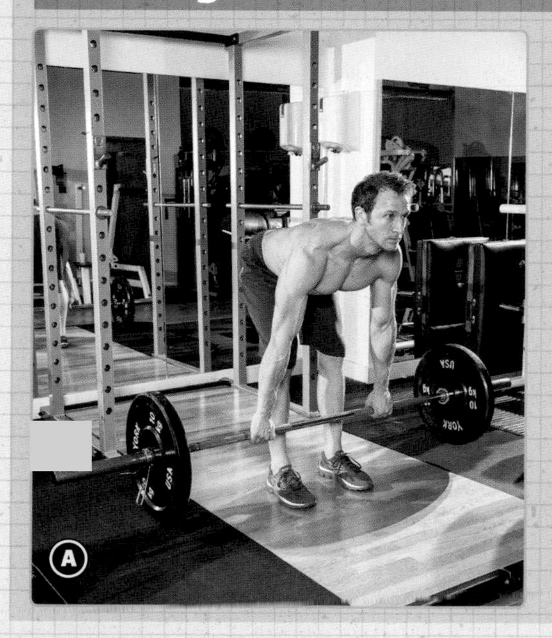

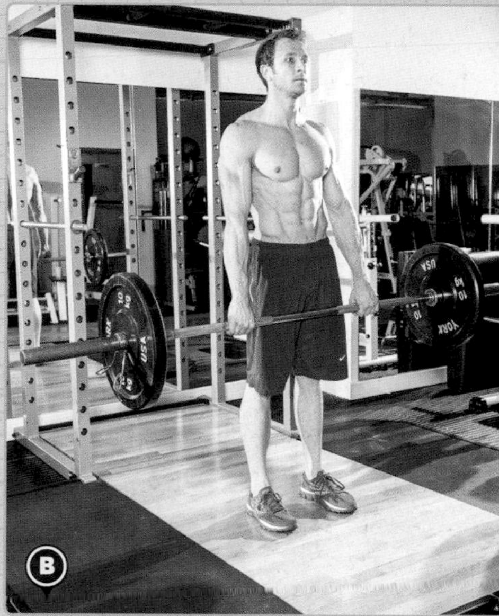

Keeping your legs straight and locked at the knees places even greater emphasis on your hamstrings but puts more pressure on your lower back.

Split dumbbell Romanian deadlift

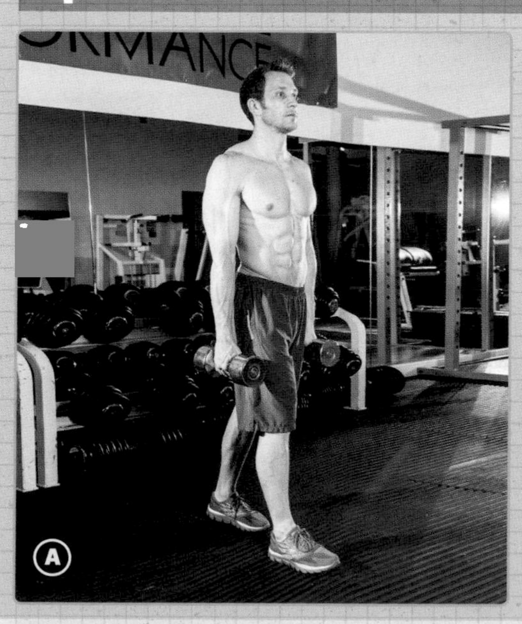

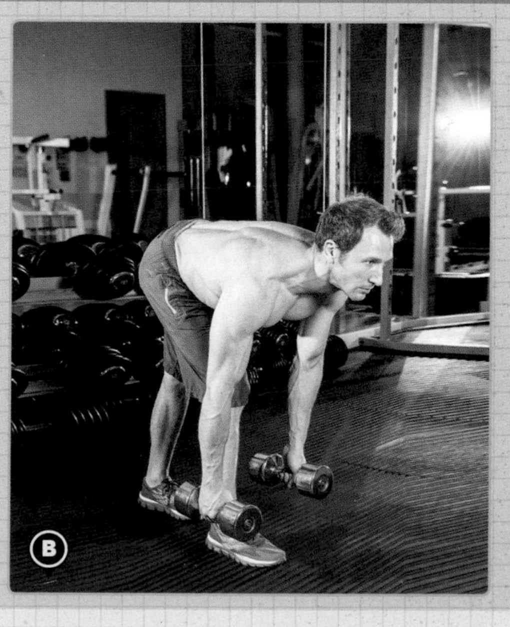

As well as working each leg separately, this move replicates the way you pick up objects from the ground, making it a great injury-preventing move.

KETTLEBELL GOBLET SQUAT

***Targets** Quads, glutes, hamstrings*

Make a bodyweight squat harder and work the target muscles more by holding a kettlebell with both hands at the top of your chest

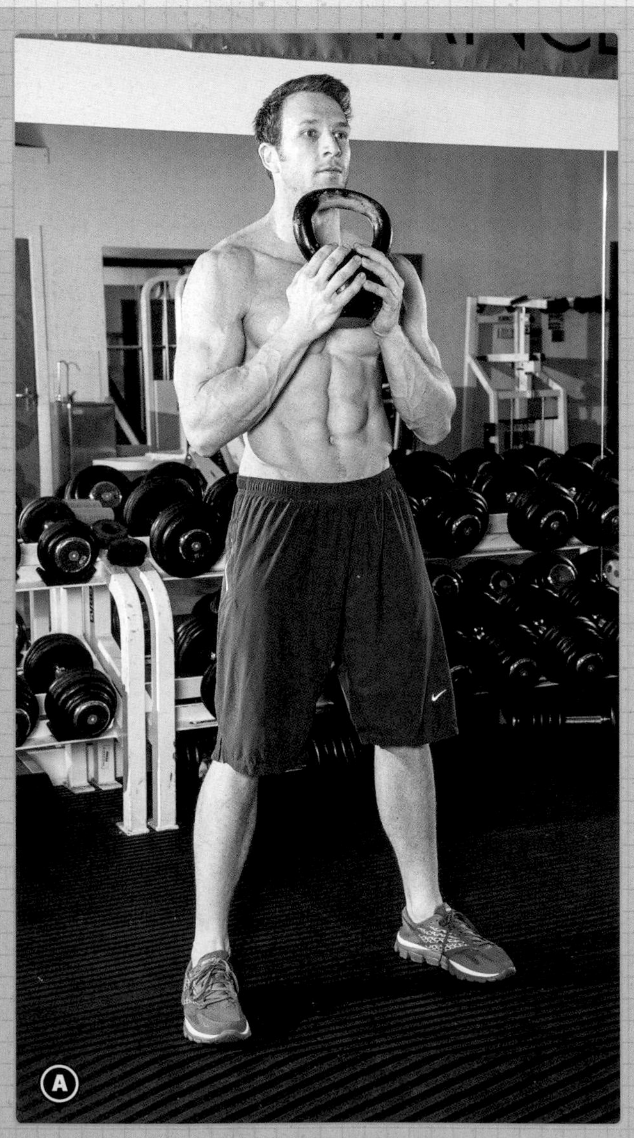

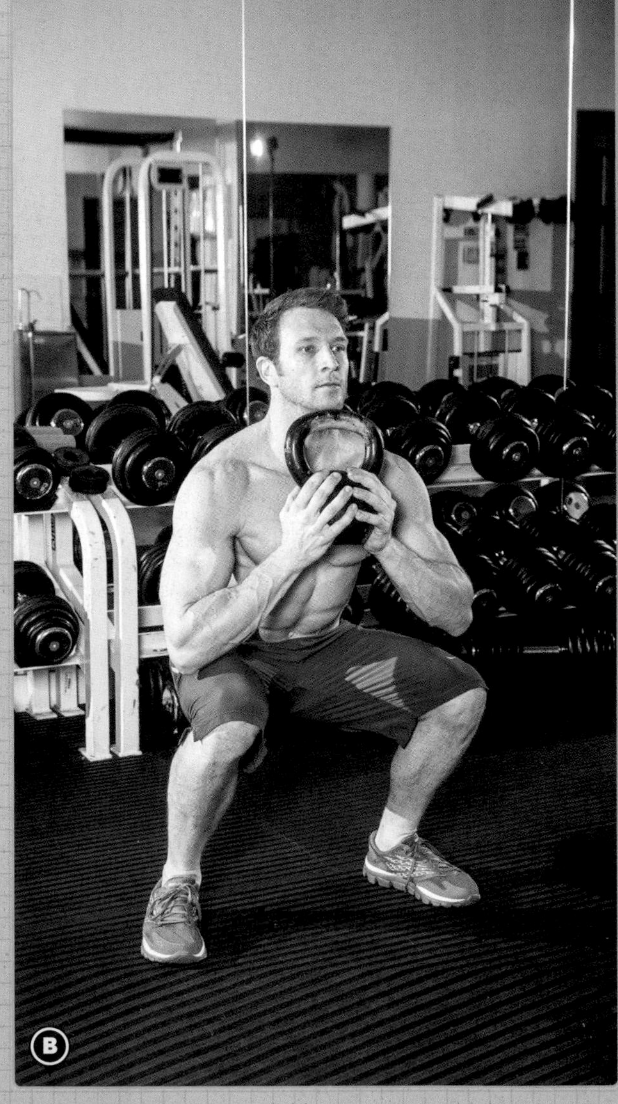

- Stand with your feet shoulder-width apart holding a kettlebell in front of your chest.
- Keeping your core braced and your knees in line with your toes, squat until your thighs are at least parallel to the floor.
- Stand back up, driving through your heels, to return to the start position.

Kettlebell pistol squat

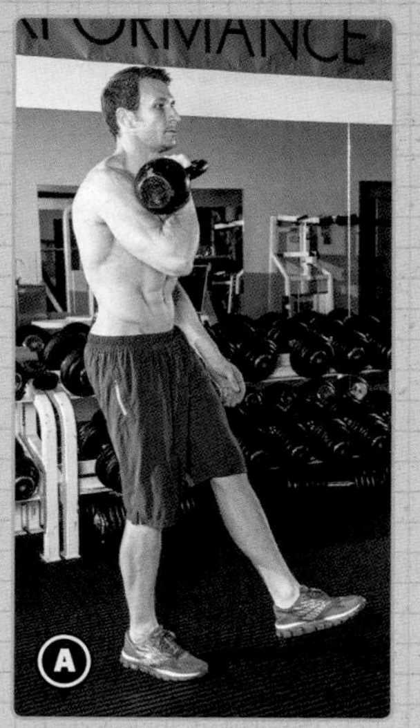

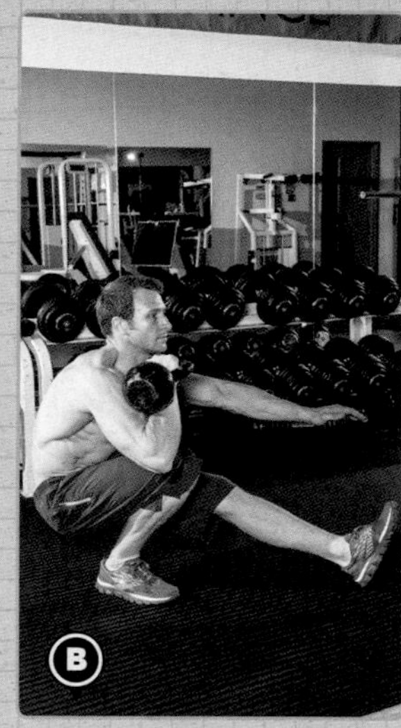

This incredibly tough move builds strength and stability, and improves balance and co-ordination.

One-leg kettlebell deadlift

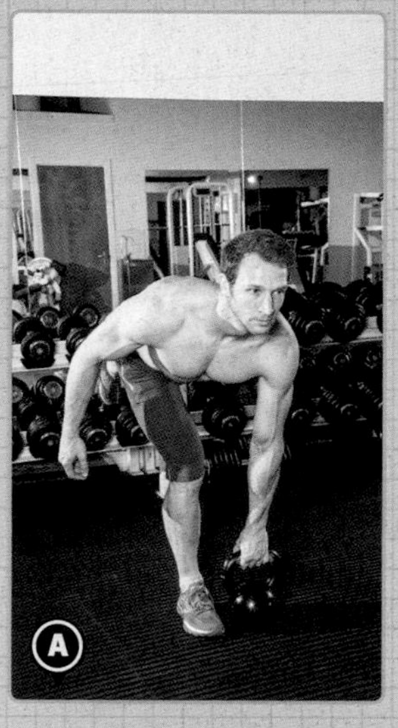

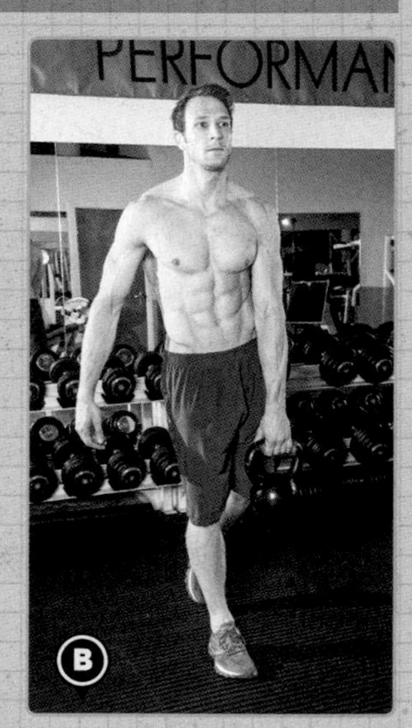

This move requires great balance and flexibility, and hits your glutes and hamstrings hard.

Kettlebell rack squat

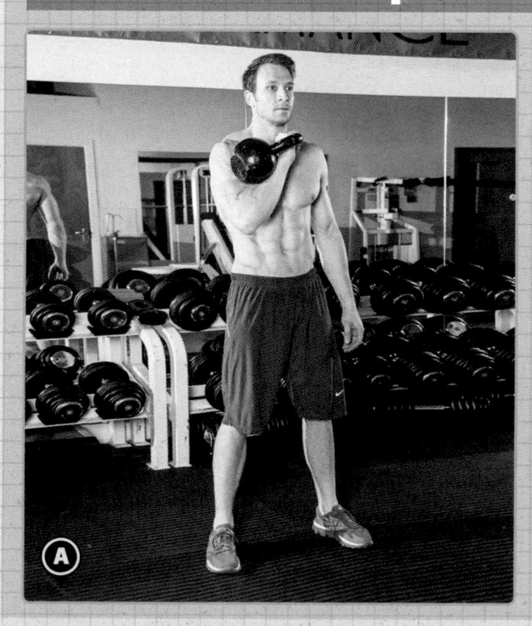

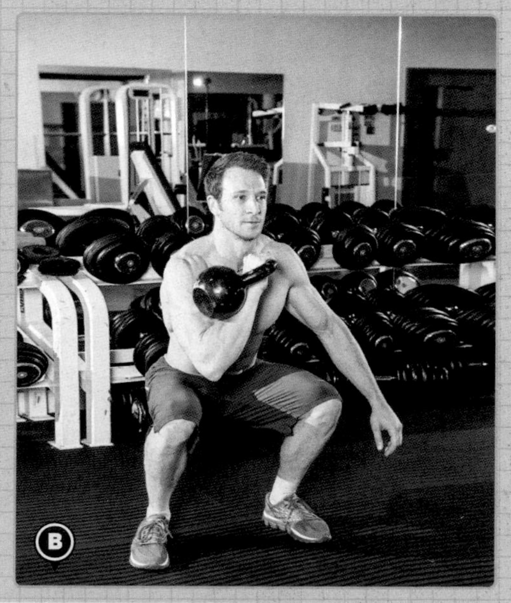

Squatting while holding the kettlebell in the rack position – resting on the front of your shoulder – makes your core work harder to stabilise your torso.

LEG PRESS

***Targets** Quads, hamstrings*

Push your quads to the limit with this standard machine move that stabilises your body so you can focus on hitting your leg muscles hard

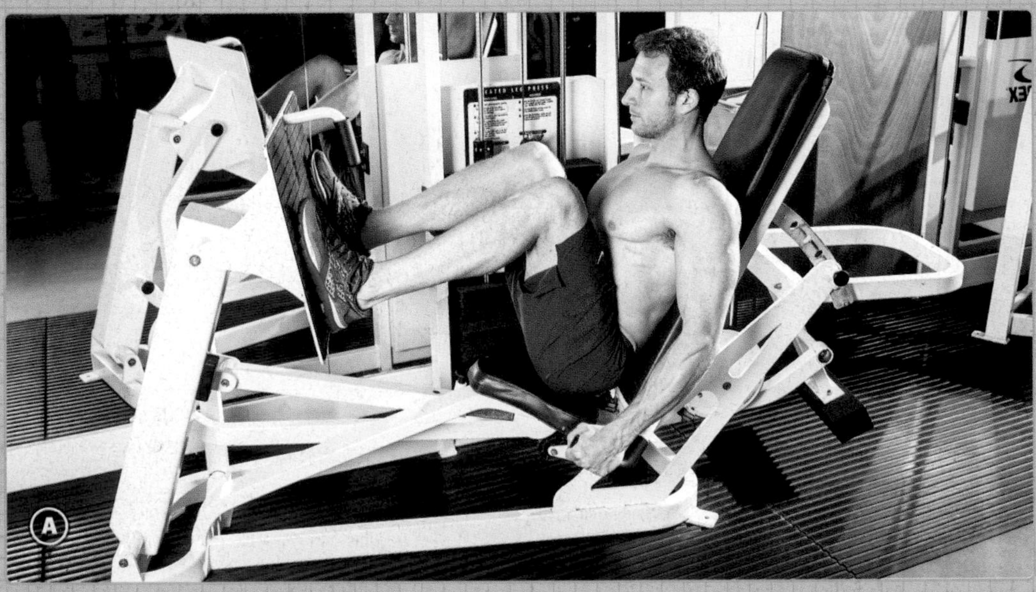

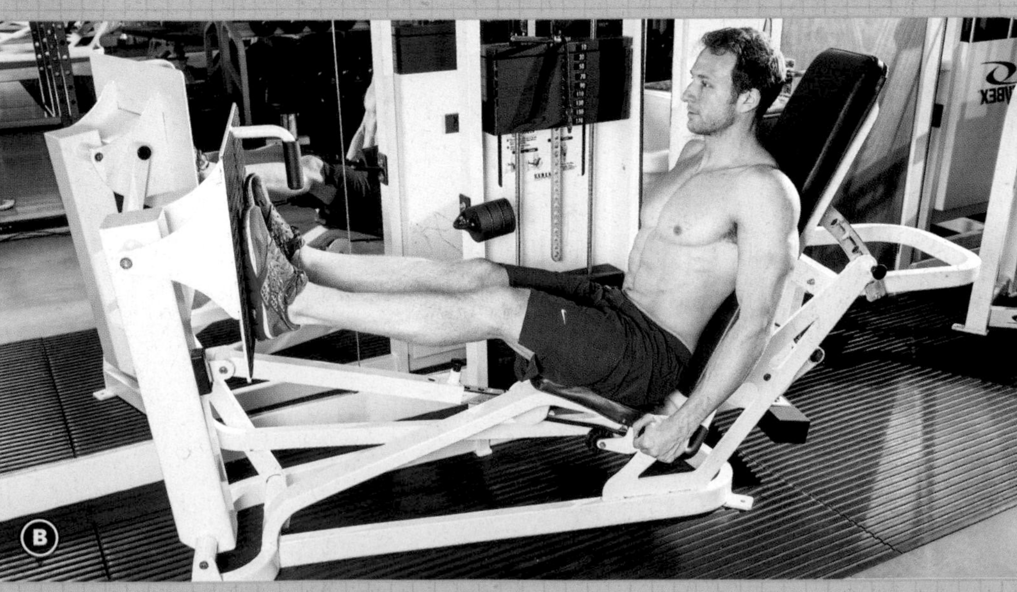

- Sit on the machine, following its instructions to position yourself correctly and safely.
- Release the lock then slowly lower the platform towards you by bending your knees.
- Pause briefly at the bottom, then push through your heels to straighten your legs and return to the start.

Wide-stance leg press

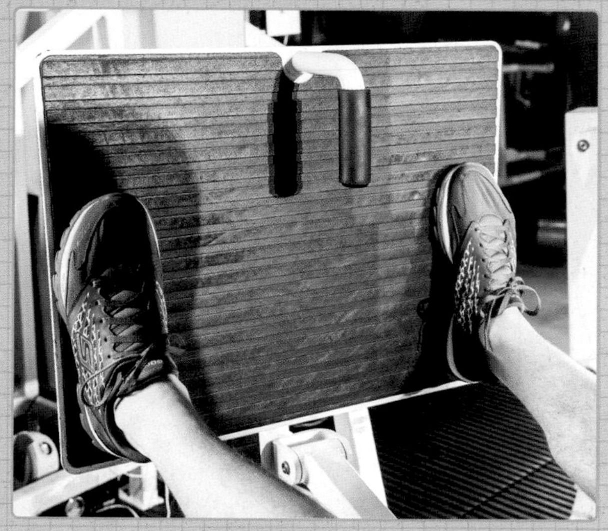

Placing your feet further apart on the platform works your abductors more.

Narrow-stance leg press

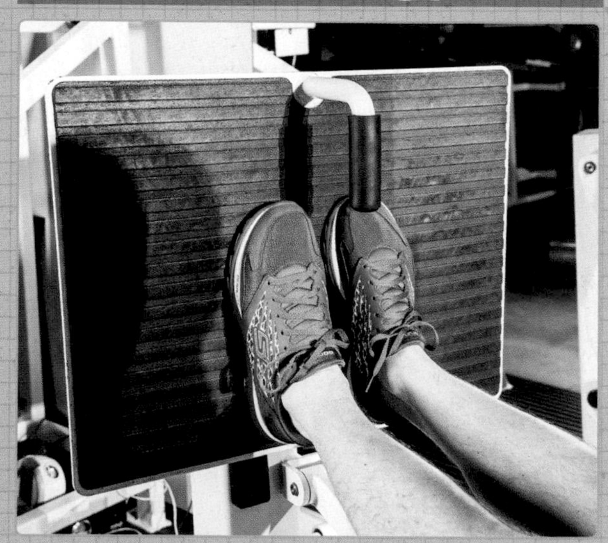

Placing your feet closer together on the platform hits the outer muscles of your quads more.

Leg extension

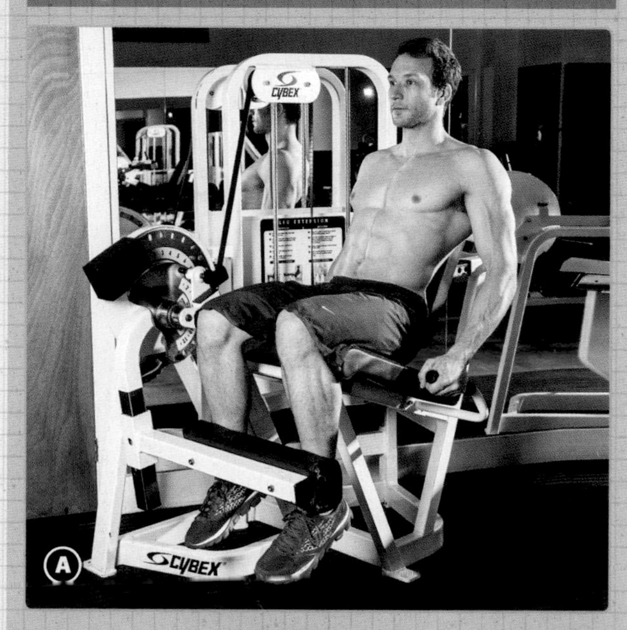

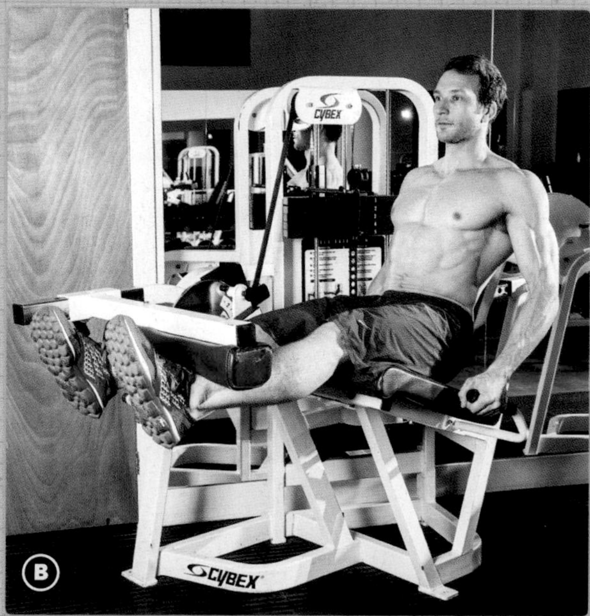

Work your quads in isolation by straightening your legs from a seated position. Just ensure you are positioned correctly to avoid straining your knee joints.

LYING HAMSTRING CURL

Targets *Hamstrings*

Work your hamstrings in isolation with this move that allows you to lift heavy weights safely

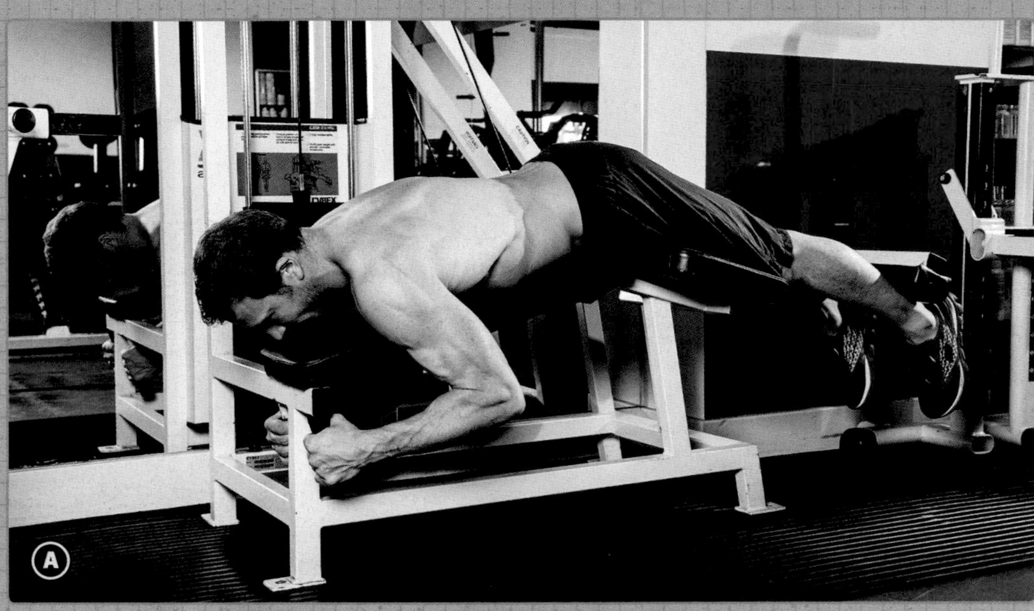
A

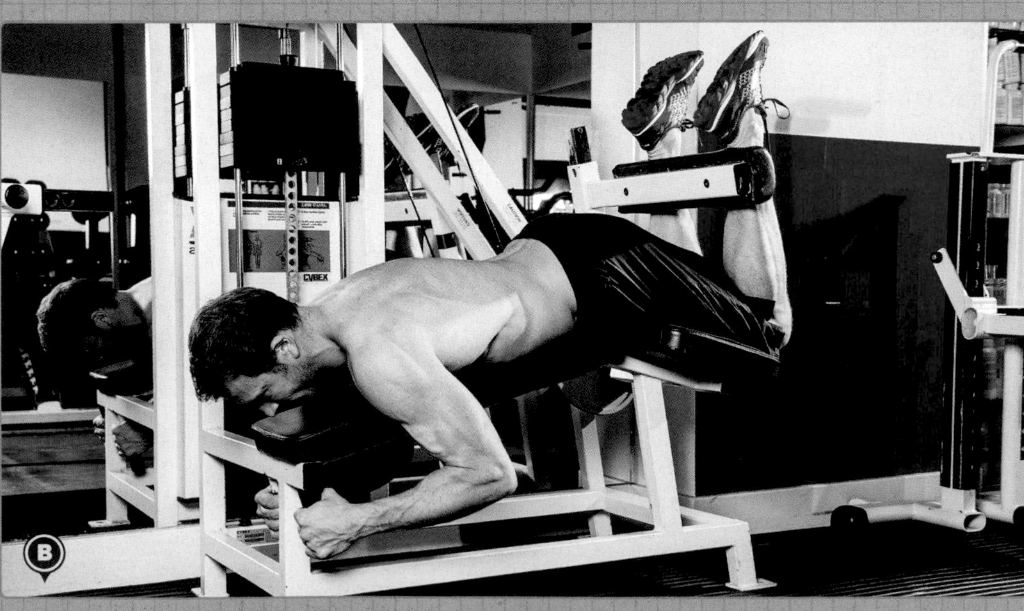
B

- Lie on the machine, following its instructions to position yourself correctly and safely.
- With the pad against the back of your lower calves, raise it up by contracting your hamstrings.
- Return slowly to the start.

Gym ball hamstring curl

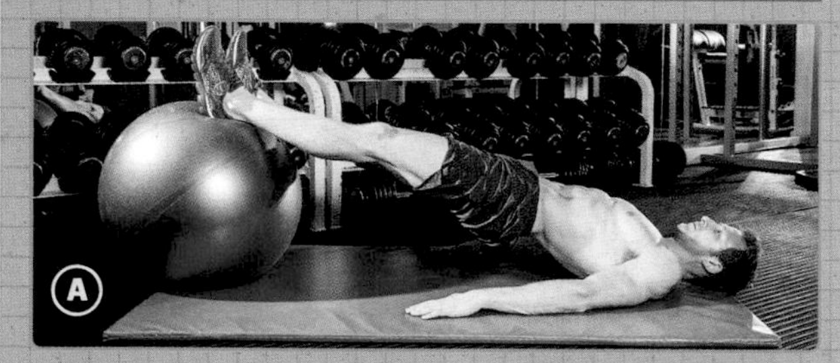

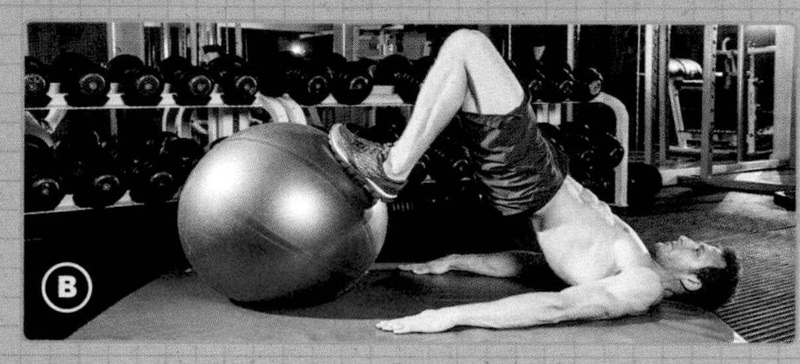

Use your bodyweight to work your hamstrings in this harder-than-it-looks move.

Glute bridge

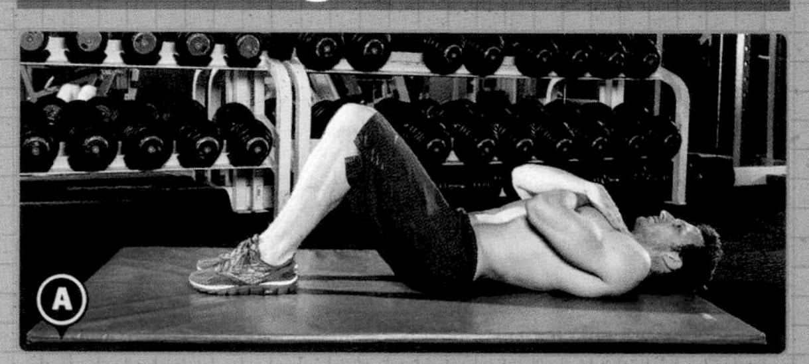

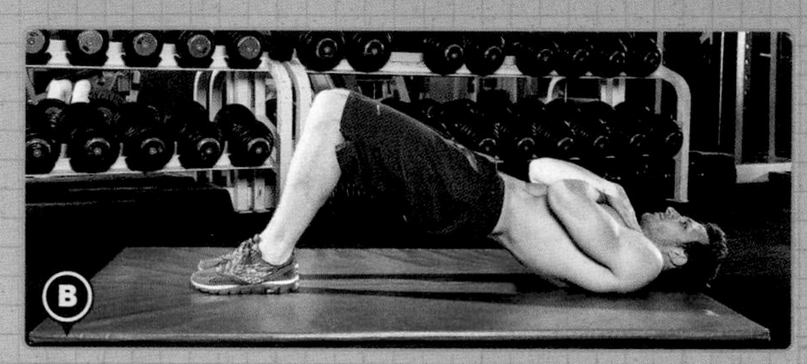

Isolate your all-important glutes with this simple but effective move.

Gym ball glute bridge

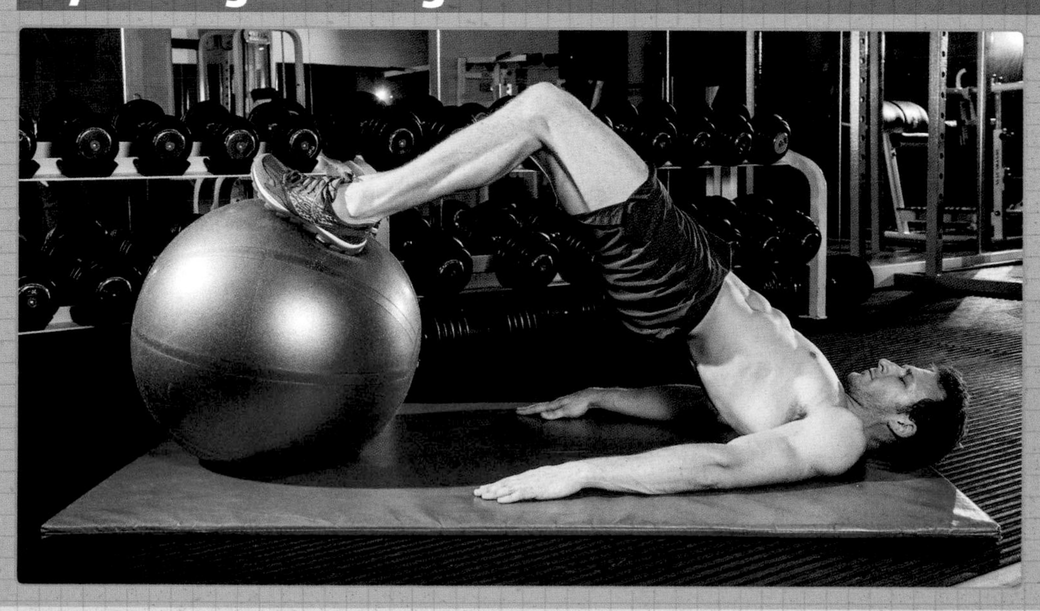

Resting your feet on a gym ball adds instability to the move so your glutes and core have to work harder.

STANDING CALF RAISE

***Targets** Calves*

Your calves are among the hardest-to-grow muscles because they are used to working hard every day. Go heavy with this isolation lift to force them into getting bigger and stronger

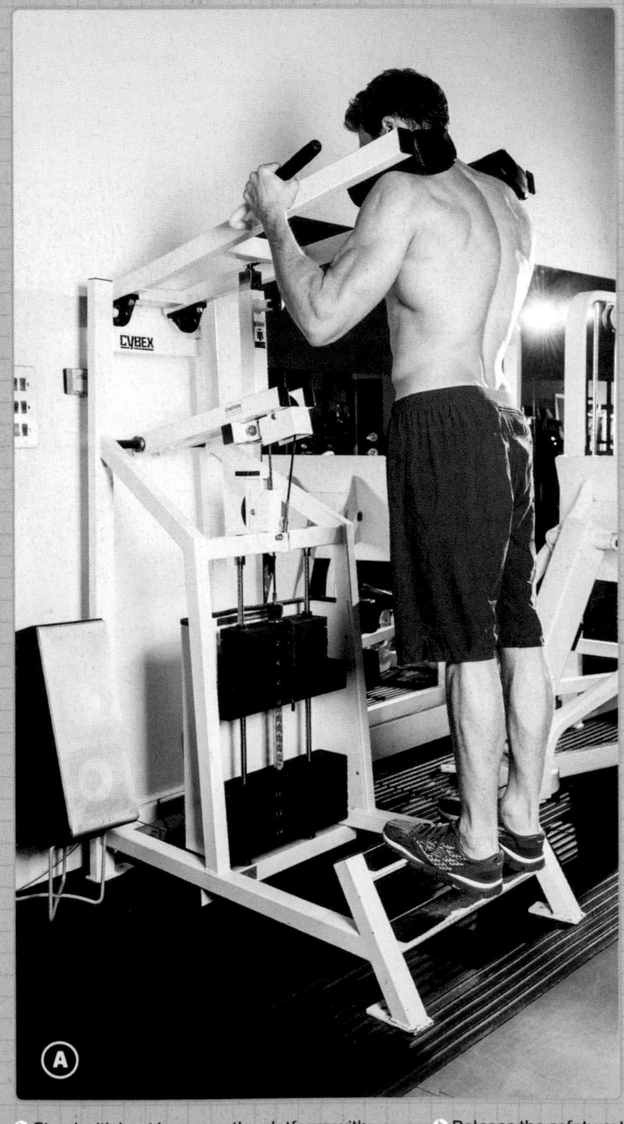

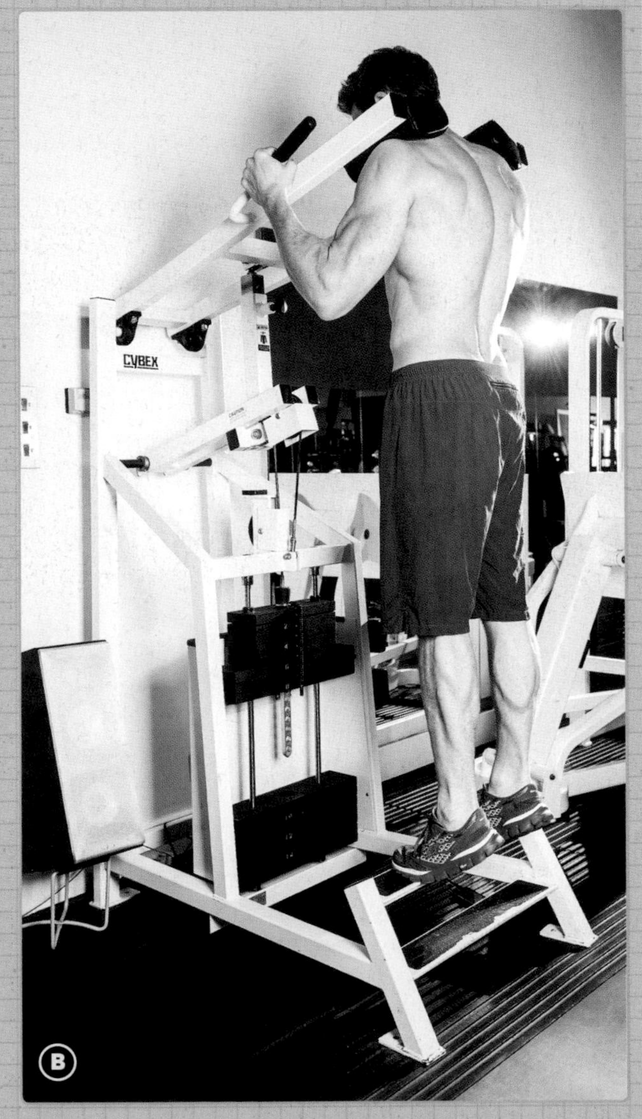

- Stand with bent knees on the platform with the padded bars resting comfortably over each shoulder.
- Release the safety catch and rise on to your tiptoes, keeping your body stable.
- Pause briefly then lower back to the start, ensuring your heel goes below the platform for a full range of motion.

Standing dumbbell calf raise

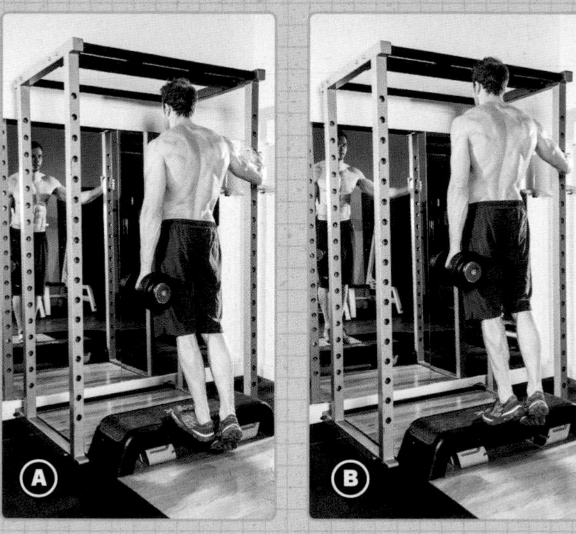

Using a platform and a dumbbell works your calves while recruiting your abs and other stabilising muscles to keep your body balanced.

Supine gym ball calf raise

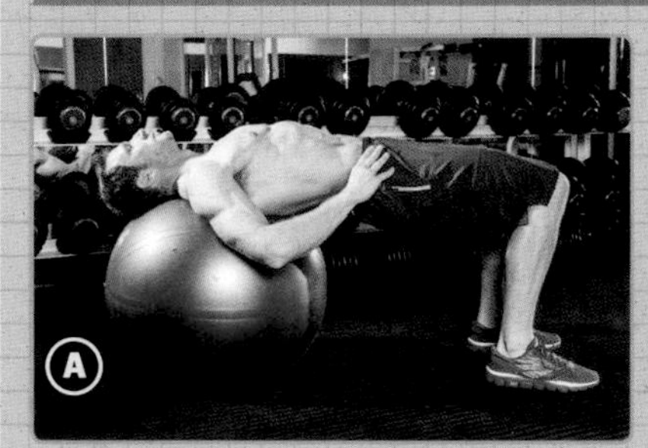

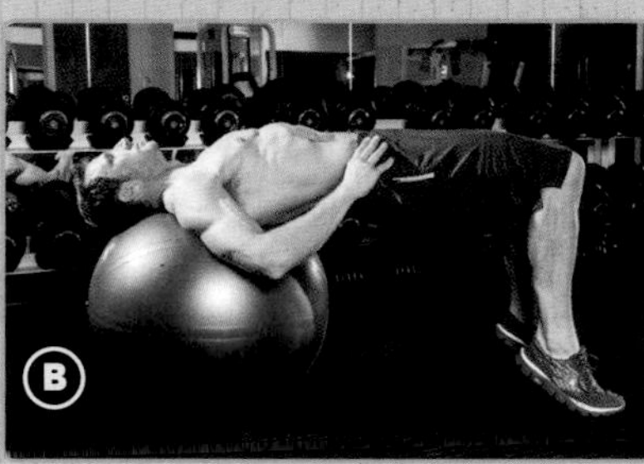

Lying with your upper back supported on a gym ball will work your abs and glutes as well as your calves.

Seated calf raise

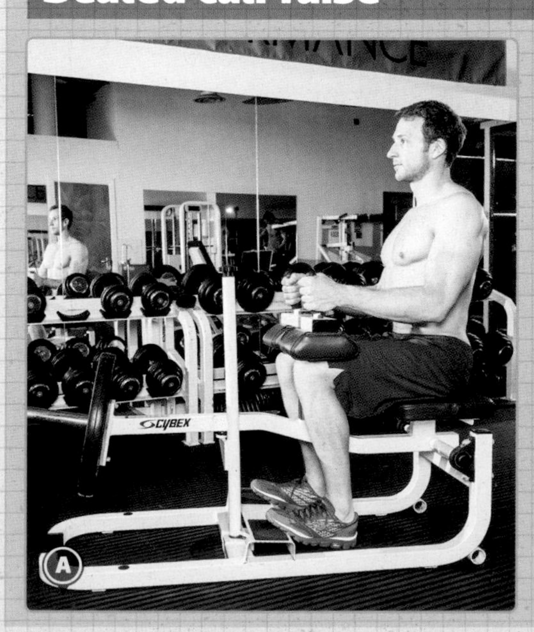

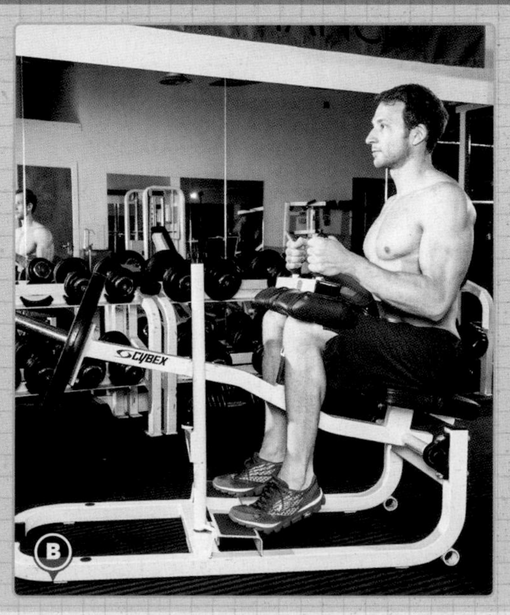

Performing the move whilex sitting down targets the soleus, which forms lower part of the calf muscles.

SHOULDERS

Build big shoulders and create a wide, V-shaped torso

Strong shoulders are essential to improving muscular size and strength across your upper body because the shoulder joint is one of the most complex and delicate in your body. Wide shoulders are also important in building a desirable V-shape torso.

The main shoulder muscles, or deltoids, are made up of three parts: one at the front of the joint, one at the side and one at the back. Inside the joint is a group of four small but crucial stabilising muscles called the rotator cuff.

Weak shoulders will at best limit the amount of weight you can lift in all upper-body moves and at worst result in injury. A weak rotator cuff is a leading reason for shoulder mobility problems and injury, so mastering the right moves performed in a safe and effective matter is vital for making rapid progress, whatever your training goal.

Shoulders explained

Here's how your shoulder muscles work

- The anterior deltoids, or front delts, are responsible mainly for moving your arms up and in front of your body. They also assist the chest muscles in pressing actions.
- The lateral deltoids, or side delts, are responsible mainly for moving your arms up and out to the side of your body.
- The posterior deltoids, or rear delts, are responsible mainly for moving your arms away from the chest laterally. They also work closely with the major muscles of the upper back.
- The rotator cuff is a group of four small muscles that support and stabilise the shoulder joint.

The shoulder muscles

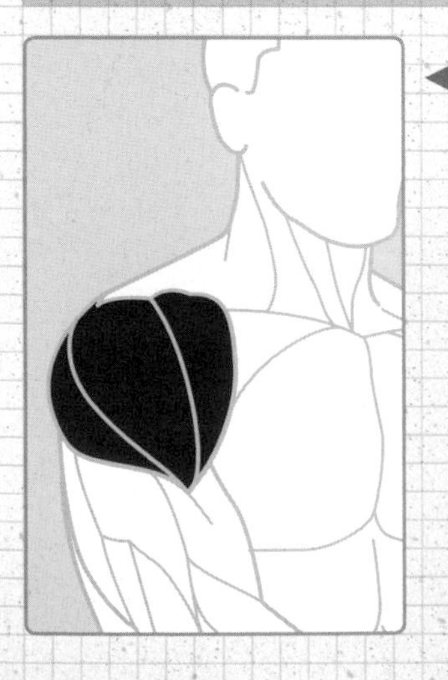

The anterior and lateral deltoids work to lift your arms out in front of you and to the side respectively.

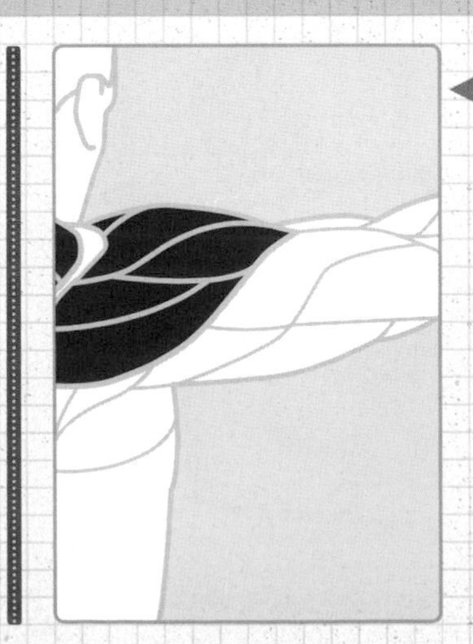

The posterior delts work with the major muscles of your upper back to move your arms.

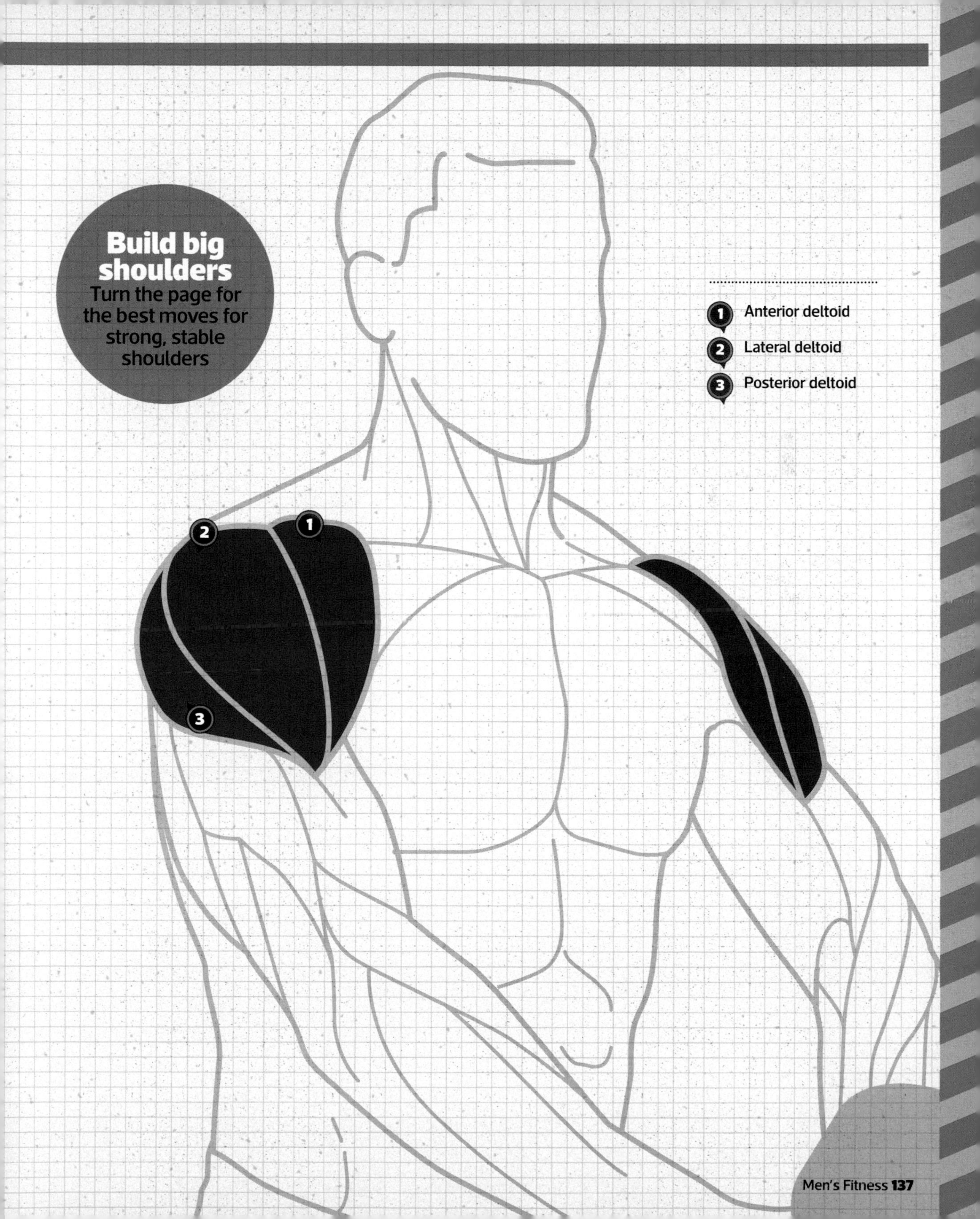
Build big shoulders
Turn the page for the best moves for strong, stable shoulders
1 Anterior deltoid
2 Lateral deltoid
3 Posterior deltoid
1
2
3

SHOULDER PRESS

***Target:* Deltoids, triceps**

The best muscle-building move to craft strong, wide and impressive shoulders

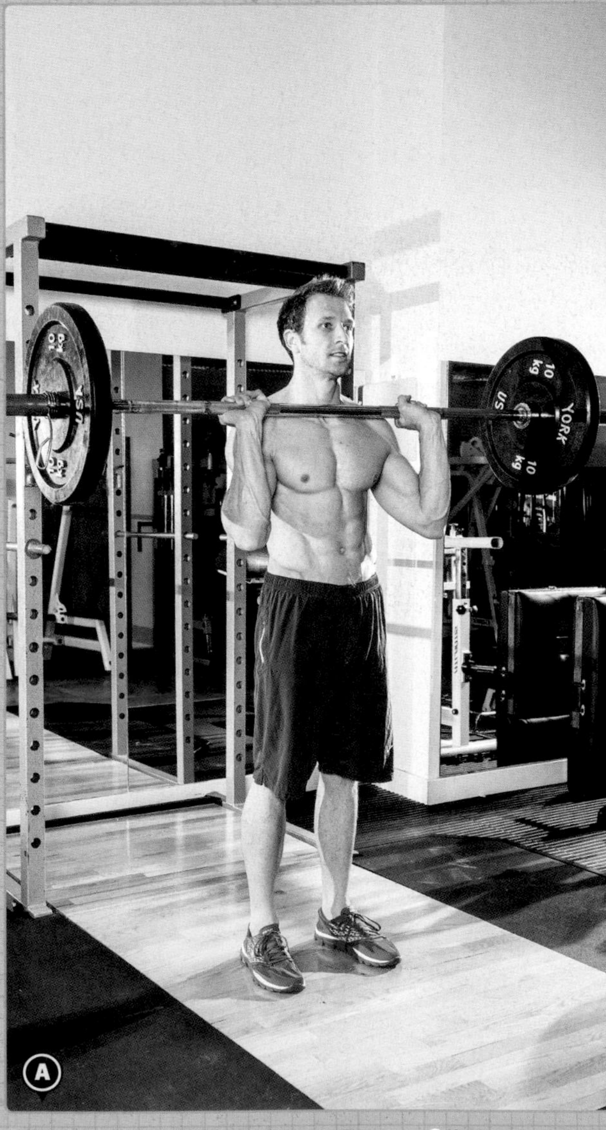

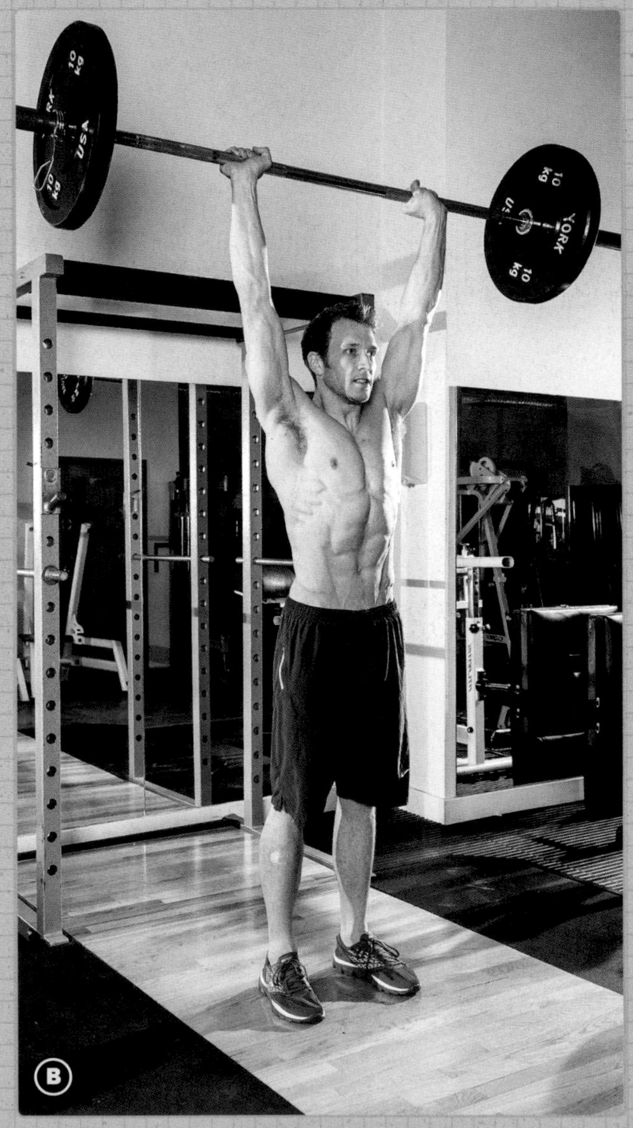

- With your feet shoulder-width apart, position a bar on your upper chest, gripping it with hands just wider than shoulder-width apart.
- Keeping your chest upright and your core muscles braced, press the bar directly upwards until your arms are extended overhead. Take care not to tilt your hips forwards.
- Lower the bar back down to your chest and repeat.

Seated behind-the-neck press

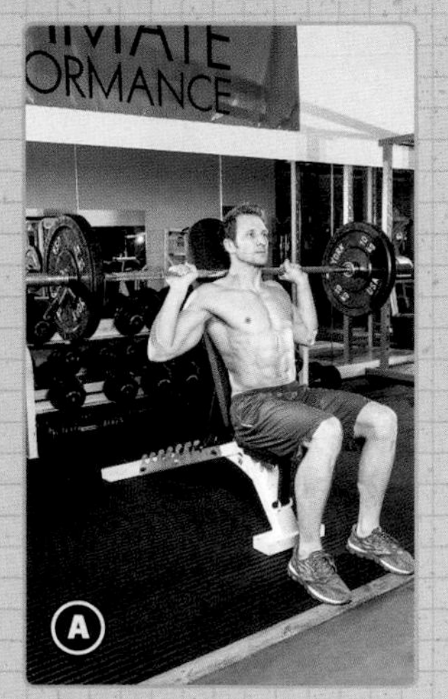

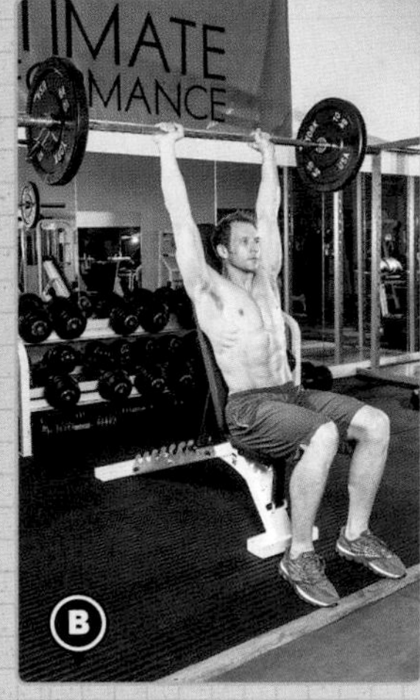

Pressing the bar up and down from behind your head hits the target muscles from a different angle.

Inverted shoulder press

This tough bodyweight move is a great way to build your shoulders outside of the gym.

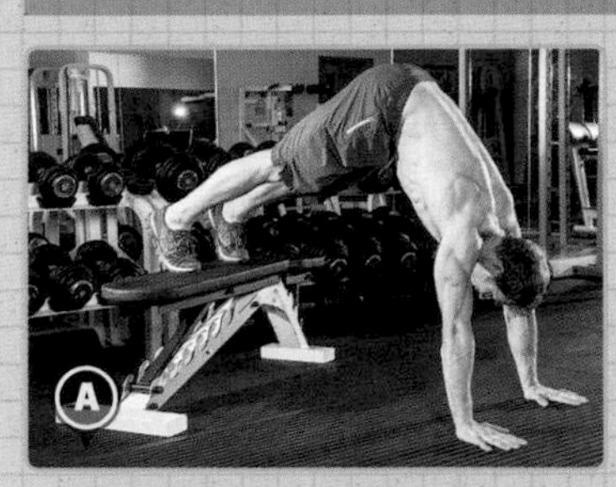

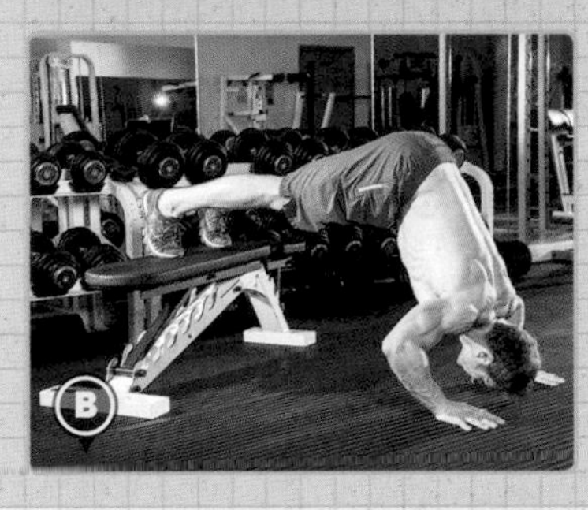

Seated shoulder press

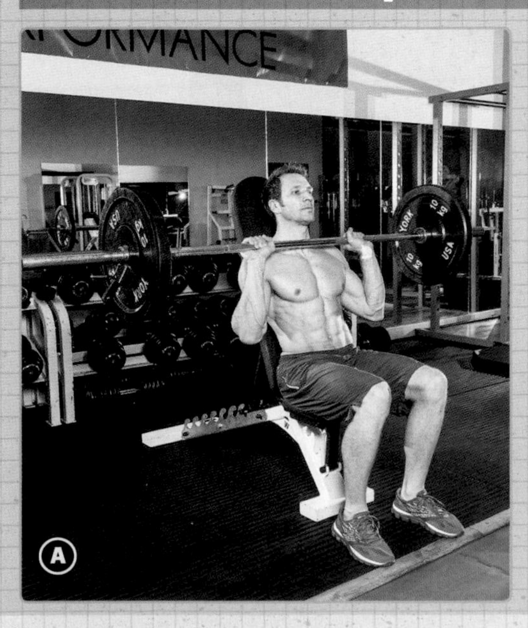

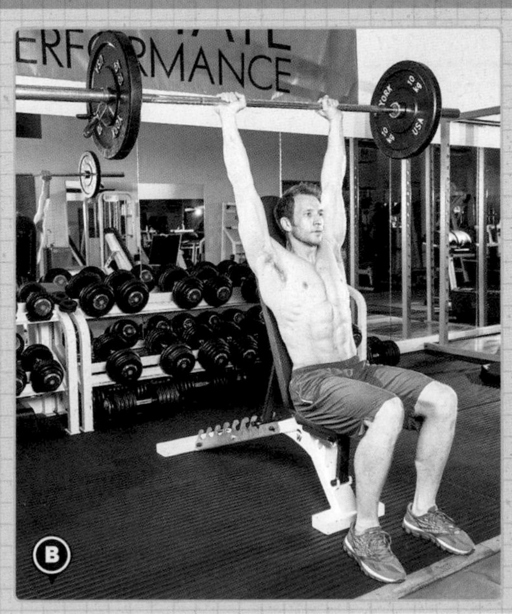

Sitting down stabilises your body so you can hit your shoulders harder.

DUMBBELL SHOULDER PRESS

***Target:** Deltoids, triceps*

Using dumbbells works each arm and shoulder joint independently for balanced gains, recruits your core for balance and allows you to press up the weights in a more natural arc

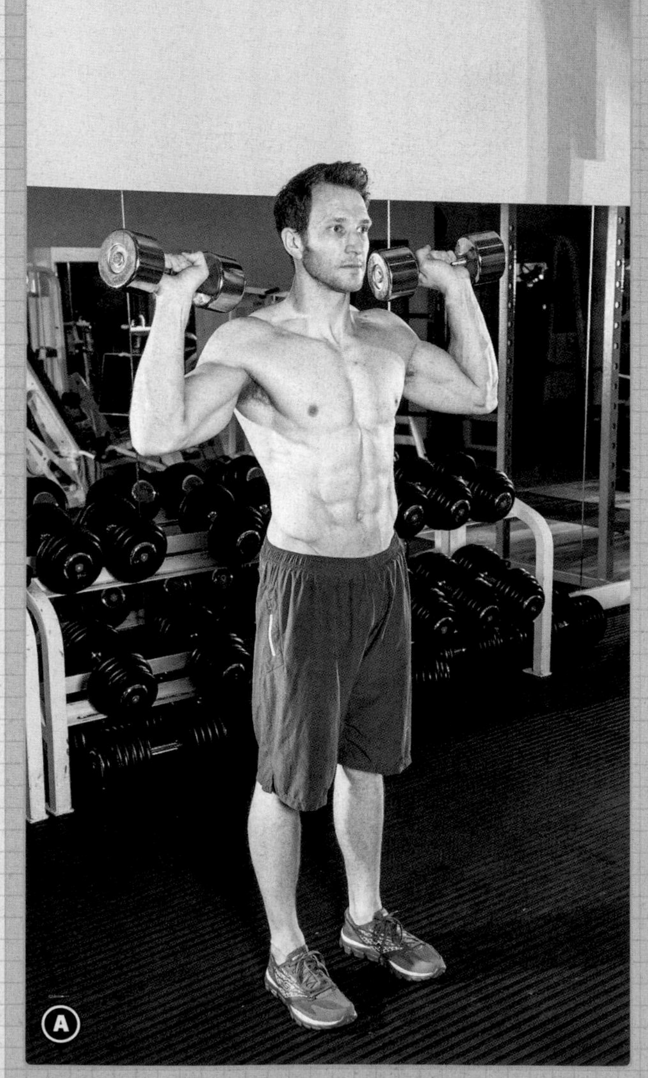

- With your feet shoulder-width apart, hold a dumbbell in each hand at shoulder height.
- Keep your chest upright and your core muscles braced.

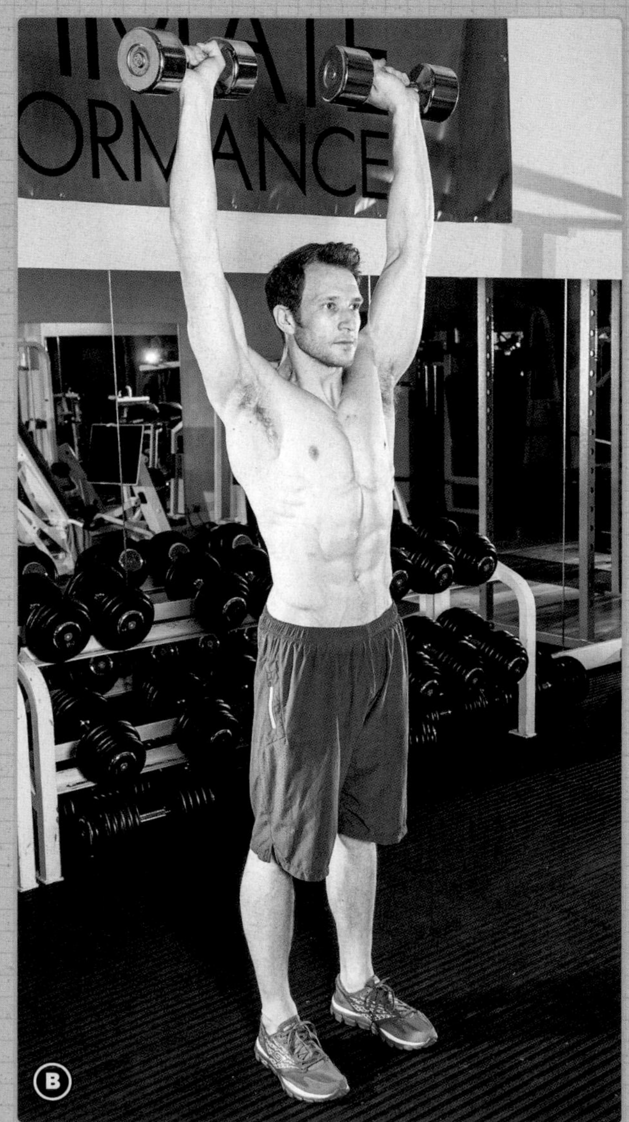

- Press the weights directly upwards, keeping your core braced, until your arms are extended overhead.
- Lower the weights back down to your shoulders.

Seated shoulder press

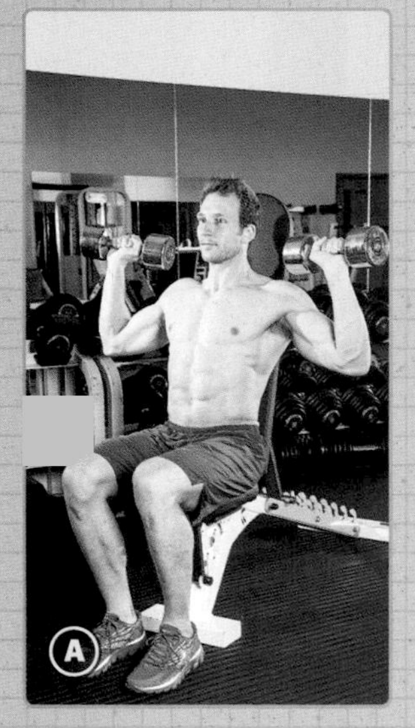

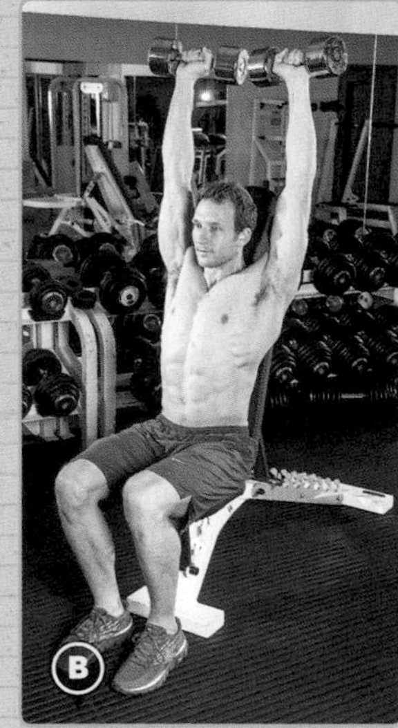

Sitting down stabilises your upper body so you are able to lift more.

Neutral shoulder press

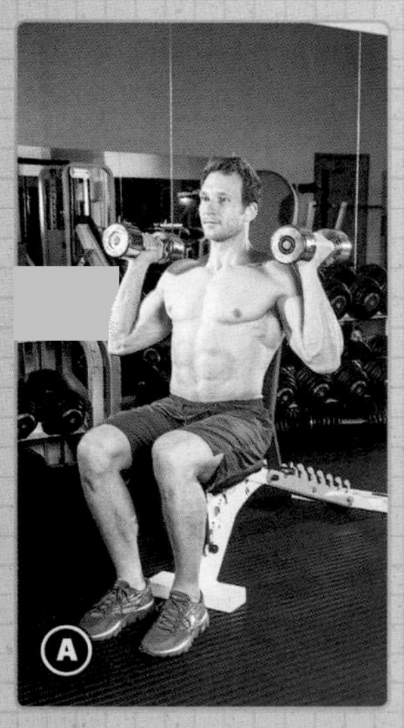

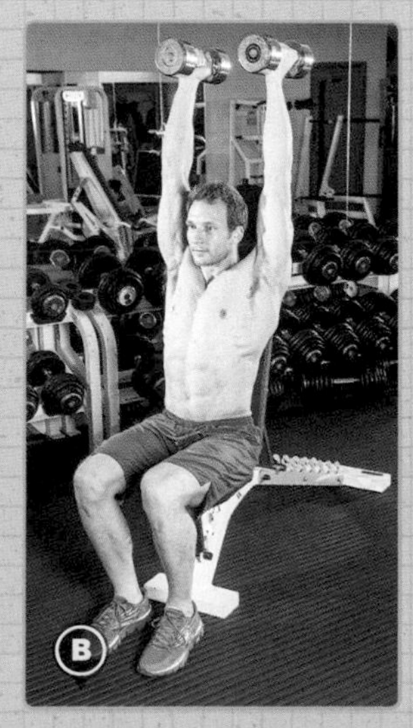

A palms-facing grip makes the move easier for those with poor shoulder flexibility, while also recruiting your chest muscles.

Arnold press

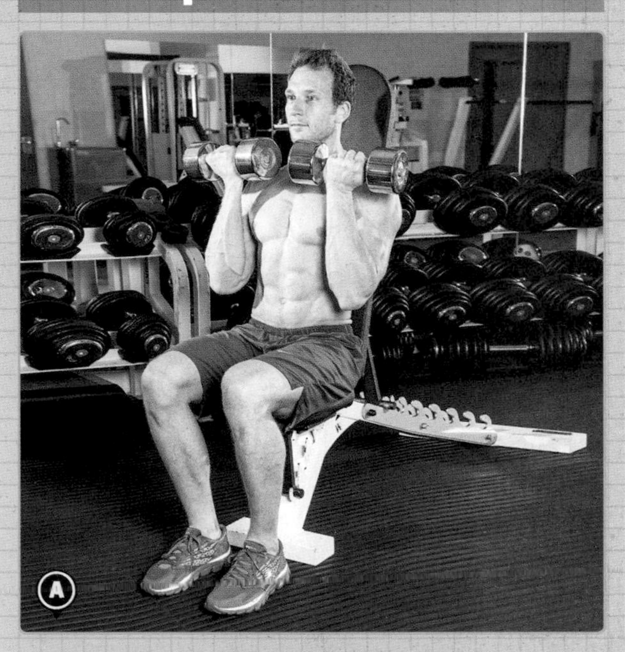

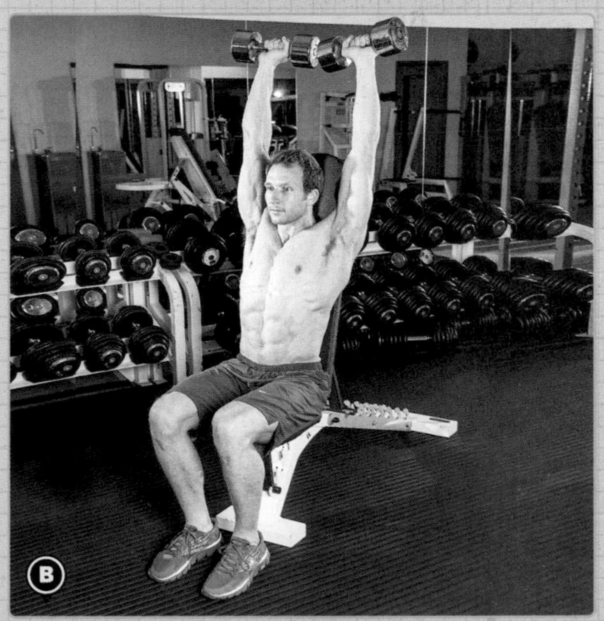

This combines a pressing motion with a rotational one – you rotate your palms from facing you at the start to facing away at the top – and therefore hits your deltoids from different angles.

ALTERNATING DUMBBELL PRESS

***Target:* Deltoids**

Work each arm independently for balanced gains

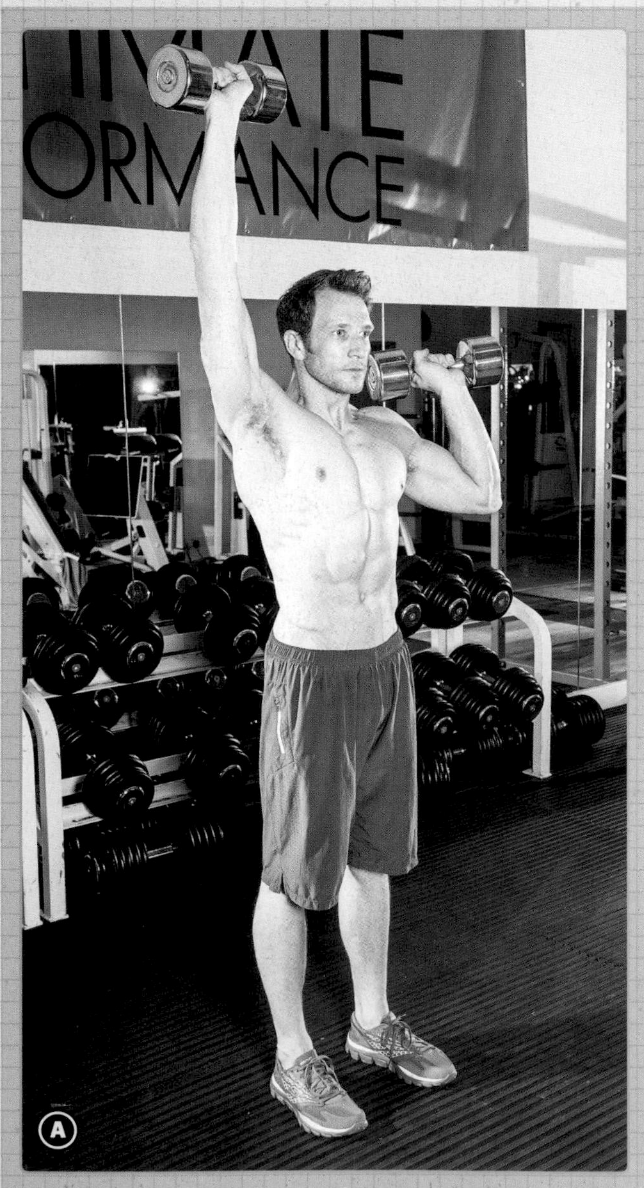

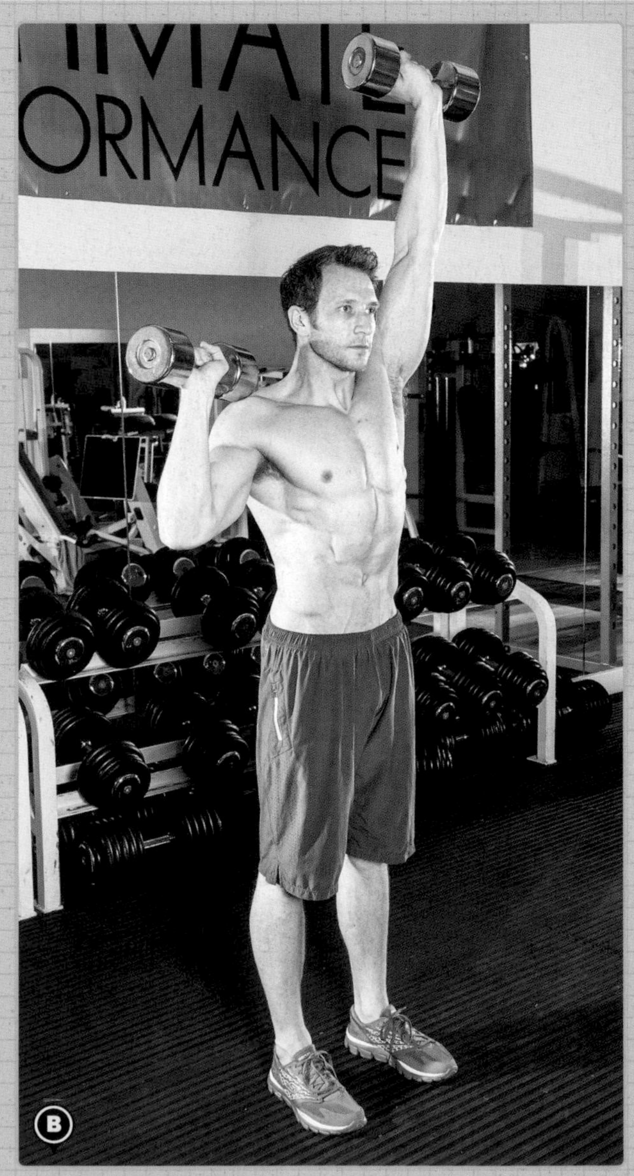

- With your feet shoulder-width apart, hold a dumbbell in each hand at shoulder height.
- Keep your chest upright and your core muscles braced.
- Press one weight directly upwards, keeping your core braced, until your arm is extended overhead.
- Lower it back down and repeat with the other arm.

Alternating wide dumbbell shoulder press

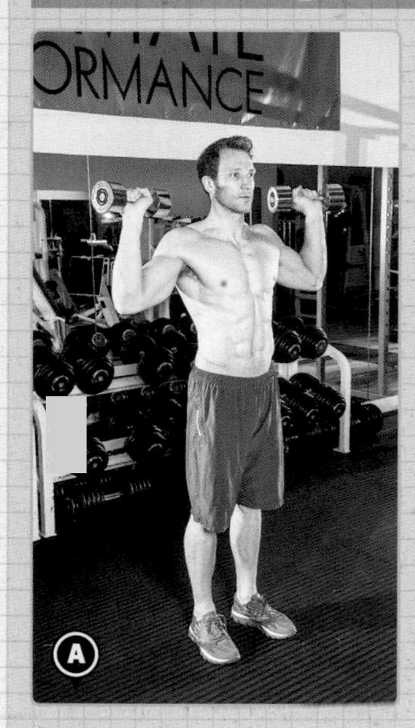

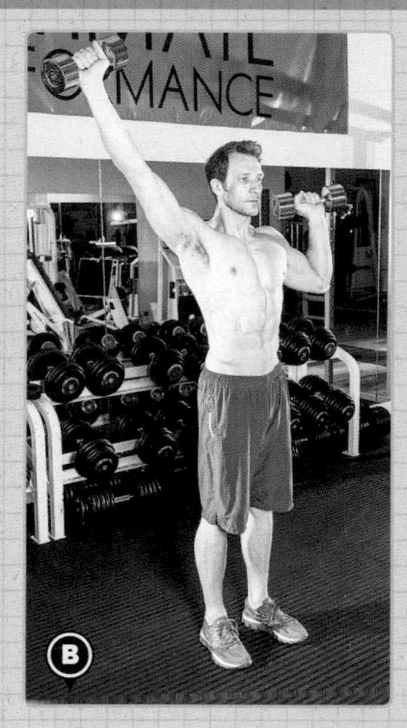

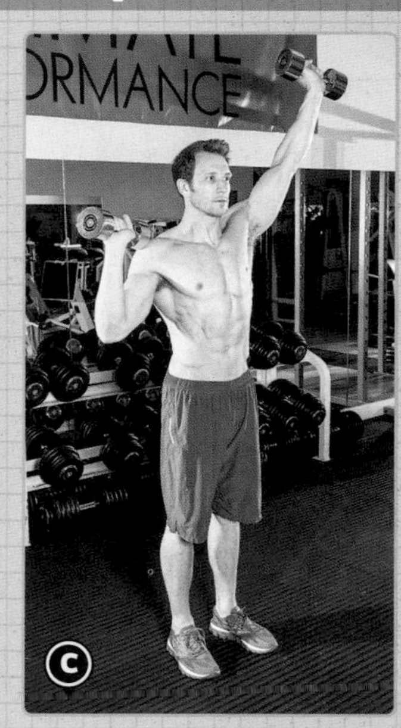

Raising your arm upwards and out to the side hits your deltoids from a new angle for increased gains.

Single-arm dumbbell press

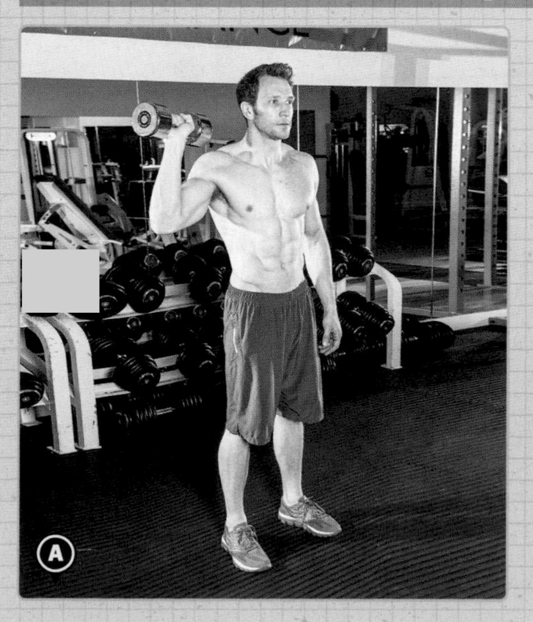

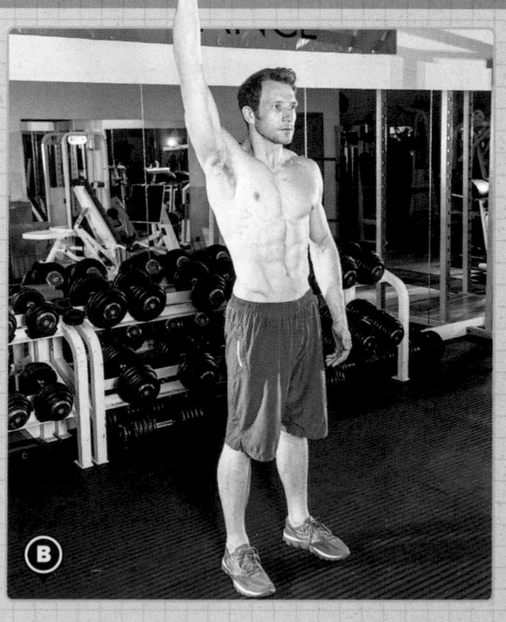

Holding and lifting only one weight at a time is a great way to improve shoulder strength and stamina.

LATERAL RAISE

***Target:* Middle deltoids**

Isolate your middle deltoid muscle with this single-joint move that will add size to your shoulders

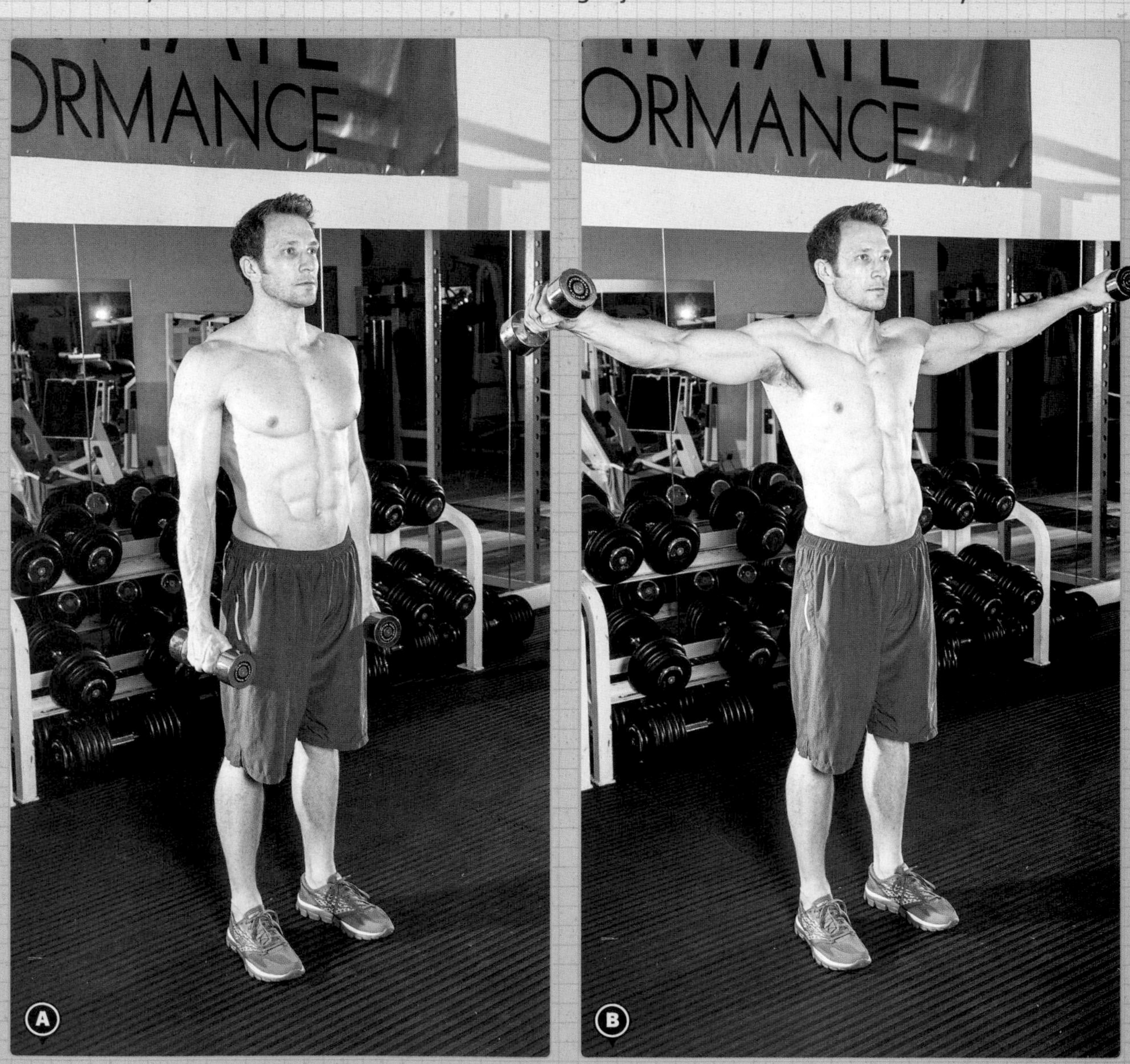

- Stand tall with your core braced and feet apart, holding a light dumbbell in each hand by your sides with your palms facing your body.
- Keeping a slight bend in your elbows, lift the weights out to the sides using your muscles and not momentum.
- Stop at shoulder height, pause for a second, then slowly return to the start.

Front raise

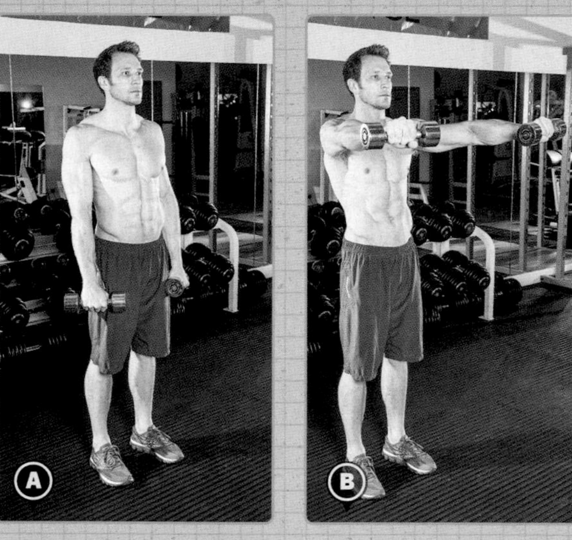

Lifting your arms out to the front will work the front deltoids.

Alternating raise

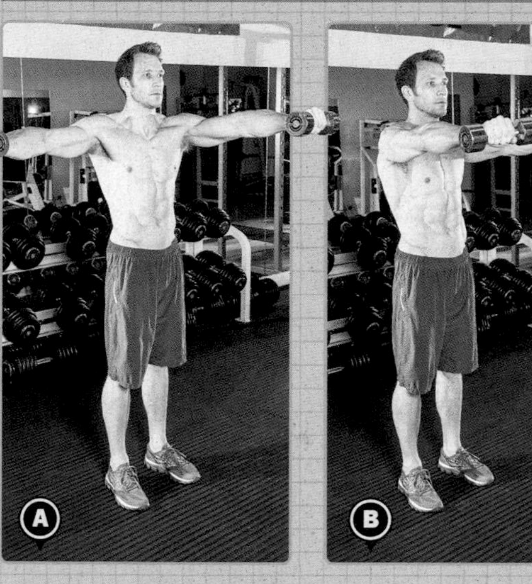

You can work both the front and middle deltoids by alternating front and lateral raises.

Cable lateral raise

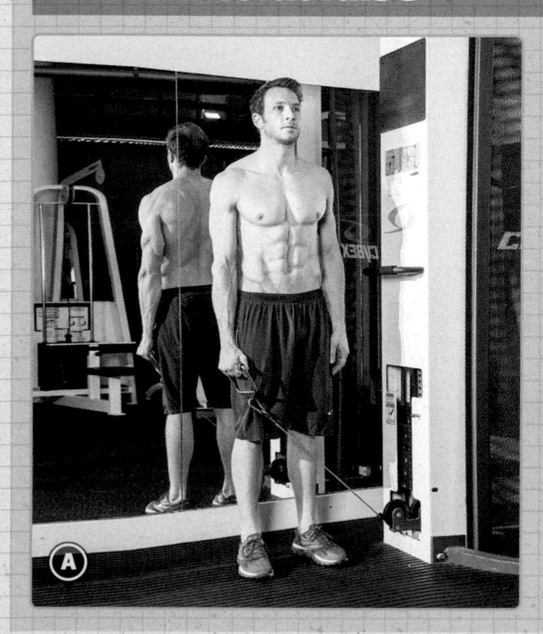

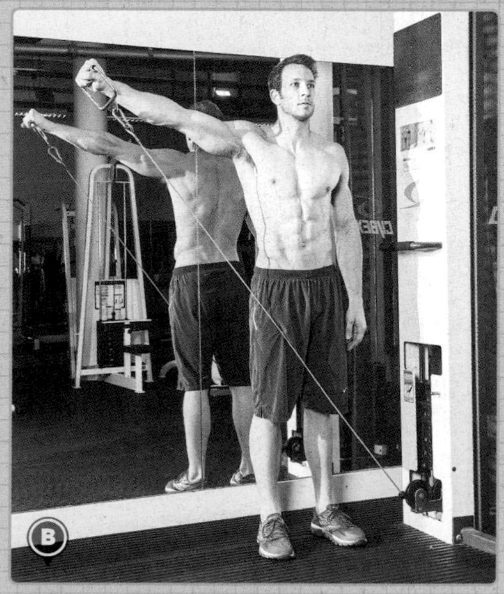

Using a cable places resistance on the target muscles throughout the move.

INCLINE REVERSE LATERAL RAISE

***Target:** Rear deltoids*

Hit the hard-to-target back shoulder muscles with this isolation lift

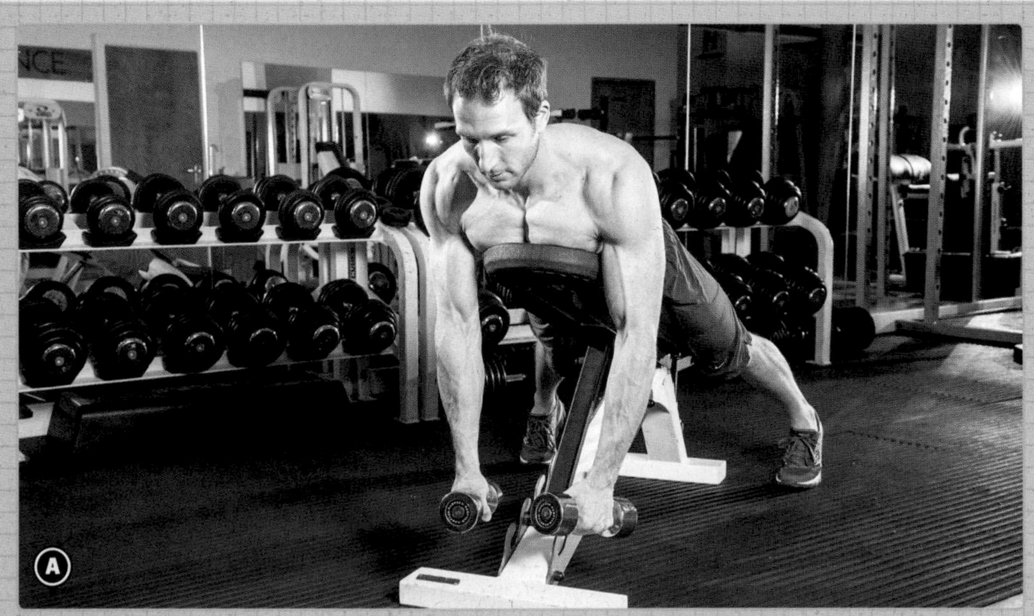

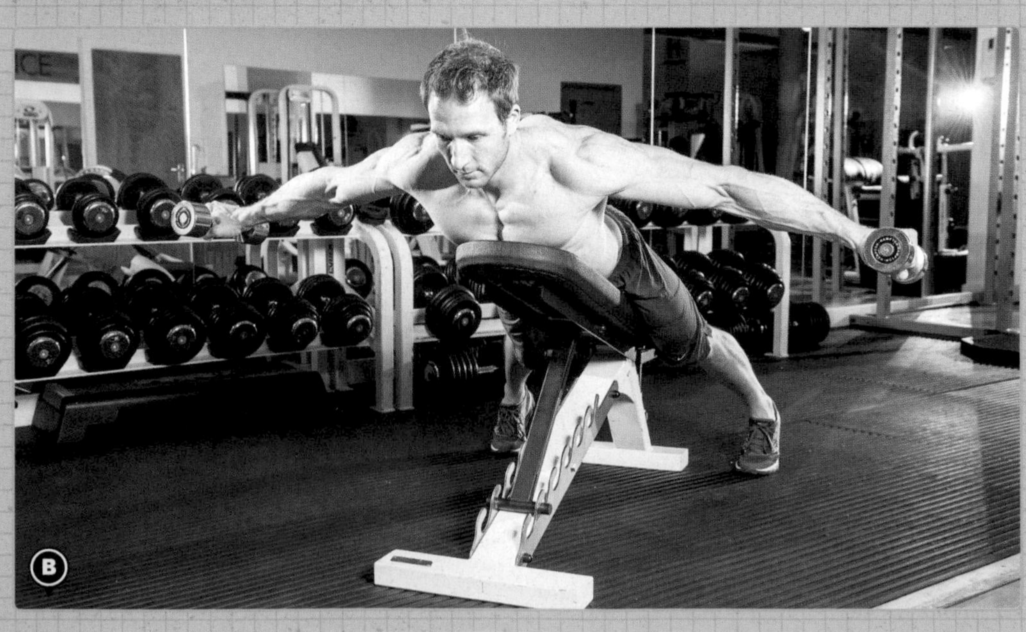

- Lie chest-down on an incline bench holding a dumbbell in each hand.
- Keeping a slight bend in your elbows, lift the weights out to your sides until they reach shoulder height.
- Return to the start.

Lying reverse lateral raise

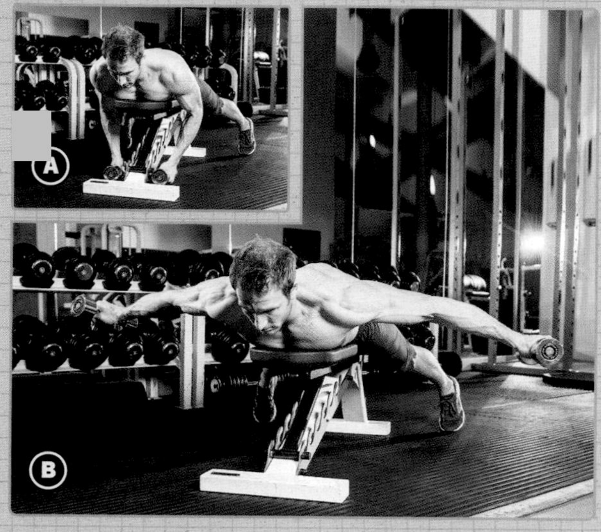

Lie on a flat bench to change the focus of the angle on your rear delts and bring in your upper back muscles.

Low-to-high cable raise

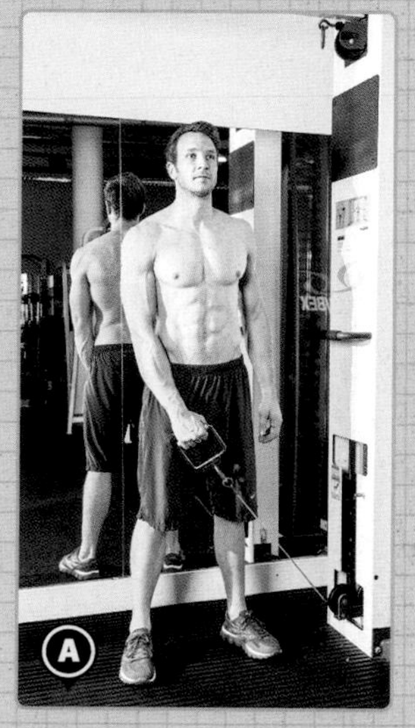

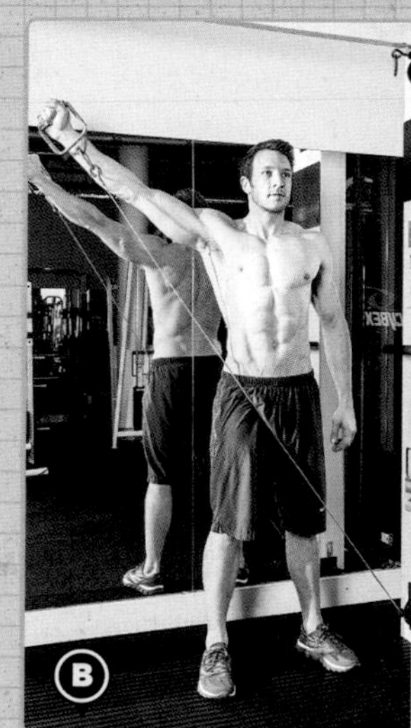

Work your muscles harder with the constant resistance of the cable.

High cable reverse flye

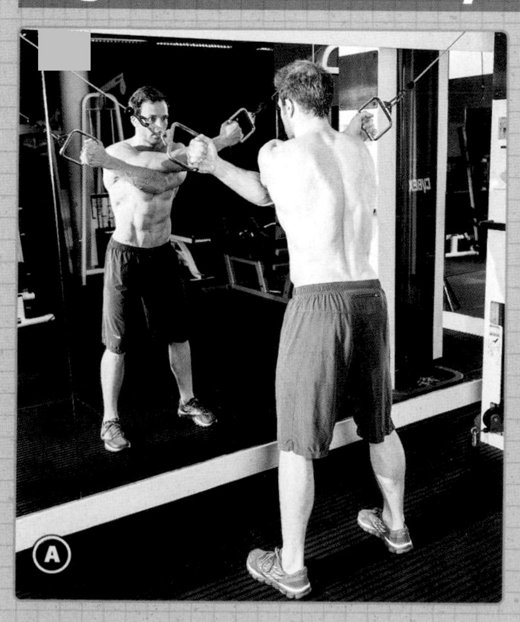

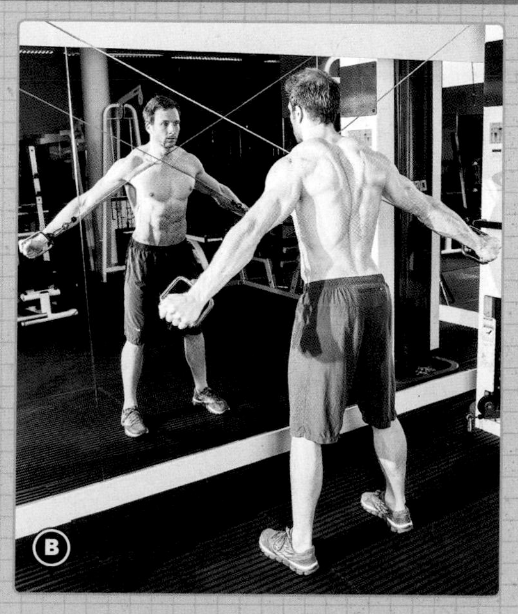

Work the target muscles and your upper back with this complex and effective cable move.

HIGH PULL

***Target:* Deltoids, traps**

Hit your shoulders and traps with this explosive lift that fires up your fast-twitch muscle fibres

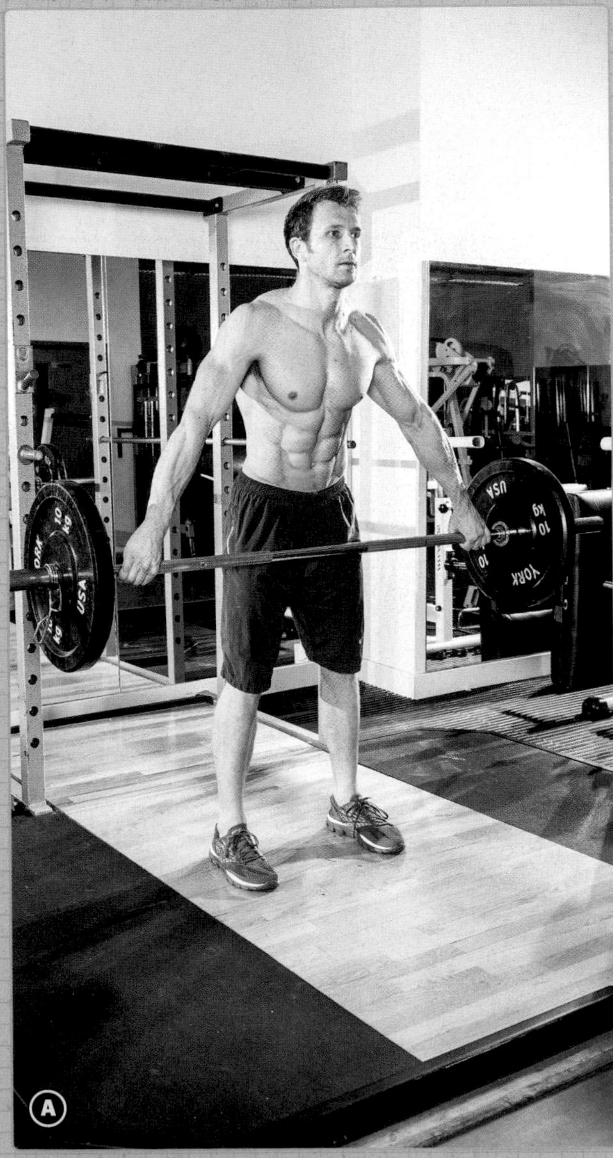

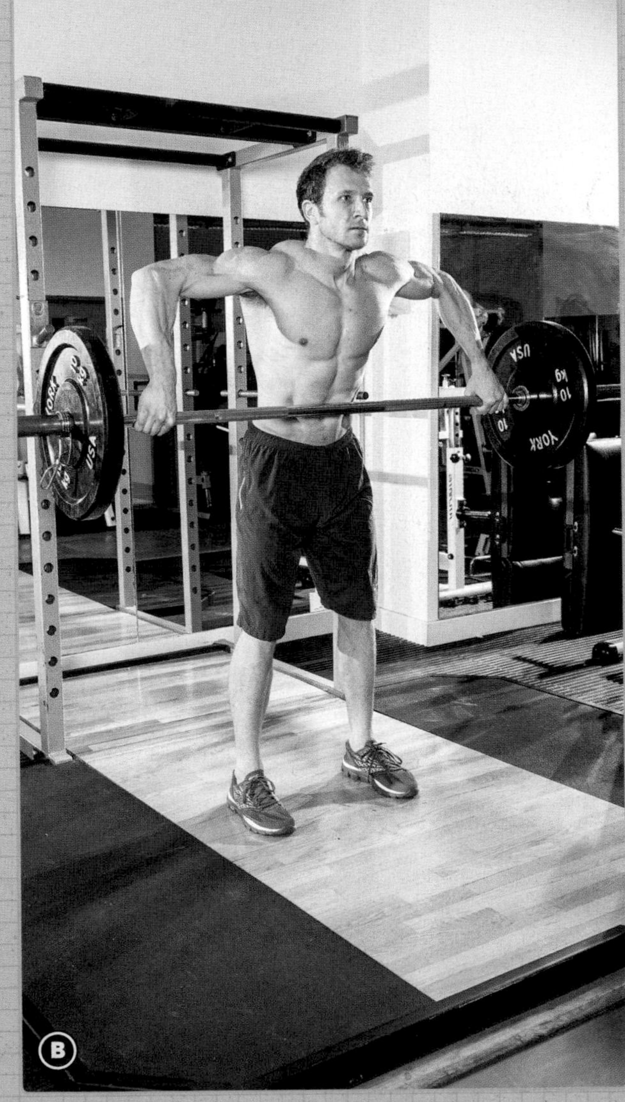

- Stand tall, holding a barbell with an overhand grip with your hands double shoulder-width apart.
- Squat slightly then straighten up, push your hips forwards and lift the bar to mid-chest height, leading with your elbows pointing to the ceiling.
- Lower the bar back to the start.

EZ-bar upright row

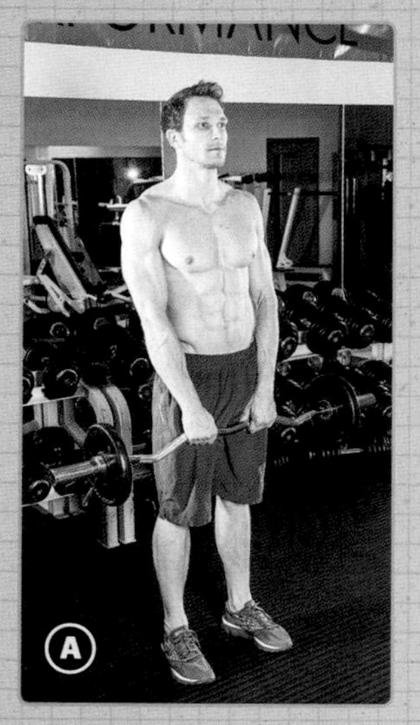

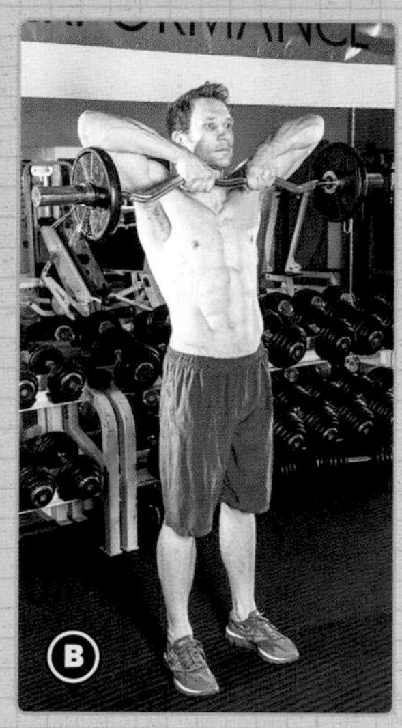

The shape of the EZ-bar reduces the strain on your joints and allows you to lift the weight to your chin.

Dumbbell upright row

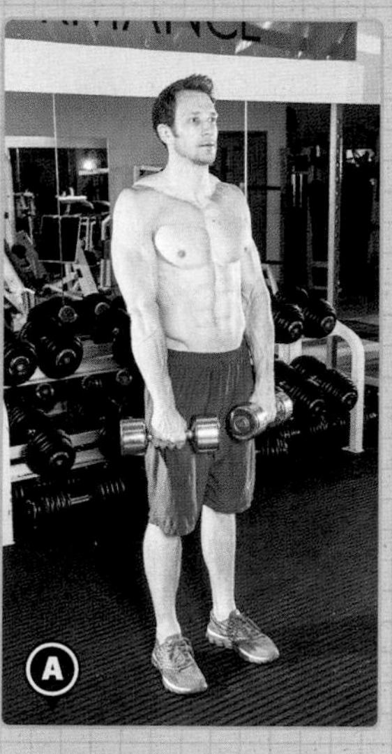

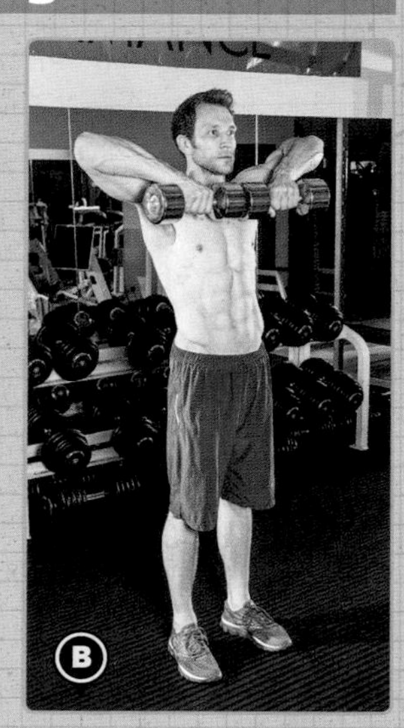

Using dumbbells works each side of your body individually to prevent your stronger side dominating.

Incline reverse bench shrug

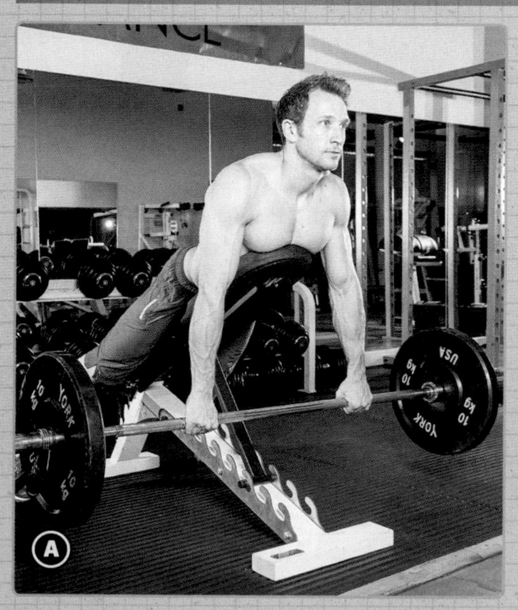

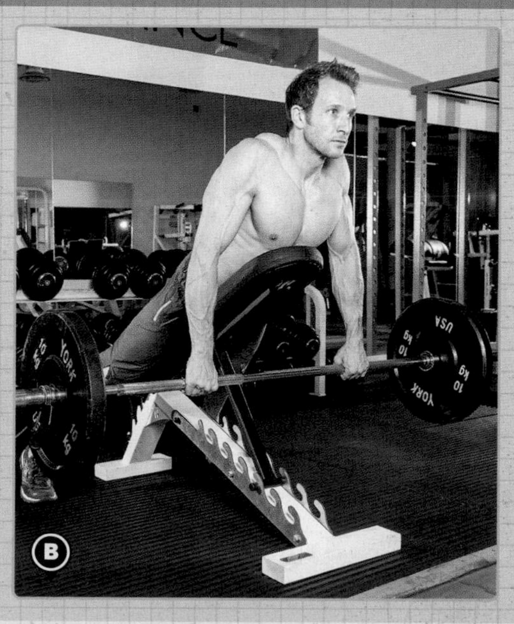

The stability of the bench and limited range of motion make it easier to lift heavier weights to shock your muscles into growth.

BARBELL CUBAN PRESS

***Target:* Rotator cuffs**

This move works the small muscles of the shoulder joint that control rotational movement. A strong rotator cuff prevents injury and allows you to lift more in most upper-body moves

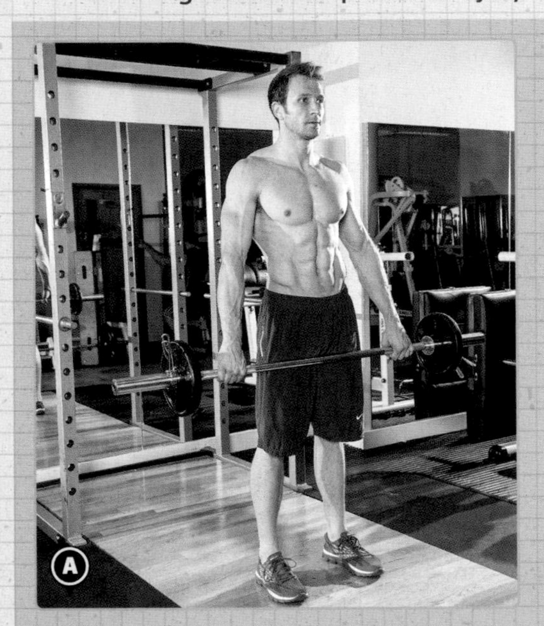

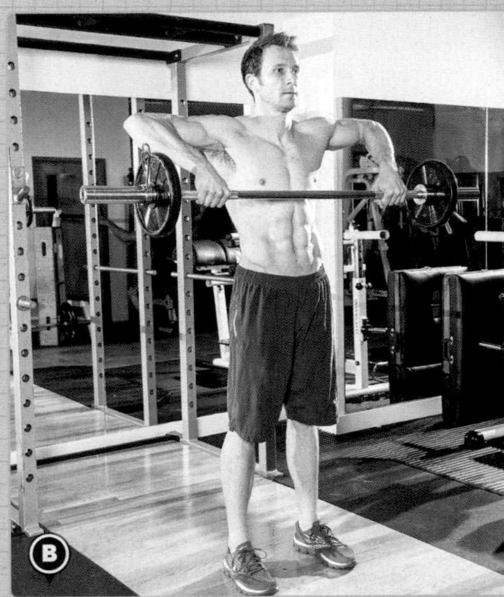

- Stand tall, holding a barbell with an overhand grip with your hands just outside your thighs.
- Lift the weight until your elbows are bent at 90°.
- Rotate your shoulders until your forearms are pointing to the ceiling, then press the weight up until your arms are straight.
- Reverse the movement to return to the start.

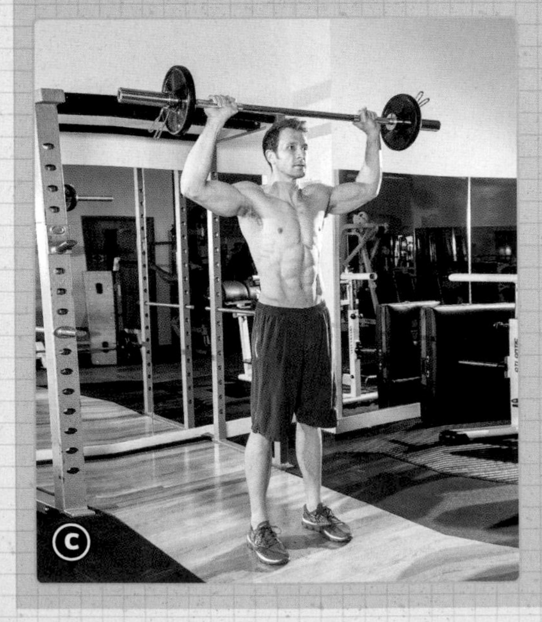

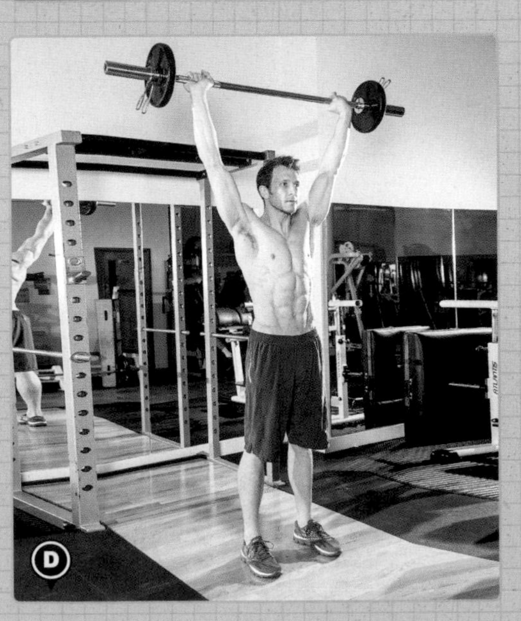

Dumbbell Cuban press

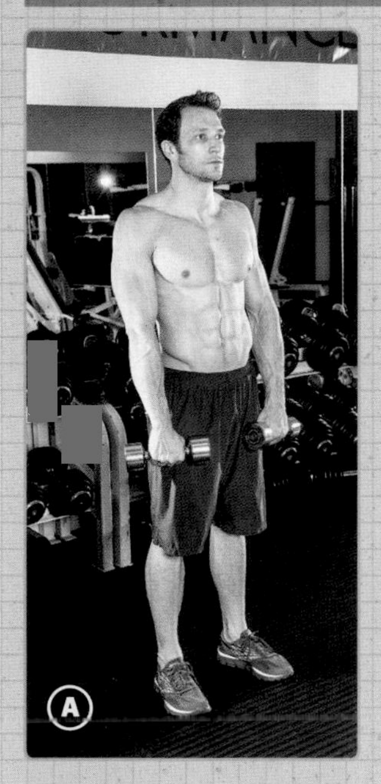

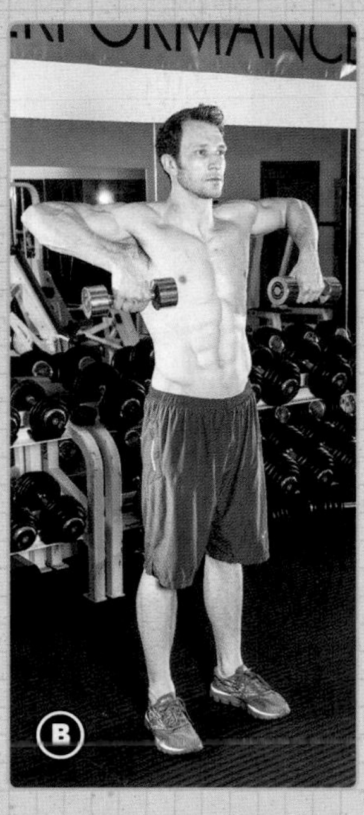

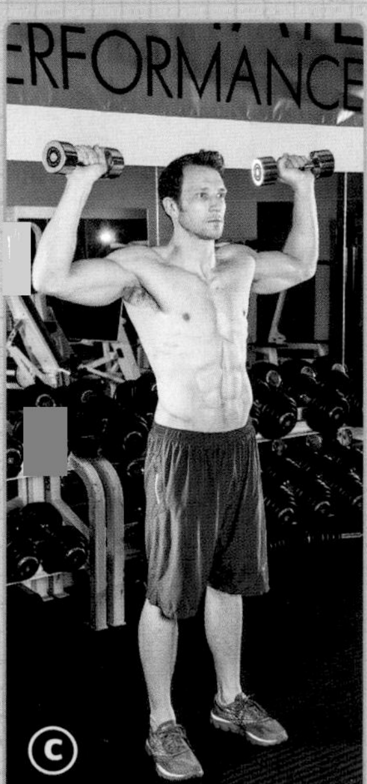

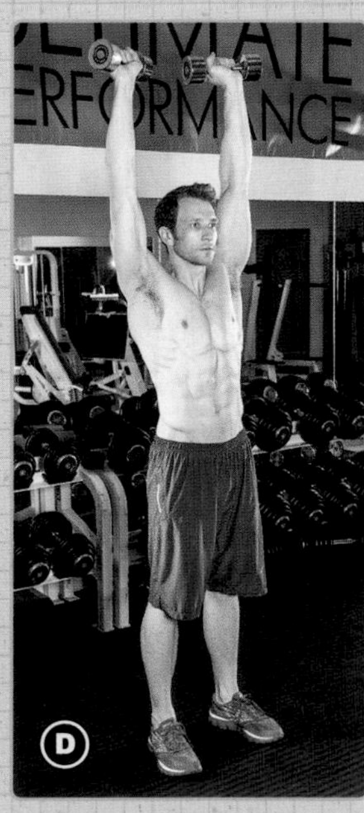

Using dumbells for this move will ensure both shoulder joints are worked independently for balanced strength and stability.

Incline Cuban press

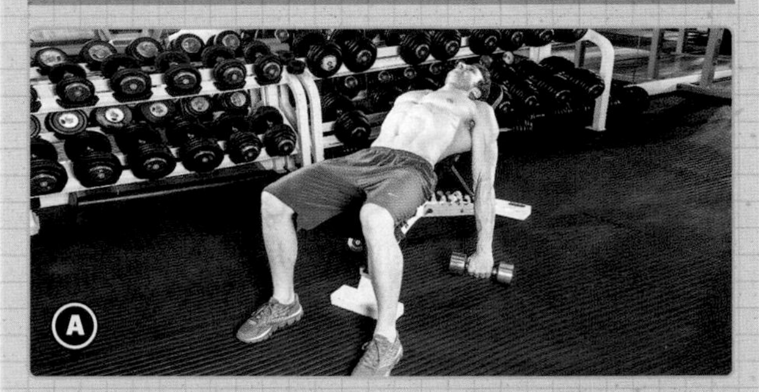

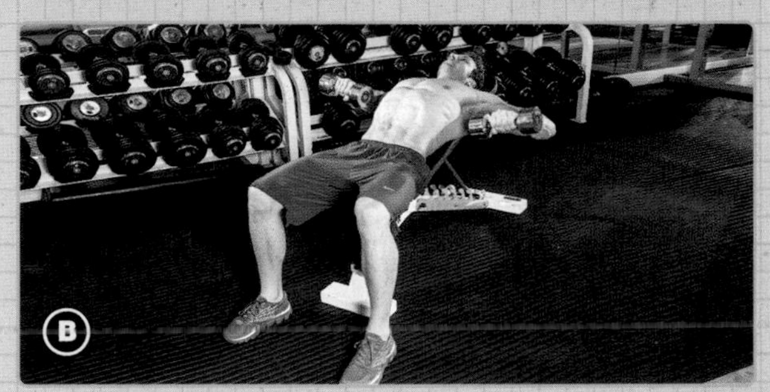

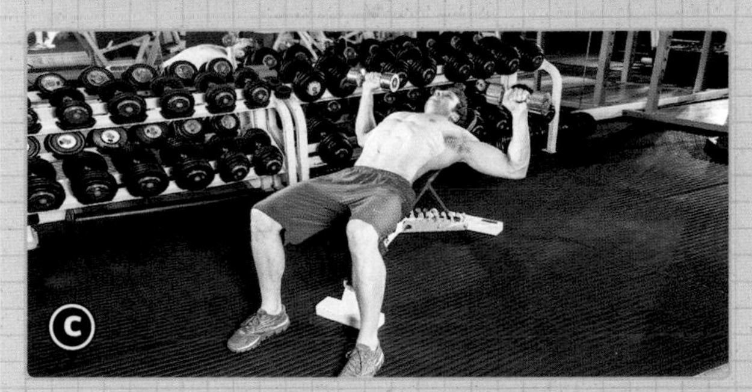

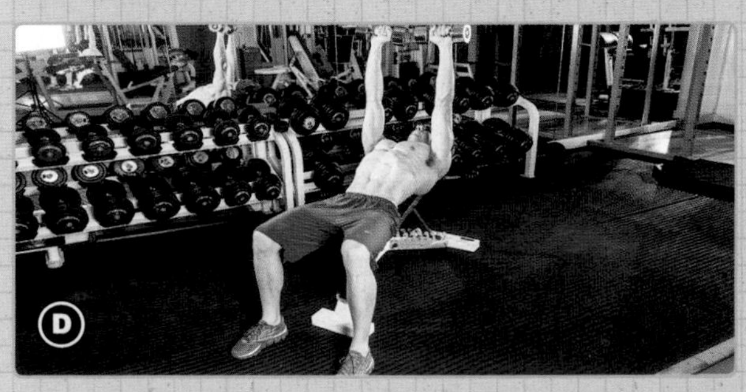

Lying on a bench changes your body position so the target muscles are worked from a different angle.

INTERNAL CABLE ROTATION

Target:* *Rotator cuffs

The cable places a different emphasis on your rotator cuff and is a beginner-friendly way to strengthen these crucial muscles

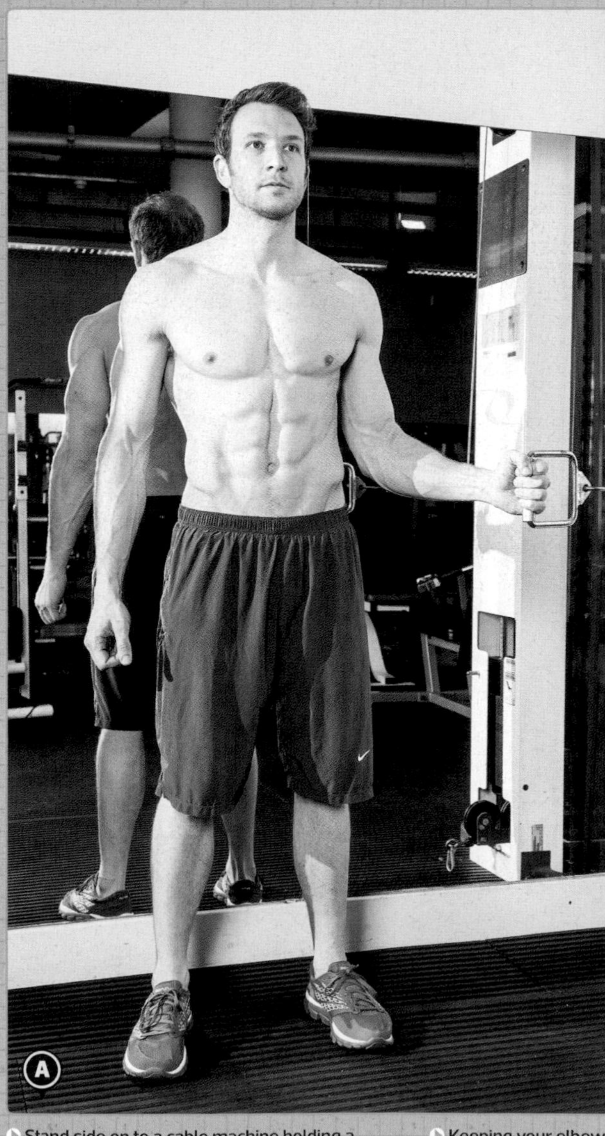

A

B

- Stand side on to a cable machine holding a D-handle attached to the middle of the machine with your closest hand.

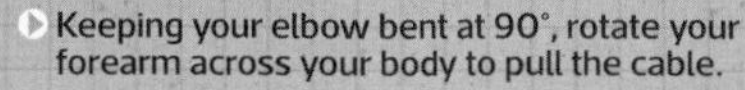

- Keeping your elbow bent at 90°, rotate your forearm across your body to pull the cable.
- Reverse the movement to return to the start.

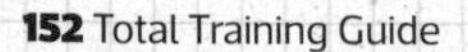

External cable rotation

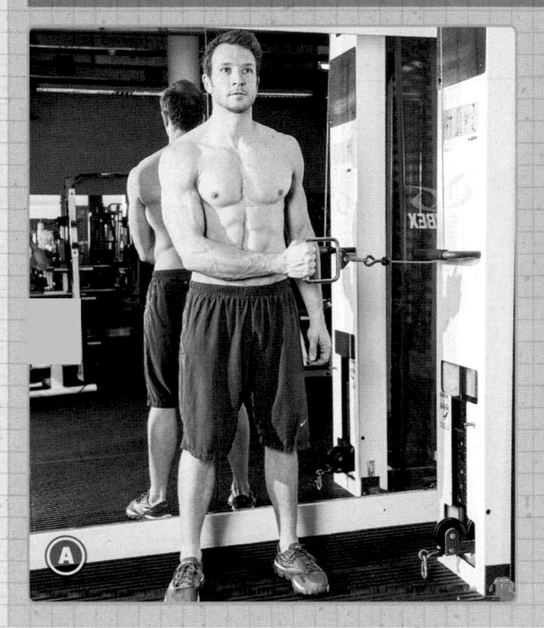

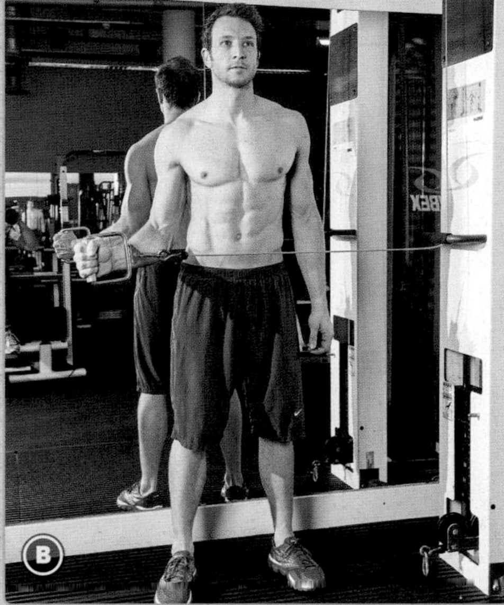

Using the hand furthest from the machine works the muscles in the opposite direction for a strong and stable shoulder joint.

Internal dumbbell rotation

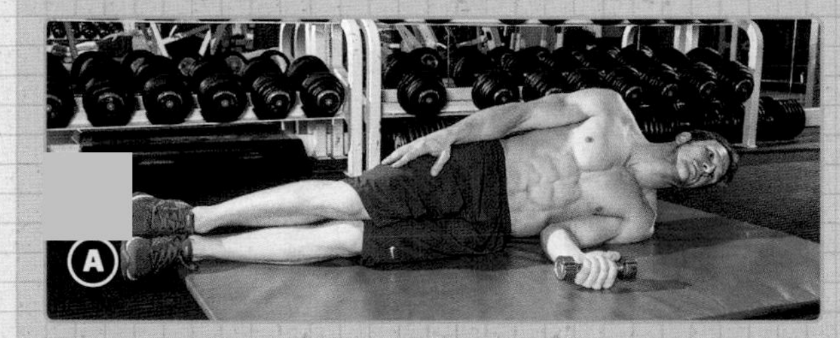

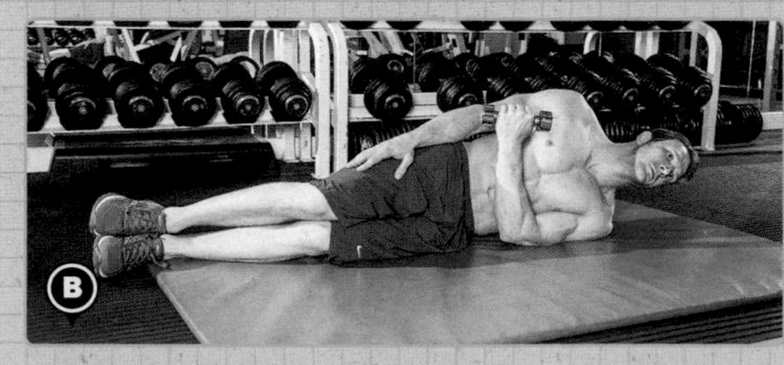

Lying on your side allows you to work your rotator cuff safely and is an ideal warm-up move.

External dumbbell rotation

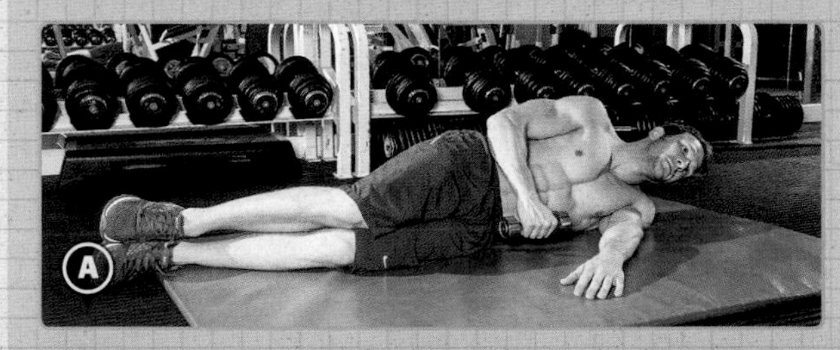

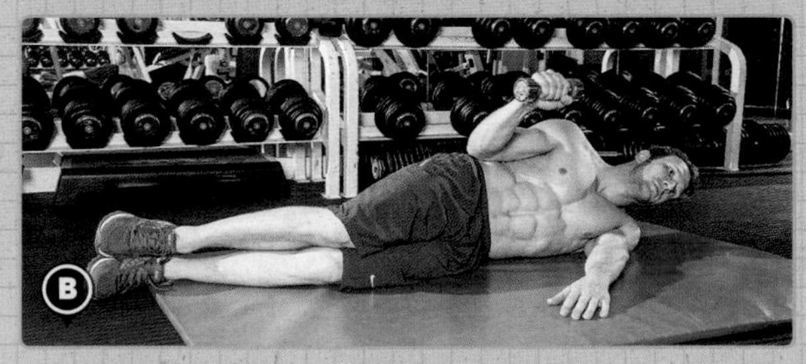

You should work your rotator cuffs in both directions to ensure your shoulder joint is as strong and stable as possible.

TOTAL BODY

Build muscle, burn fat and get bigger, stronger and leaner with these total-body moves

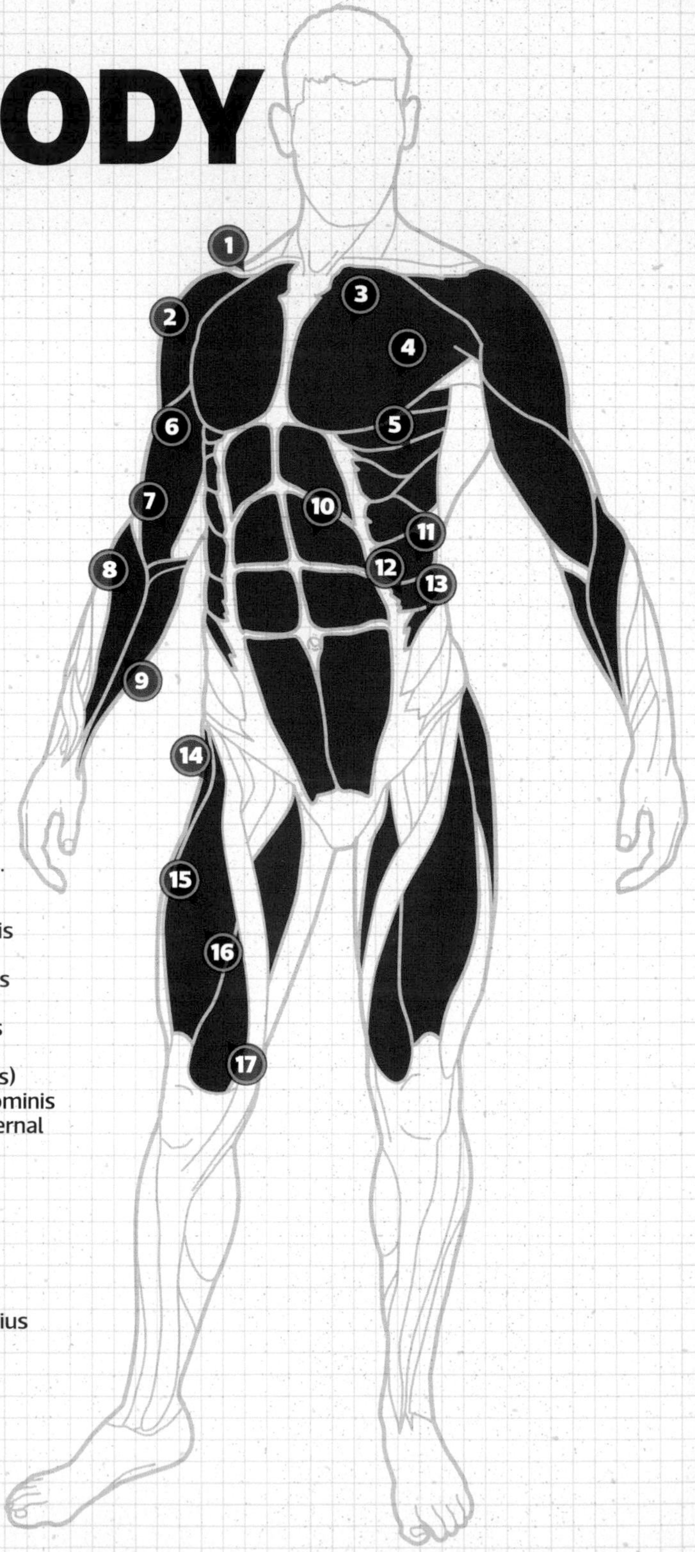

Some moves involve so many different muscle groups they can't be classified as body-part specific. These exercises deserve a chapter of their own.

Total-body moves should form a significant part of your training plan, whatever your goal, for several important reasons. Because they recruit multiple muscles they're one of the best ways to build muscle and burn fat, thanks to the growth hormones that get released after doing them. They're also a great time-saver because you can target a lot of muscles at once. Finally, they teach your different muscles to work together as a single, efficient unit, which has huge crossover benefit to sports performance and even everyday life.

Getting good at the following moves will make you bigger, stronger and leaner and help injury-proof your body.

DELTOIDS

1. Medial deltoid (middle)
2. Anterior deltoid (front)

PECTORALS

3. Pectoralis major
4. Pectoralis minor (beneath the pectoralis major)
5. Serratus anterior

BICEPS

6. Biceps brachii
7. Brachialis

FOREARMS

8. Brachioradialis
9. Flexor carpi radialis

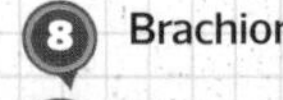

ABDOMINALS

10. Rectus abdominis
11. External obliques
12. Internal obliques (beneath the external obliques)
13. Transverse abdominis (beneath the internal obliques)

QUADRICEPS

14. Vastus lateralis
15. Rectus femoris
16. Vastus intermedius (beneath the rectus femoris)
17. Vastus medialis

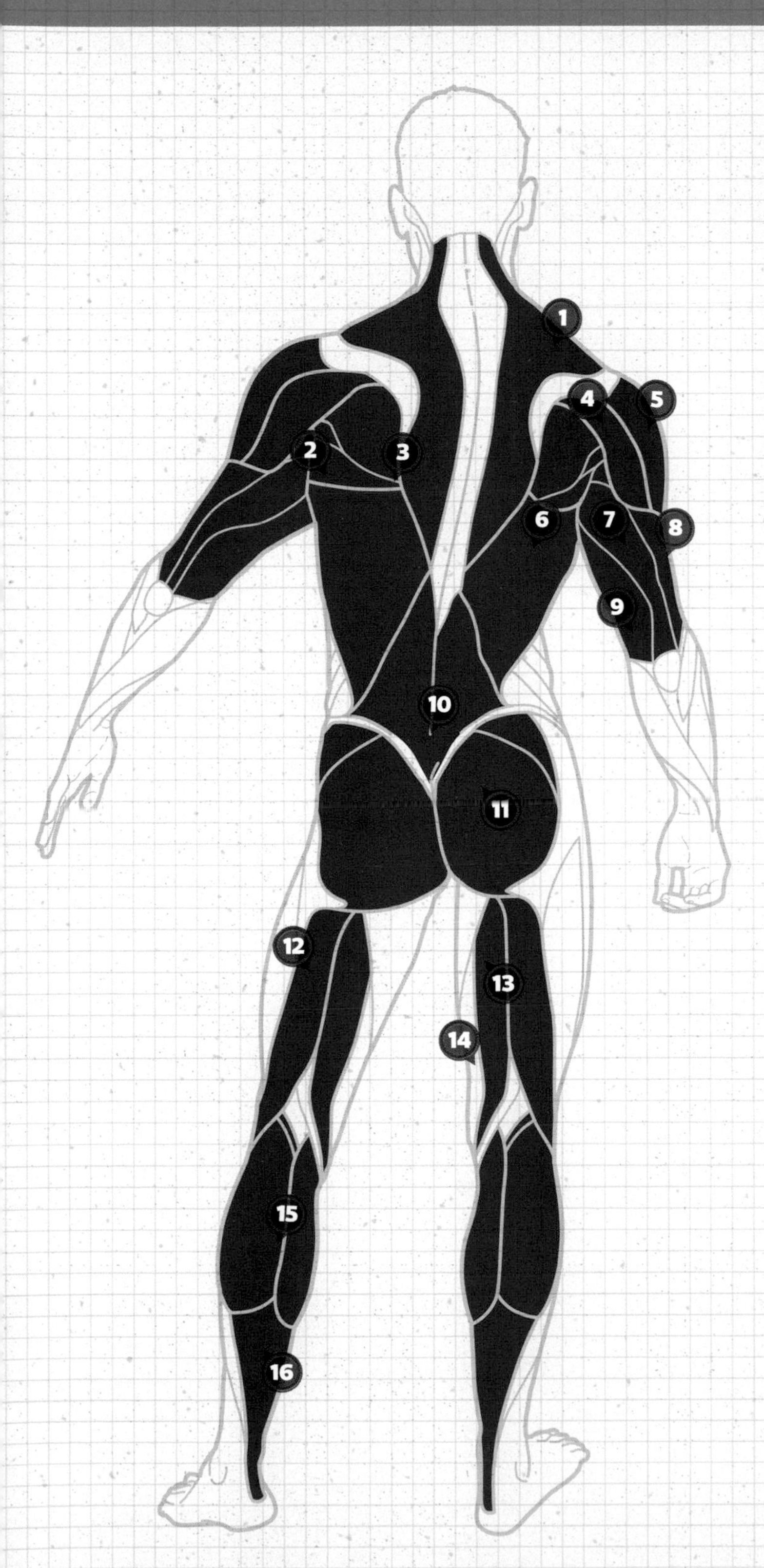

TRAPS
1. Trapezius

BACK
2. Teres major
3. Rhomboid (beneath the trapezius)

DELTOIDS
4. Rotator cuff (beneath the deltoids)
5. Posterior deltoid (back)

LATS
6. Latissimus dorsi

TRICEPS
7. Triceps brachii long head
8. Triceps brachii lateral head
9. Triceps brachii medial head

LOWER BACK
10. Erector spinae

GLUTES
11. Gluteus maximus

HAMSTRINGS
12. Biceps femoris
13. Semitendinosus
14. Semimembranosus

CALVES
15. Gastrocnemius
16. Soleus

Bigger and stronger

Turn the page for the best total-body exercises

DEADLIFT

***Targets* Total body**

The classic compound lifts works many upper- and lower-body muscles and is one of the key moves for putting on muscular size and strength all over your body

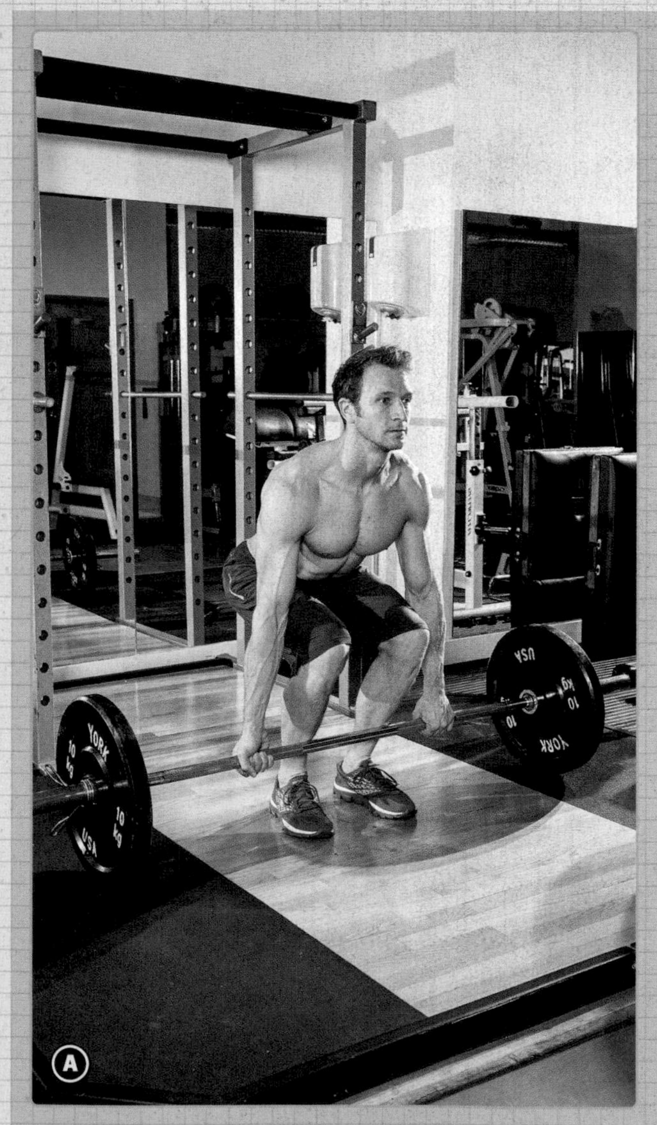

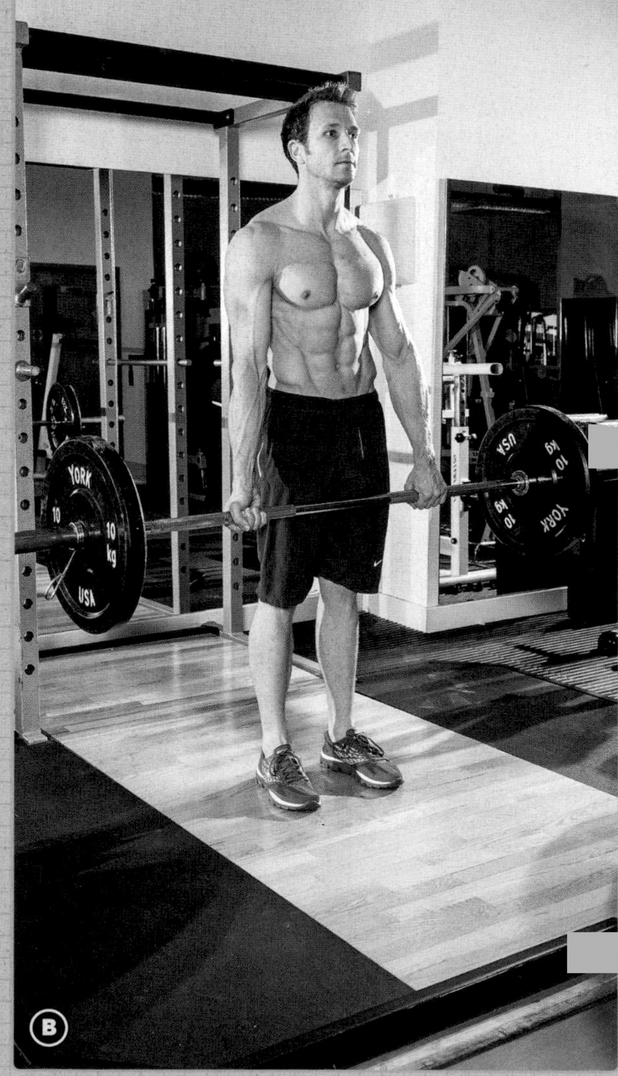

- Stand in front of a bar with your feet shoulder-width apart. Squat to take an overhand or alternate grip of the bar just outside your thighs.
- Brace your core and retract your shoulders so they're over the bar. Maintain a natural arch in your back.
- Push your heels into the floor and use your glutes to power the lift. Keep the bar close to your body.
- As the bar passes your knees, push your hips forwards until you're standing tall. Reverse the movement back to the start.

Rack pull

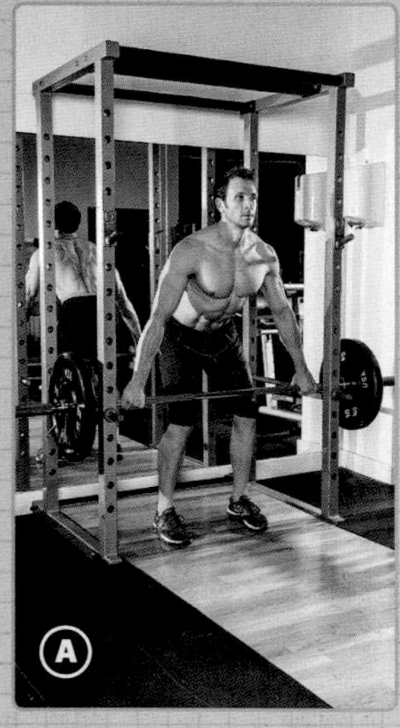

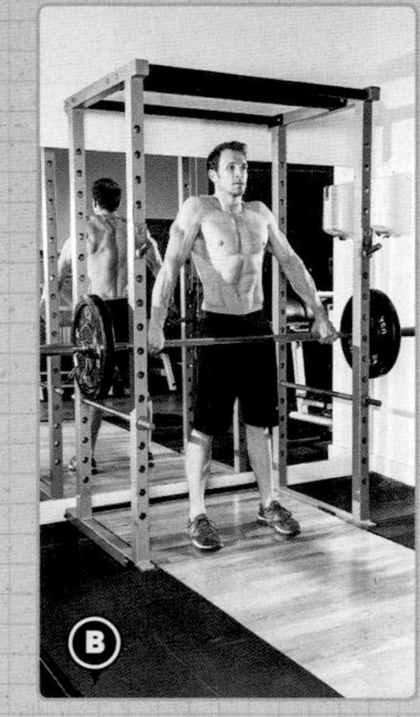

Starting the move on safety bars set at mid-level increases the focus on your upper back and shoulders.

Deficit deadlift

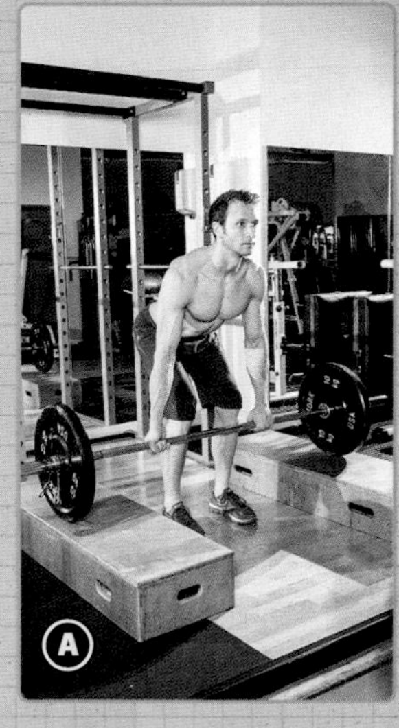

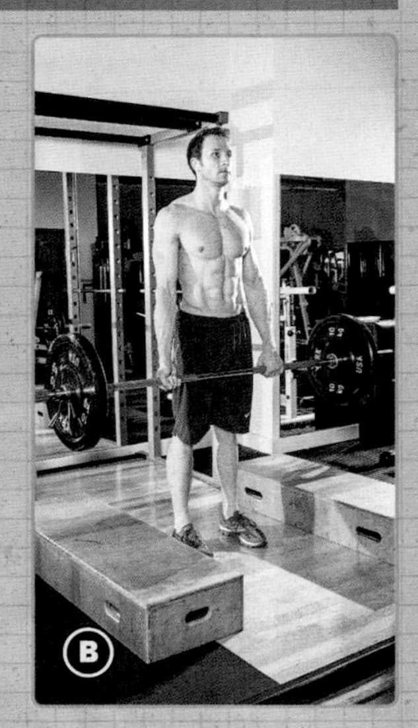

Starting with the weights on range blocks is good for those with poor flexibility or a weak lower back.

Snatch-grip deadlift

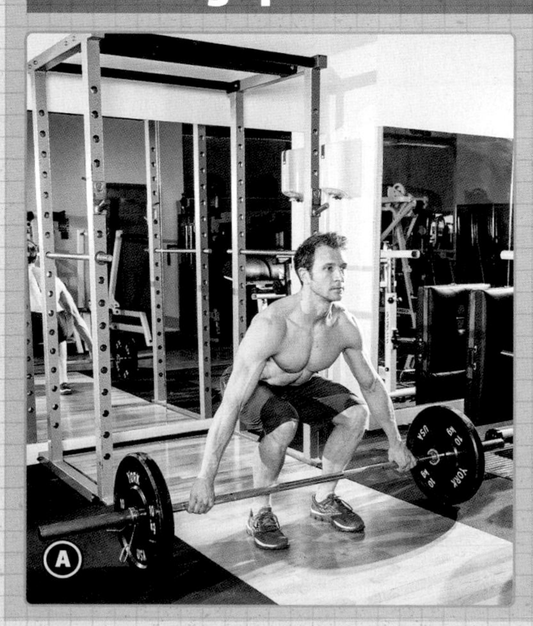

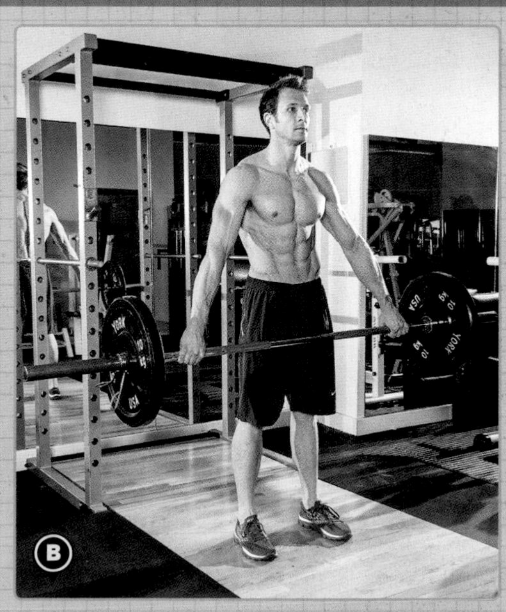

A wide grip on the bar places more emphasis on your upper back.

CLEAN

***Targets* Total body**

This complex and dynamic total-body move works all the major muscles of your legs and posterior chain, or those muscle groups down the back of your body

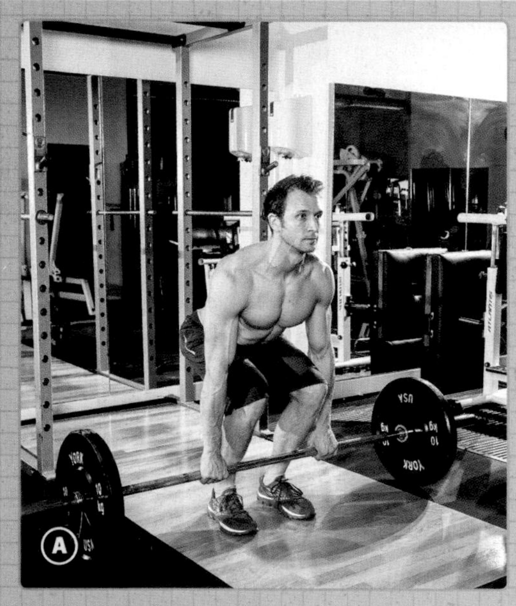

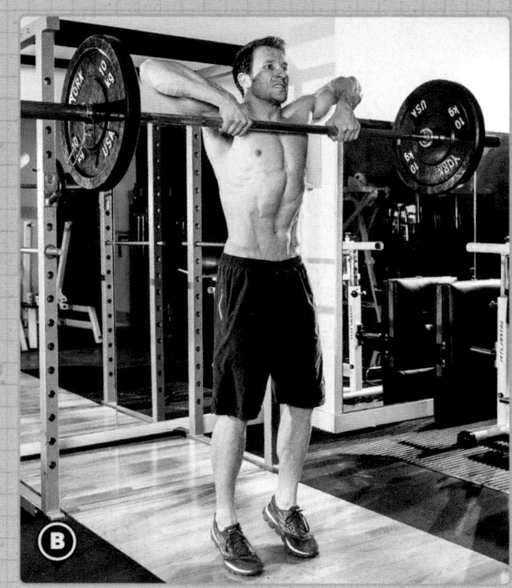

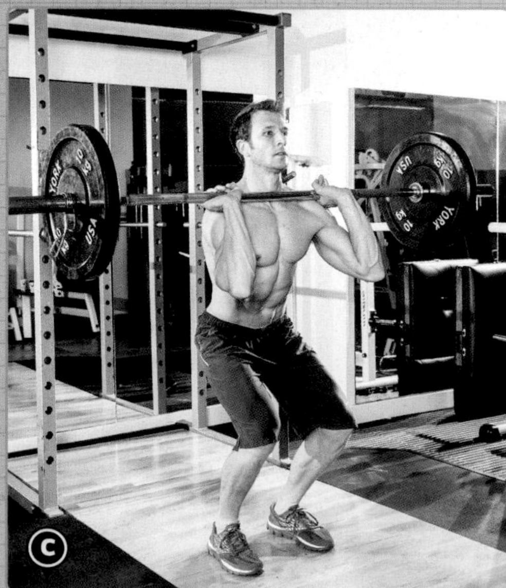

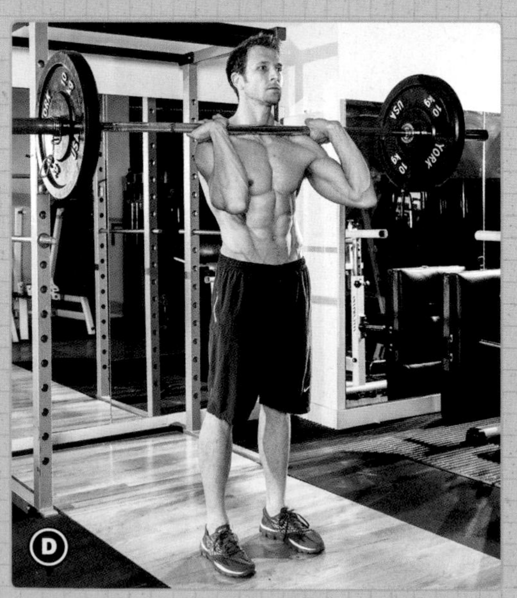

- Stand with your shins touching the bar and feet shoulder-width apart.
- Squat and hold the bar with an overhand grip.
- Keeping your core braced, your chest up and a natural arch in your back, drive through your heels and lift the bar off the ground.
- Once the bar reaches your hips, rise up on tiptoes, shrug your shoulders powerfully and pull the bar up higher, leading with your elbows.
- As the bar travels towards shoulder height, squat under the bar and rotate your elbows forwards so you catch it on your fingers and the front of your shoulders.
- Stand tall, then reverse the move back to the start.

Snatch

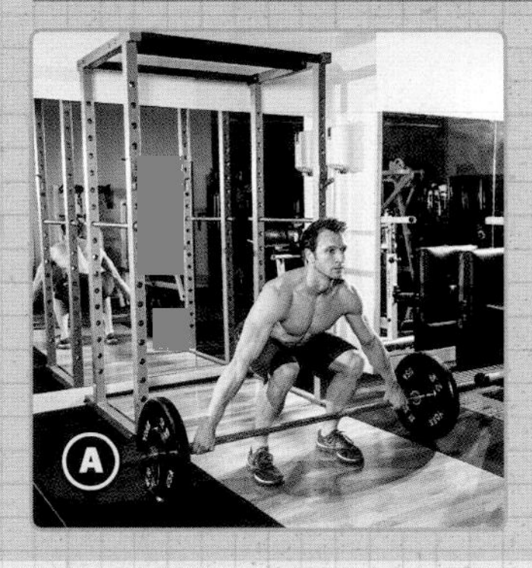

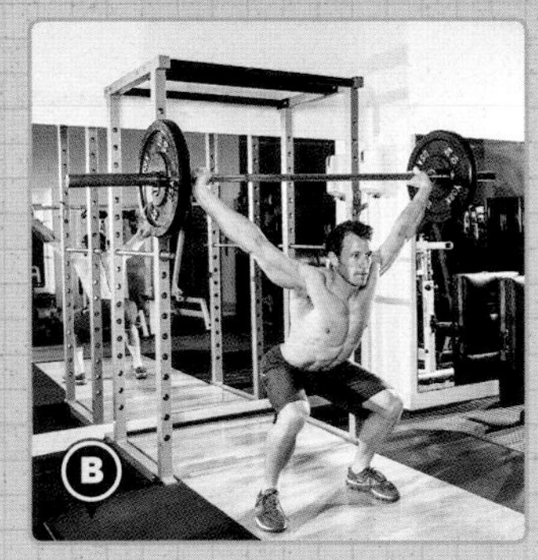

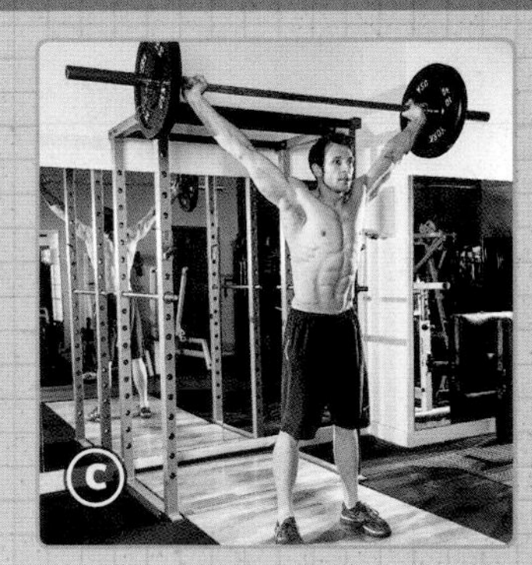

Lifting the bar from the floor to above your head by ducking under it is a highly complex and explosive move that requires strength, balance, co-ordination and flexibility.

Hang clean

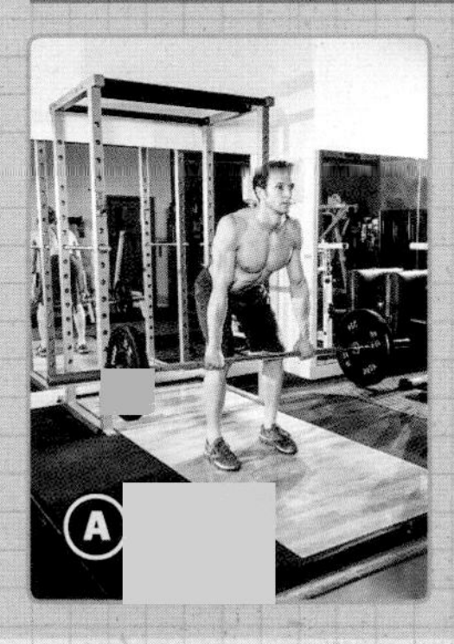

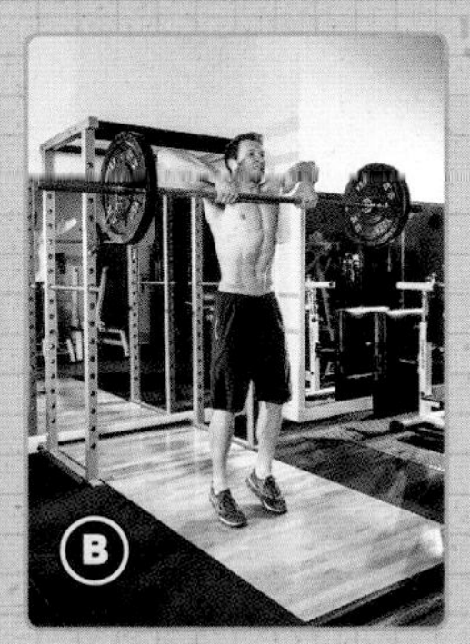

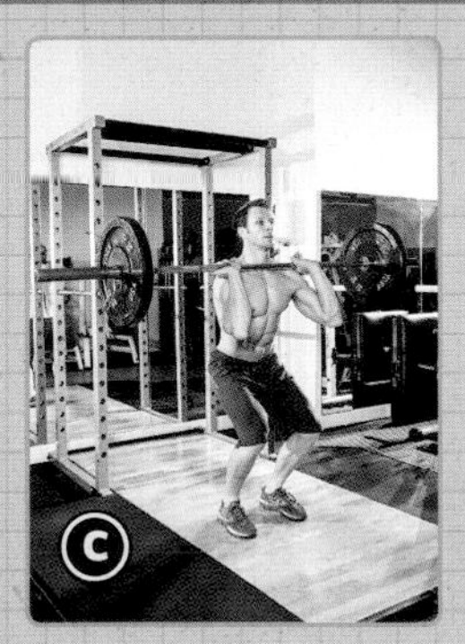

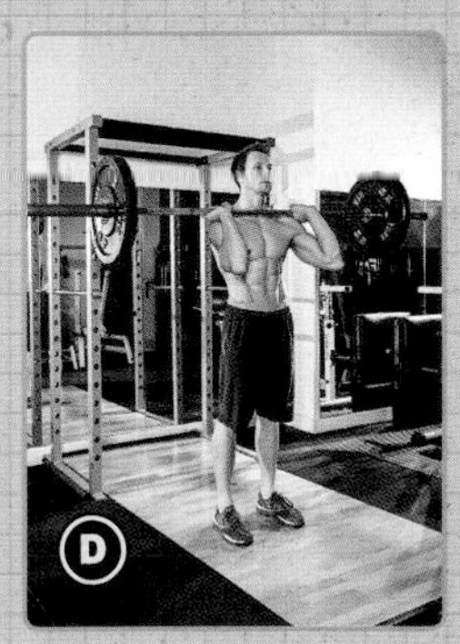

Starting with the bar at mid-thigh level is an easier variation but still requires strength and co-ordination.

Clean and jerk

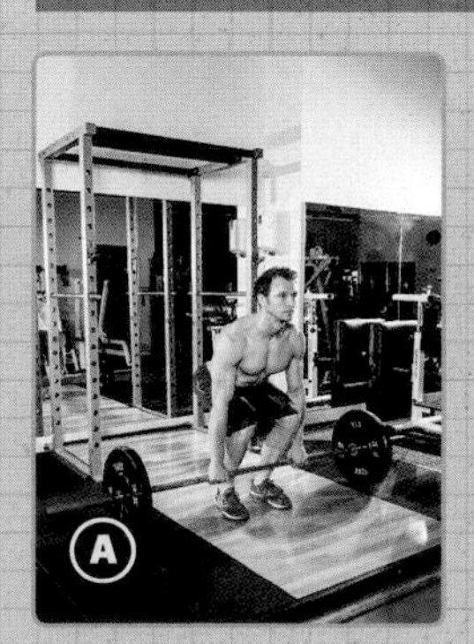

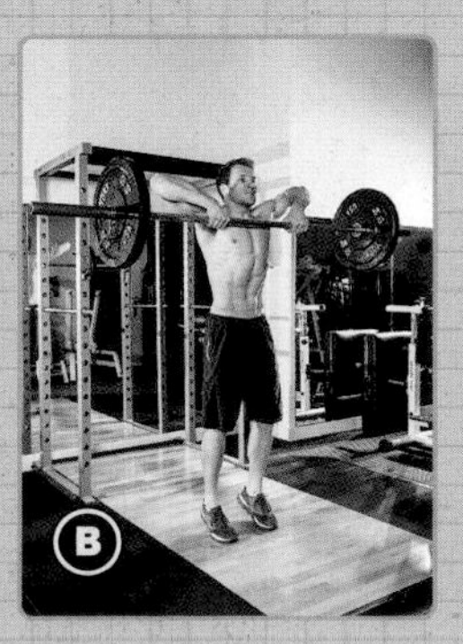

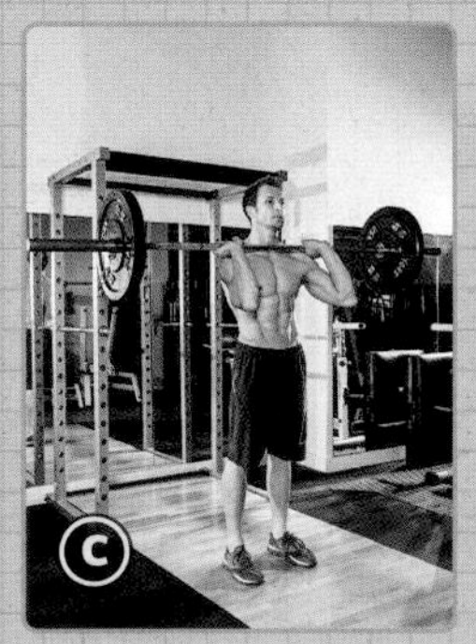

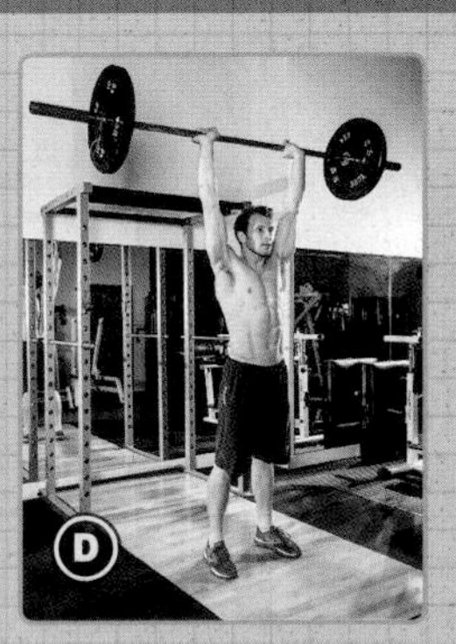

This advanced move, which requires you to press the bar overhead at the top of the clean, works your shoulders and upper back.

BURPEE

***Targets* Total body**

One of the hardest and most intense bodyweight moves, this will work all your major muscle groups and get your heart rate soaring

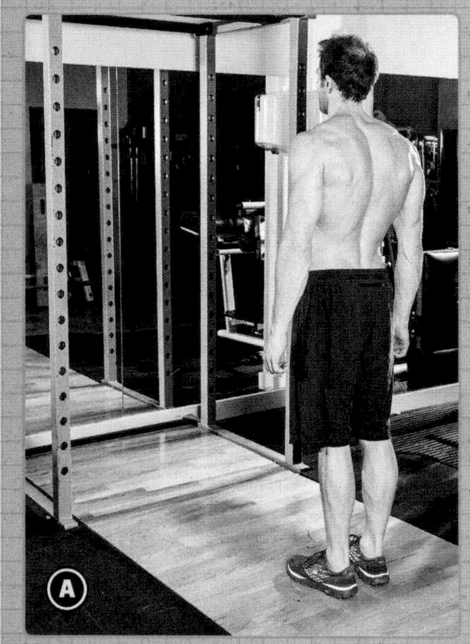

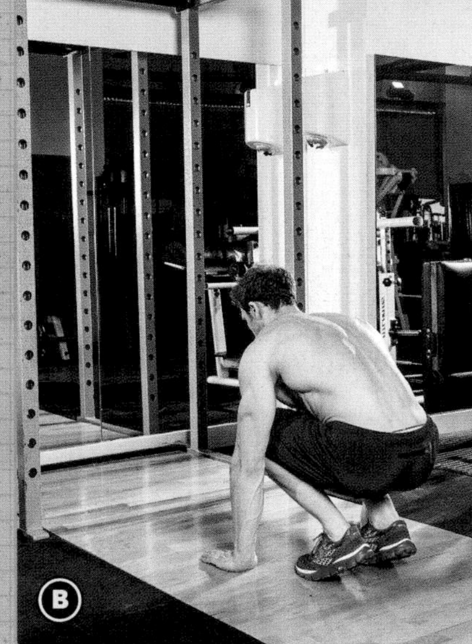

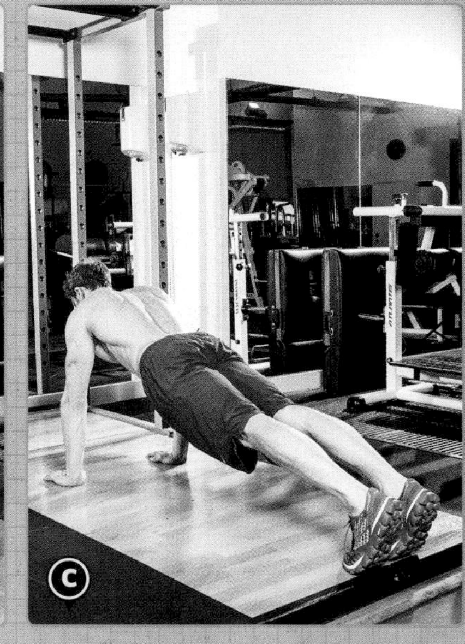

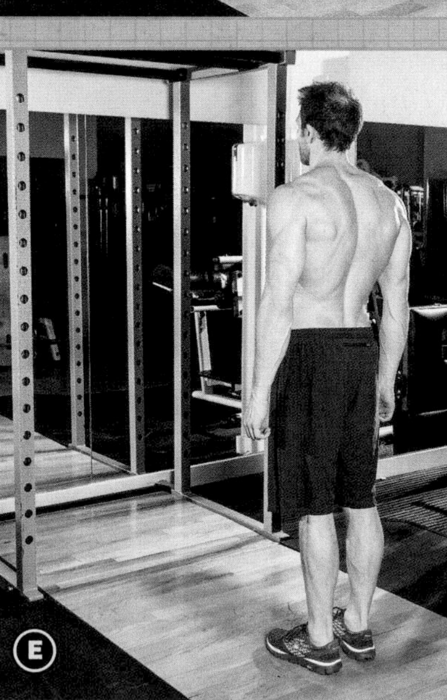

- Stand tall with your feet hip-width apart.
- Squat, place your hands on the floor and kick your legs backwards until you're in a press-up position.
- Bring your legs back underneath you and jump back up to return to the start position.

Bastard burpee

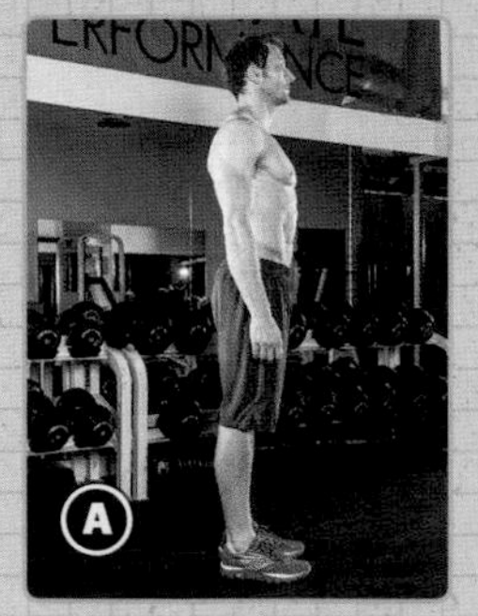

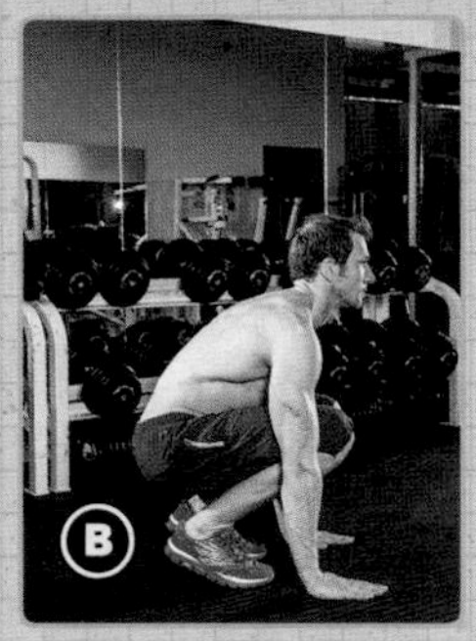

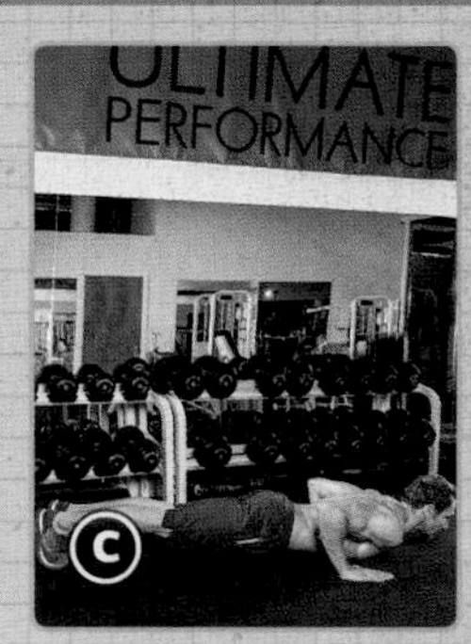

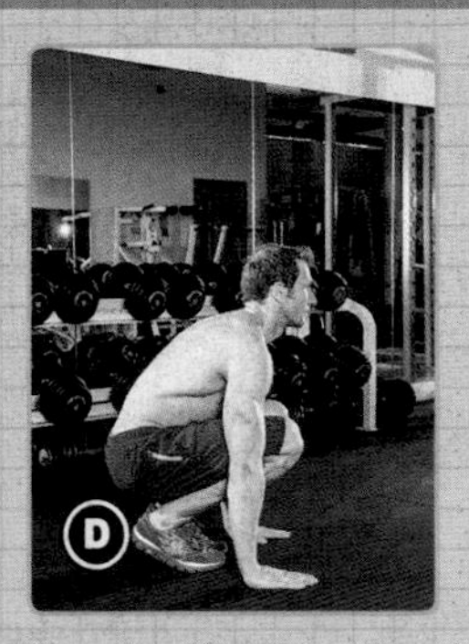

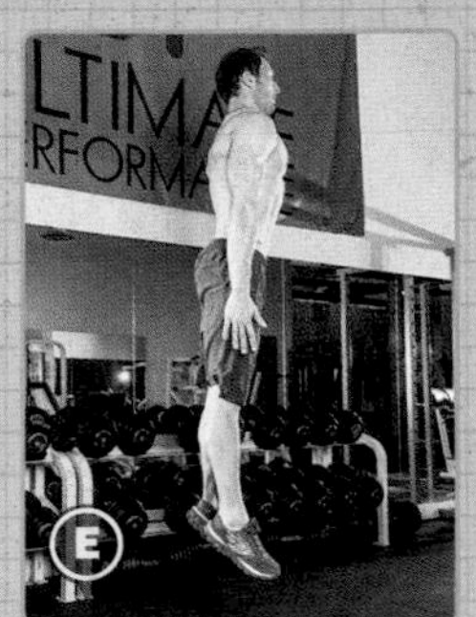

Adding a press-up will work your chest and triceps even harder.

Tuck-jump burpee

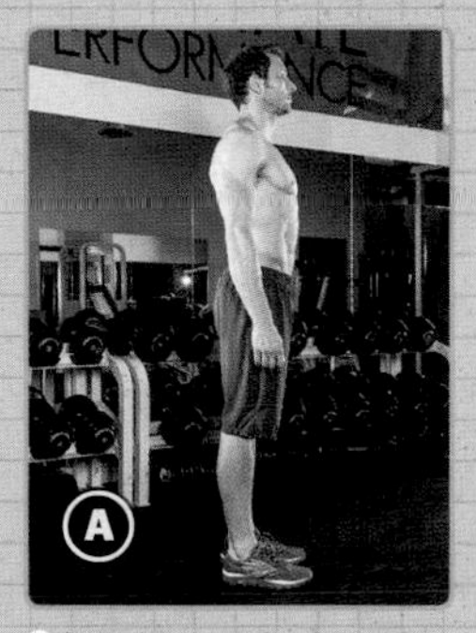

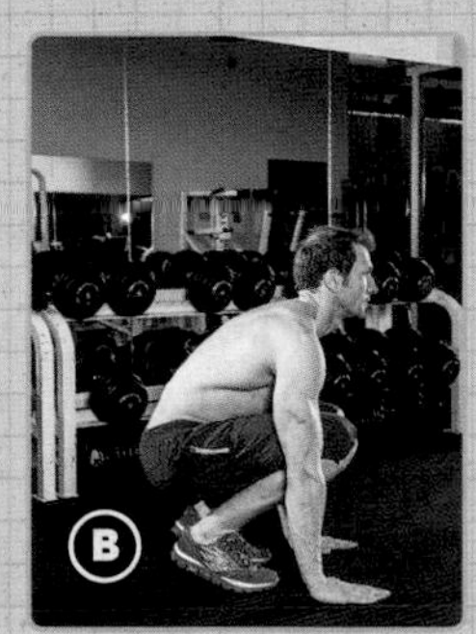

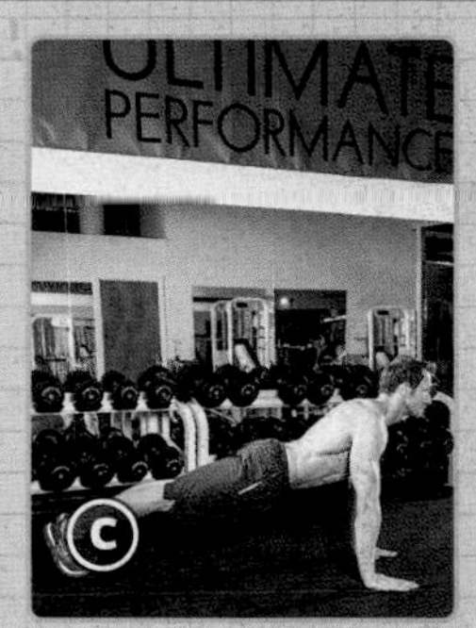

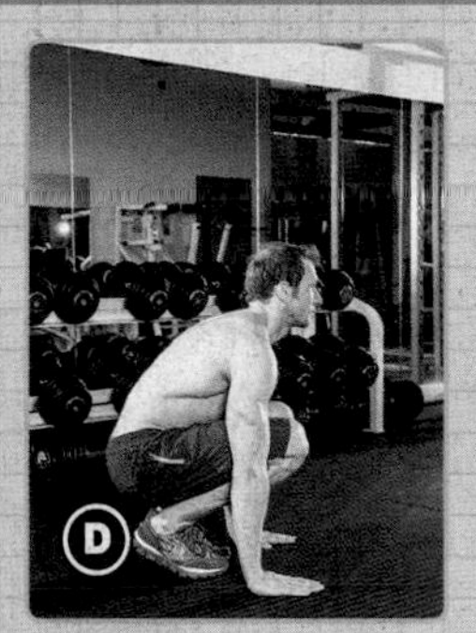

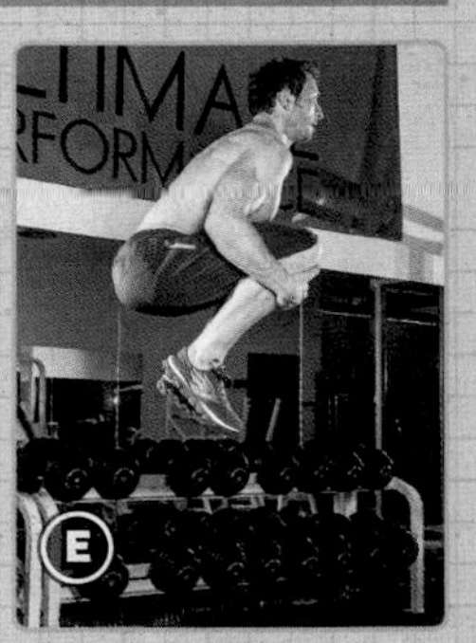

Jumping into the air and grabbing your knees at the end of the move will send your heart rate through the roof while also building explosive power.

Pull-up burpee

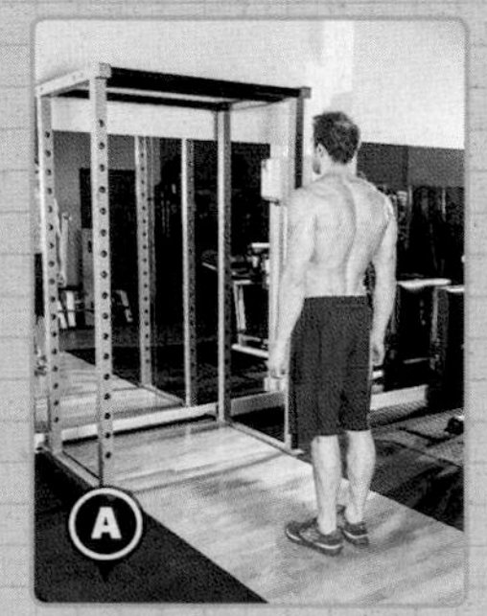

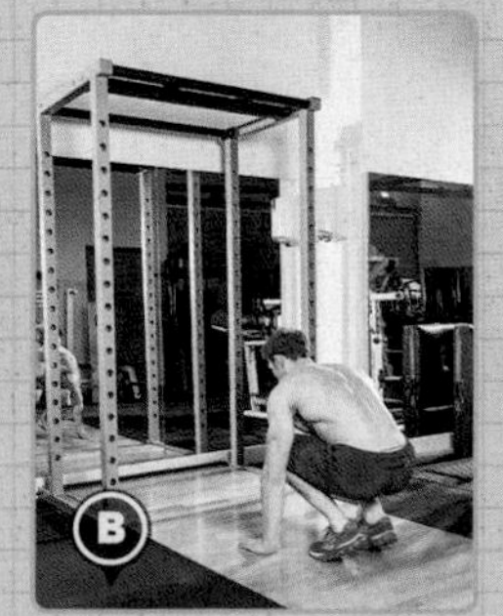

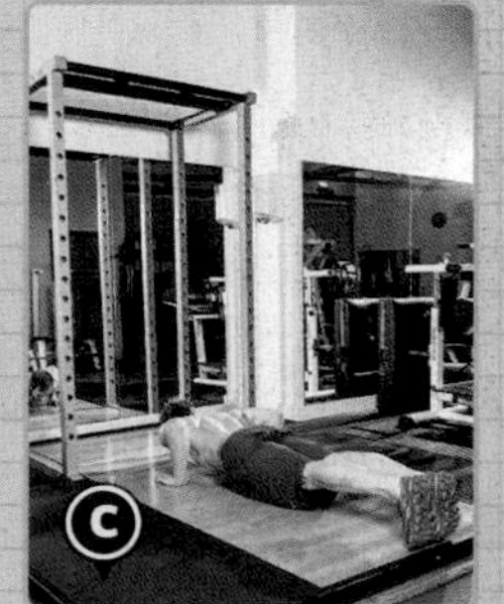

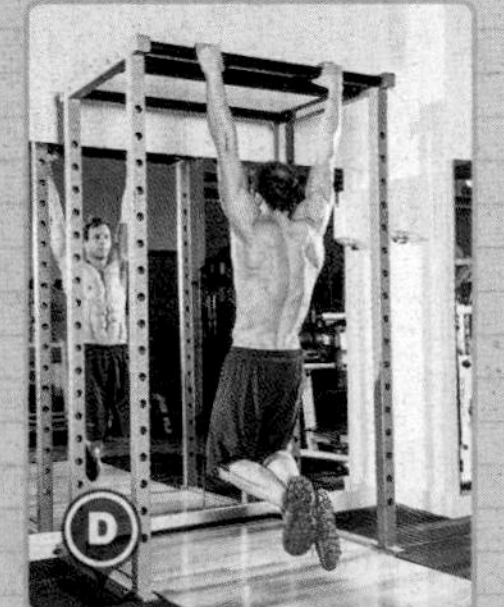

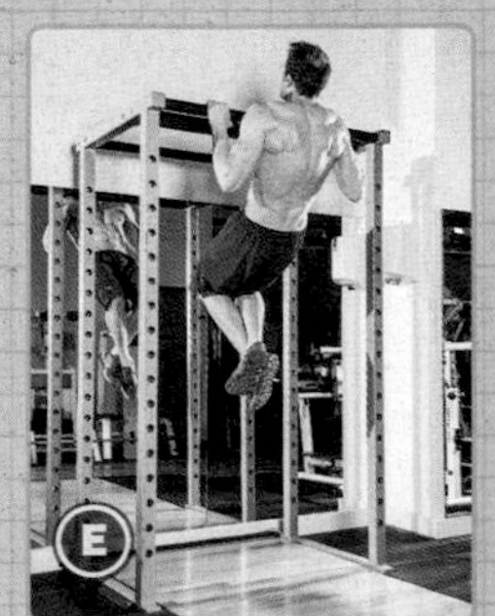

Adding a pull-up at the end of this hard move makes it even tougher by recruiting your upper back, core and arms.

ONE-ARM DUMBBELL CLEAN

***Targets** Total body*

Holding a dumbbell in one hand works that side of the body for balanced gains and is a great option ahead of advancing to the barbell version

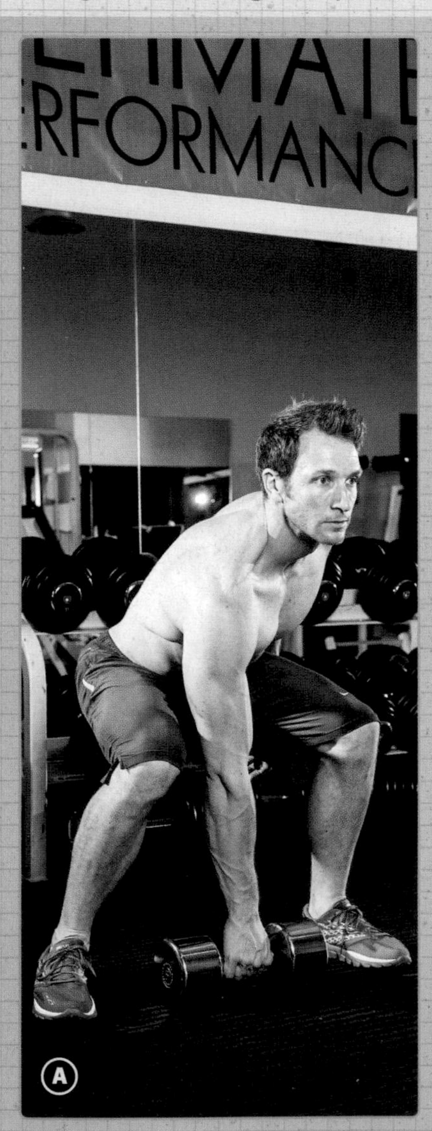

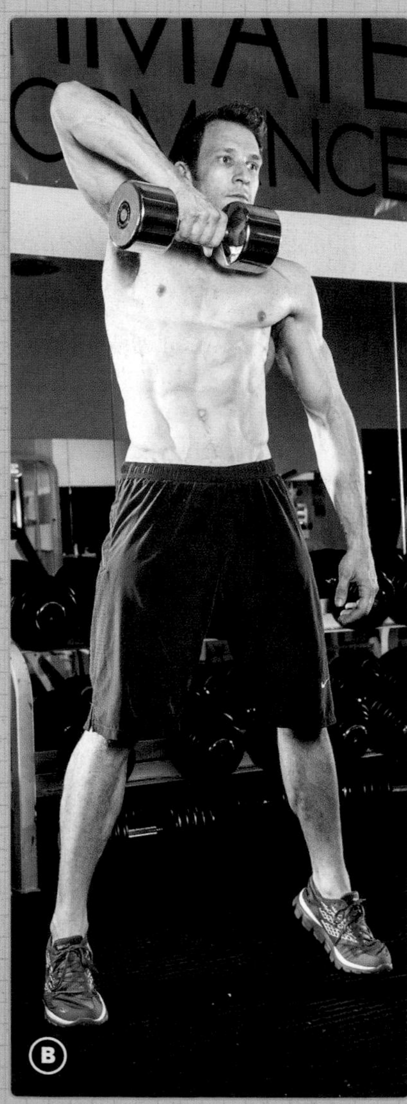

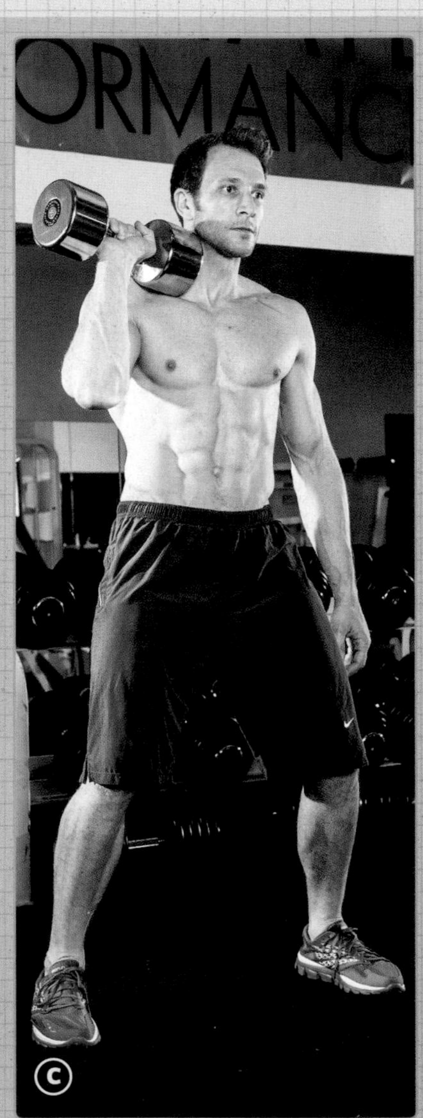

- Stand with your feet shoulder-width apart. Squat and pick up the dumbbell.
- Keeping your core braced, your chest up and a natural arch in your back, lift the weight off the ground by driving up through your heels.
- Once the dumbbell reaches your hips, rise up on tiptoes, shrug your shoulders and pull it higher, leading with your elbow.
- As the weight reaches shoulder height, squat under it and rotate your elbows so you catch it on the front of your shoulders.

One-arm dumbbell clean and press

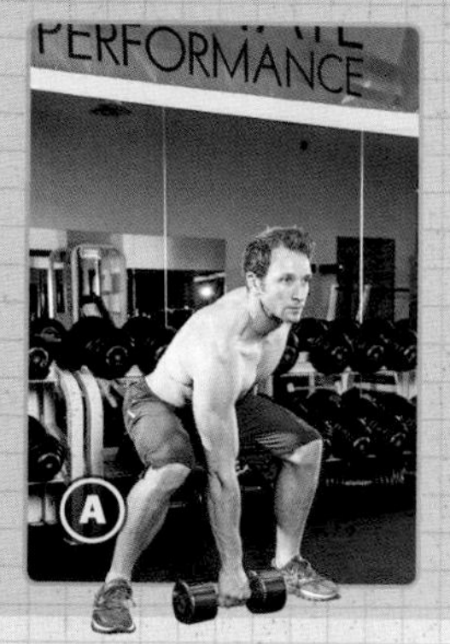

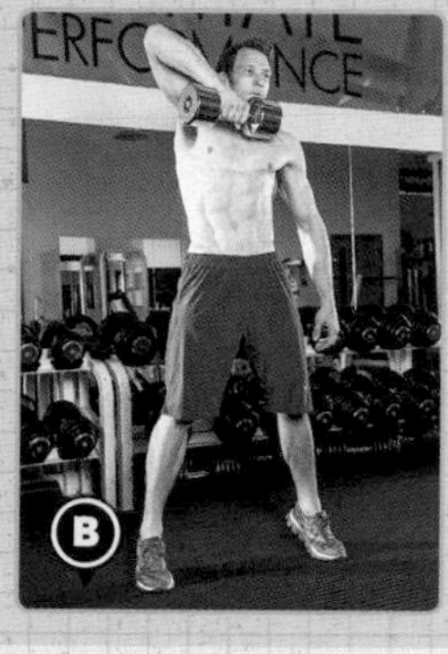

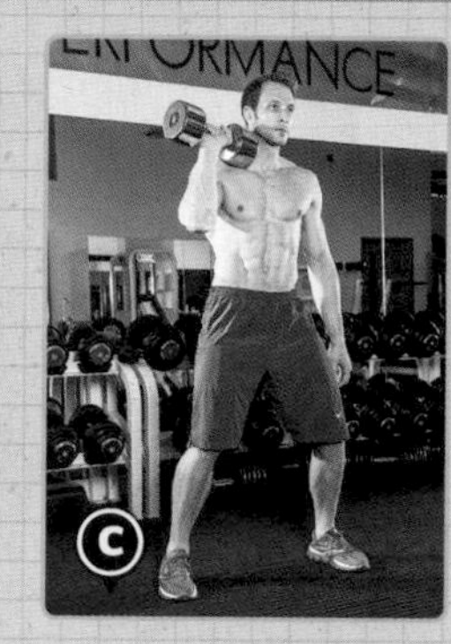

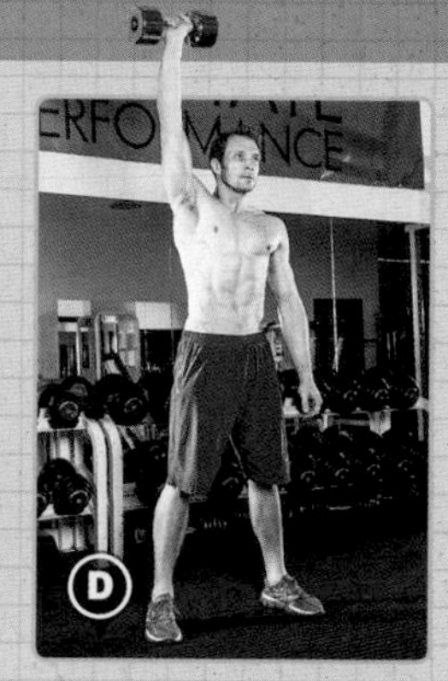

This variation is great for getting your body used to working as a single unit while still building explosive strength and power.

One-arm dumbbell snatch

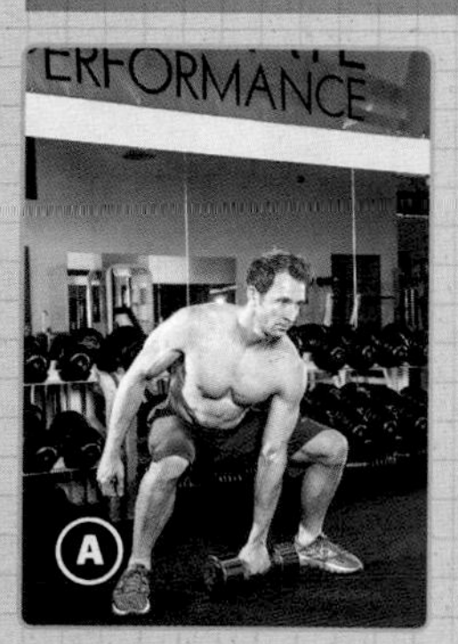

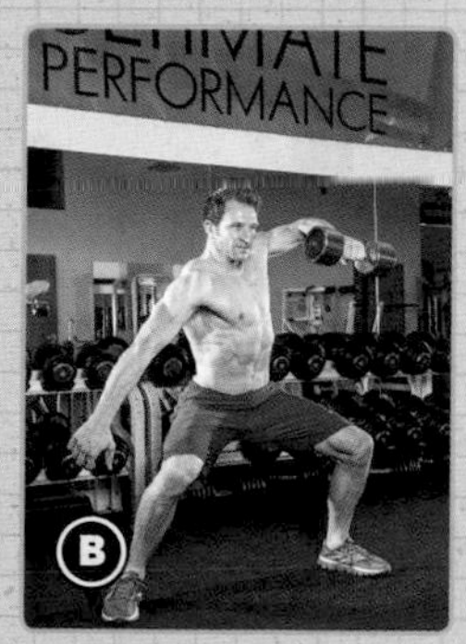

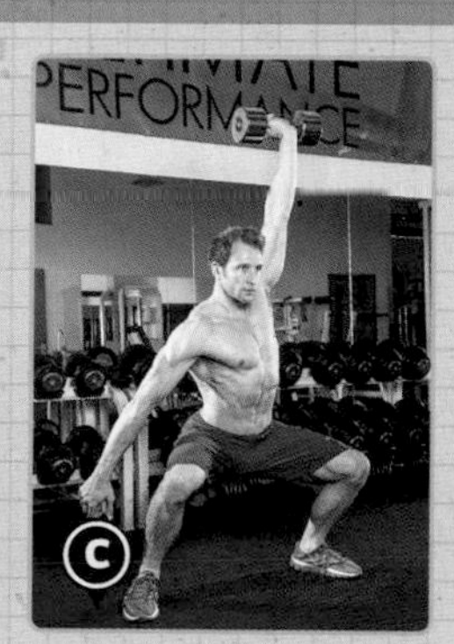

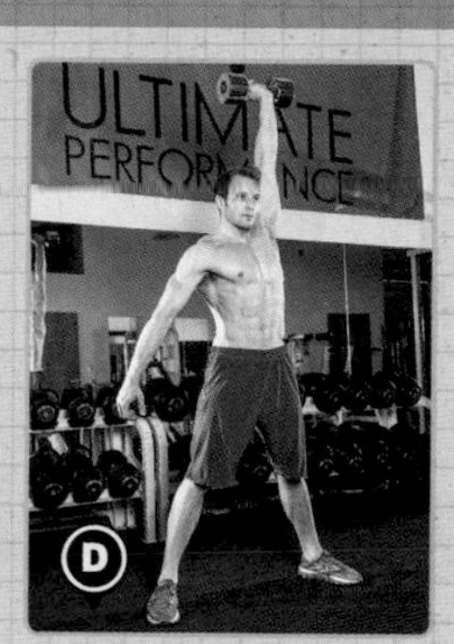

This is a great alternative to master the complex movement patterns of the main move while still working each side of your body hard.

One-arm dumbbell swing

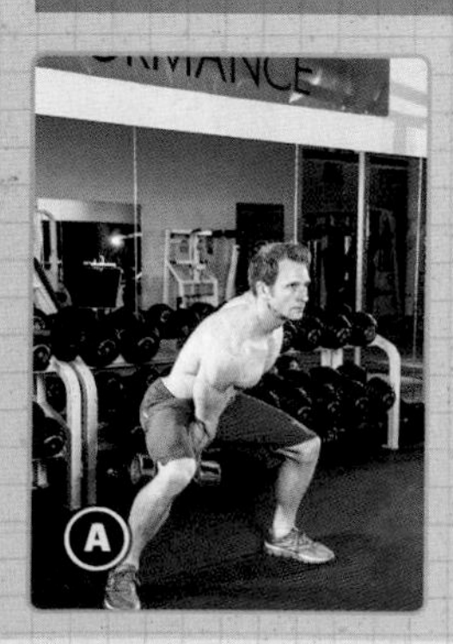

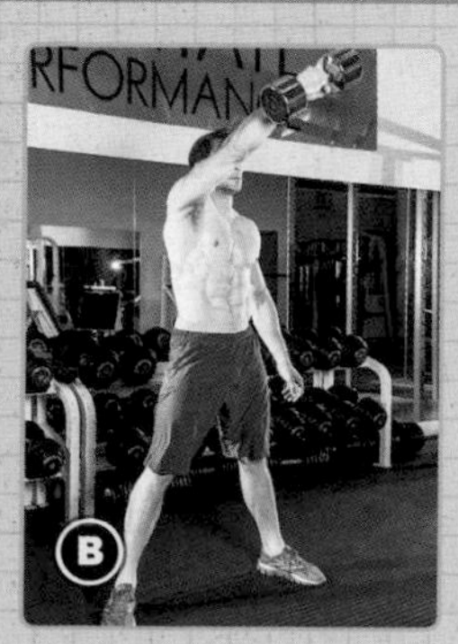

Swinging a dumbbell instead of a kettlebell is a great option if your gym doesn't have the latter.

PUSH PRESS

***Targets** Deltoids, quads, glutes, core*

Generate more power by descending into a quarter-squat then exploding powerful upwards to raise the bar overhead

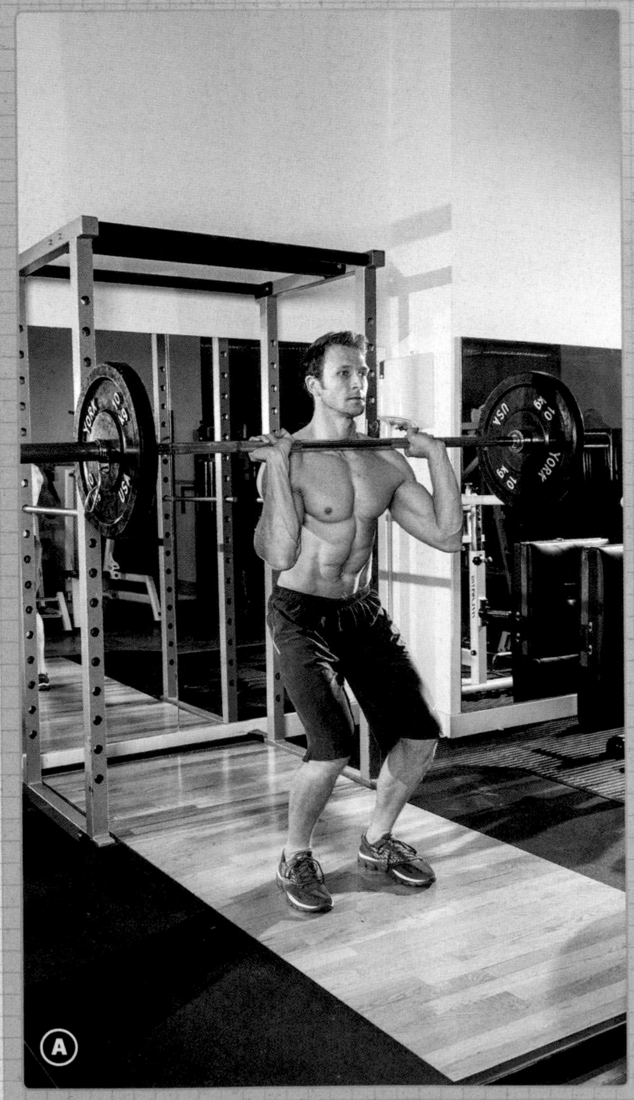

- With your feet shoulder-width apart, position a bar on your upper chest, gripping it with hands just wider than shoulder-width apart.
- Keep your chest upright and your core muscles braced.

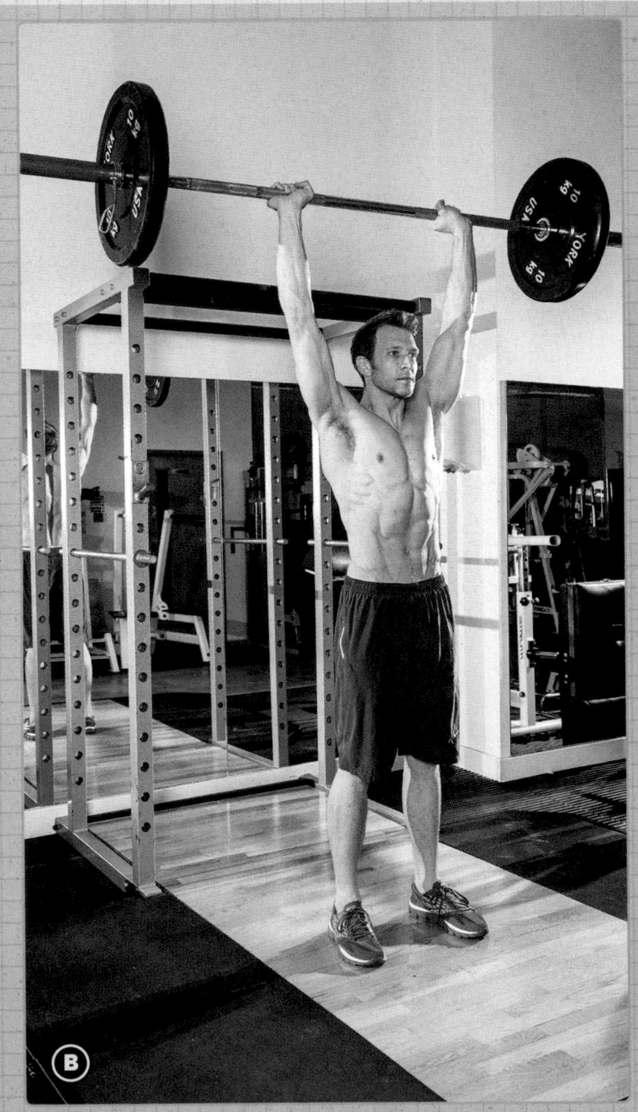

- Drop into a quarter-squat then straighten powerfully while pressing the bar upwards until your arms are extended overhead.
- During the lifting phase, don't tilt your hips forwards. Lower the bar back to return to the start.

Dumbbell lunge to press

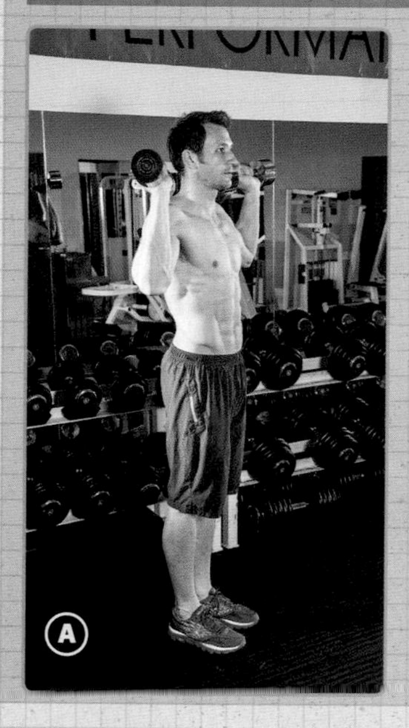
A

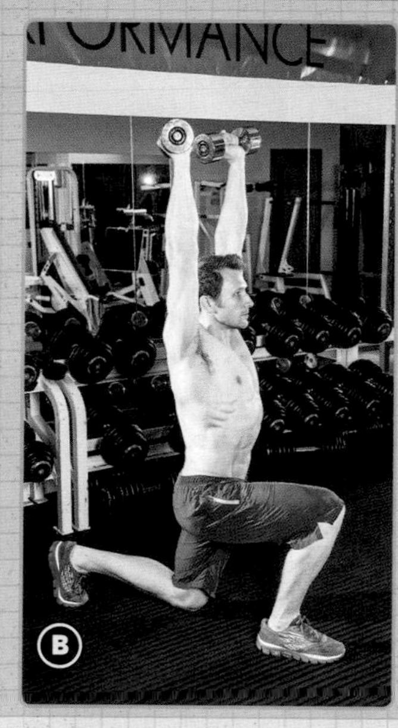
B

Combine a lunge with a shoulder press to work many major muscle groups at once.

Dumbbell squat to curl to press

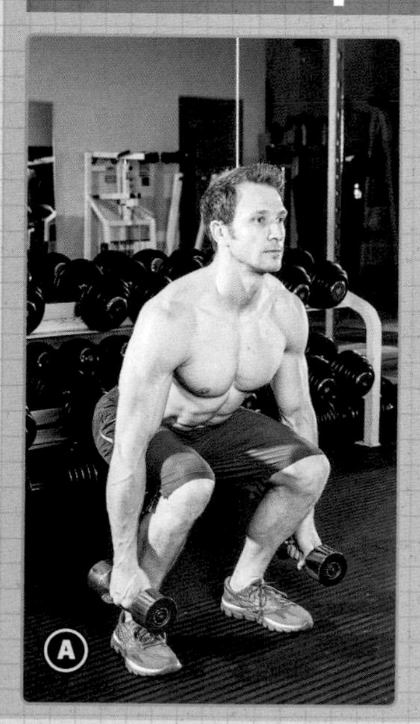
A

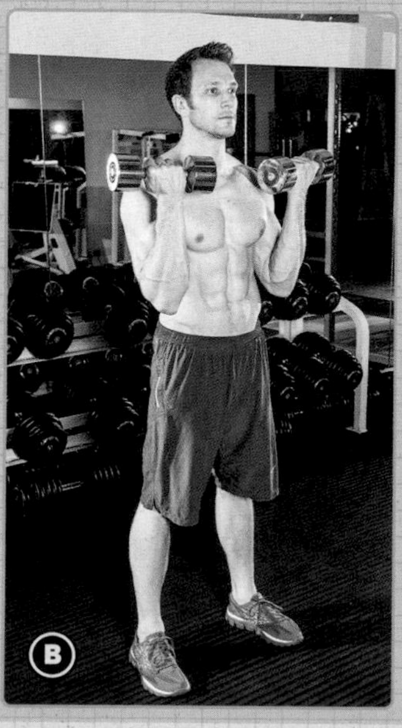
B

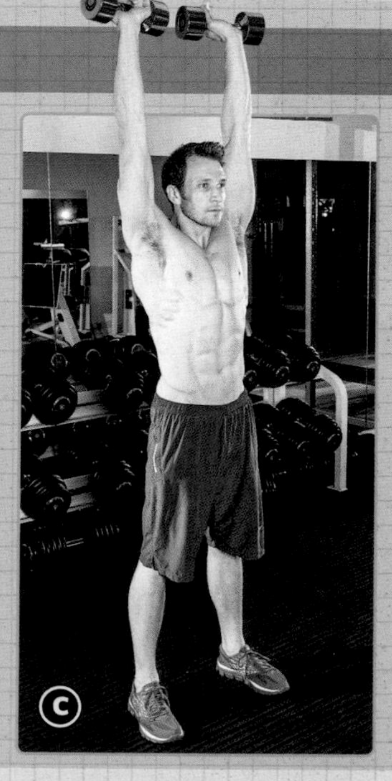
C

This works your legs, core, biceps and shoulders in one simple yet effective muscle move.

TWO-HAND KETTLEBELL SWING

***Targets** Total body*

The classic kettlebell move requires perfect form to hit the major muscle groups and to get your heart rate high

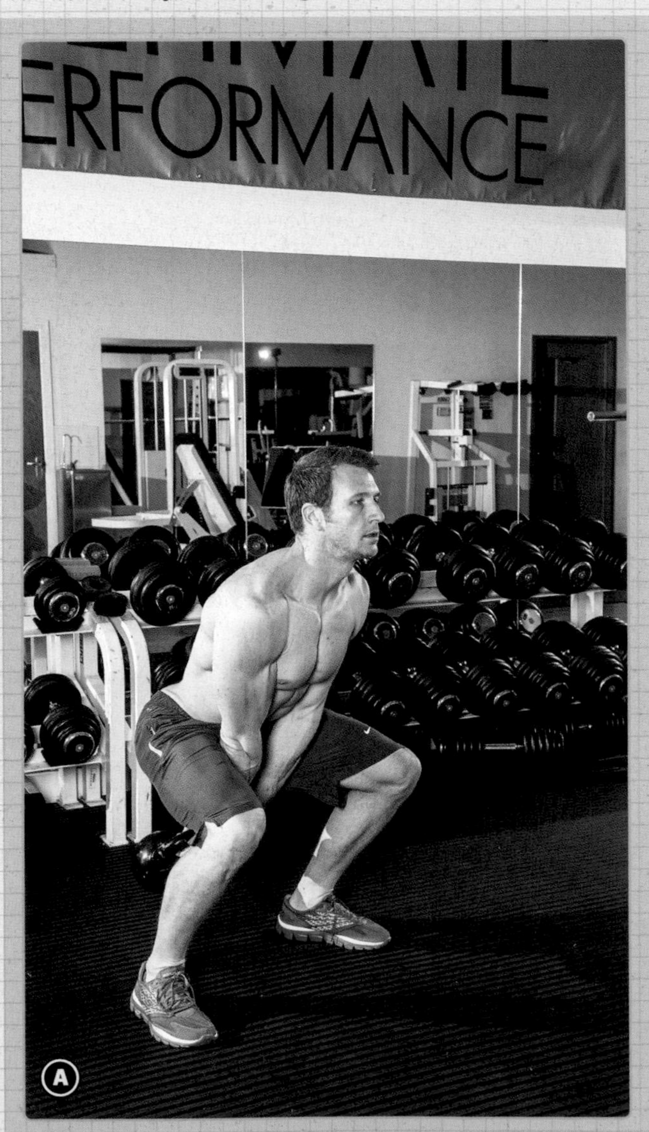

- Stand with your feet shoulder-width apart and hold a kettlebell in both hands.
- Keeping your back straight and your knees in line with your feet, bend at the knees and move the kettlebell between your legs.
- Stand and snap your hips forwards to propel the kettlebell up to shoulder height. The power comes from your hips, not your arms.
- Breathe out at the top of the movement and in during the kettlebell's descent. Continue the swing in a fluid movement.

One-hand kettlebell swing

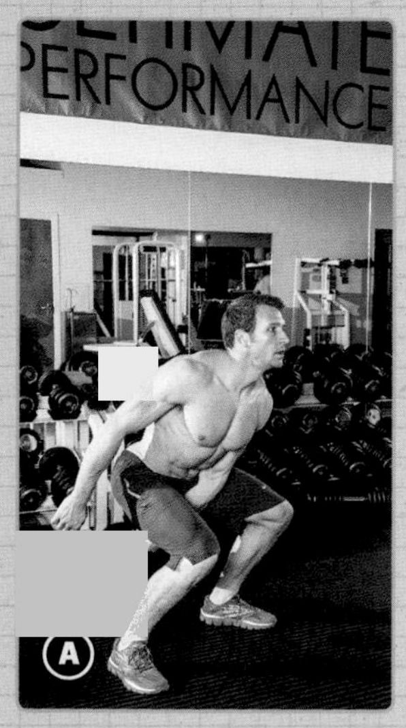

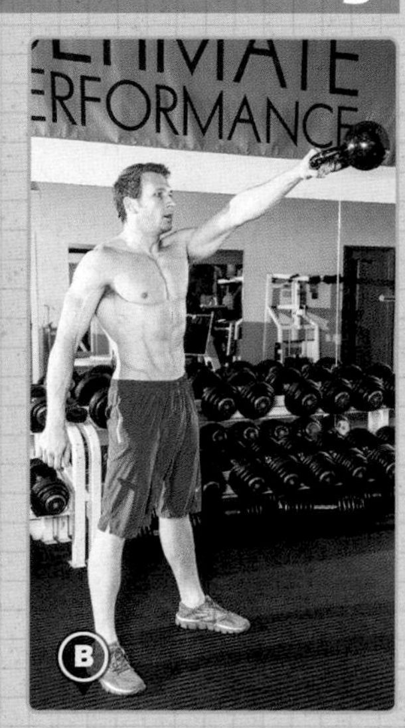

Make the swing harder and work one side of your upper body at a time by holding the kettlebell in one hand.

American kettlebell swing

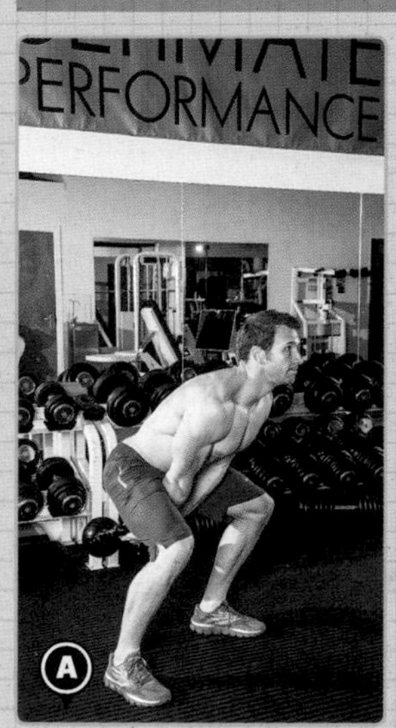

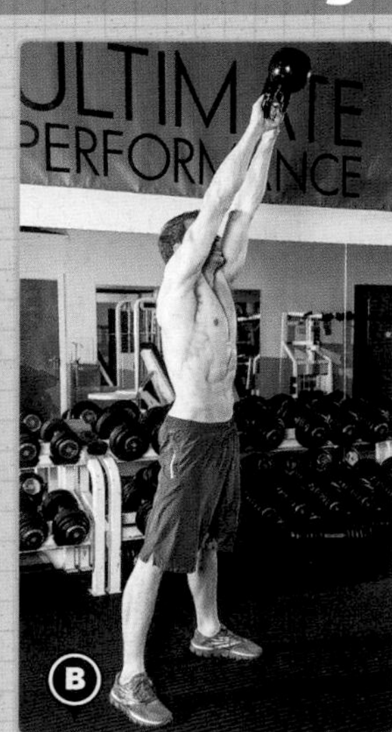

Control the weight all the way up until it's directly above your head.

Kettlebell hand switch

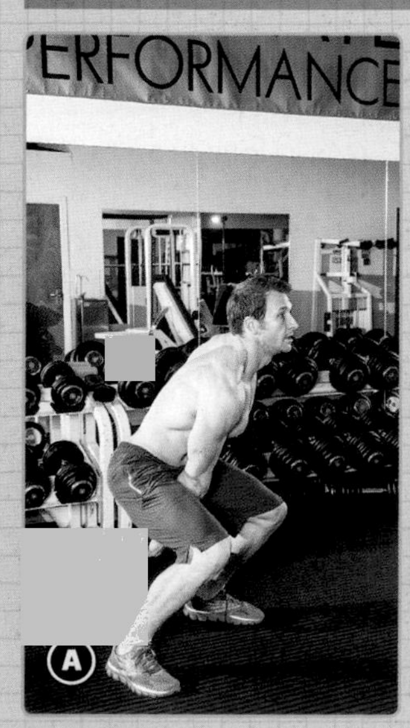

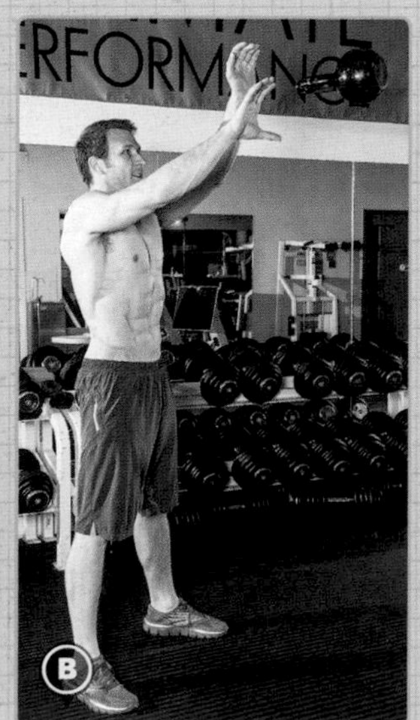

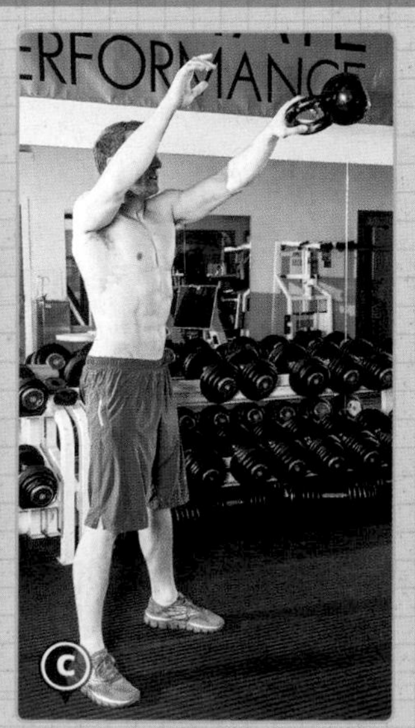

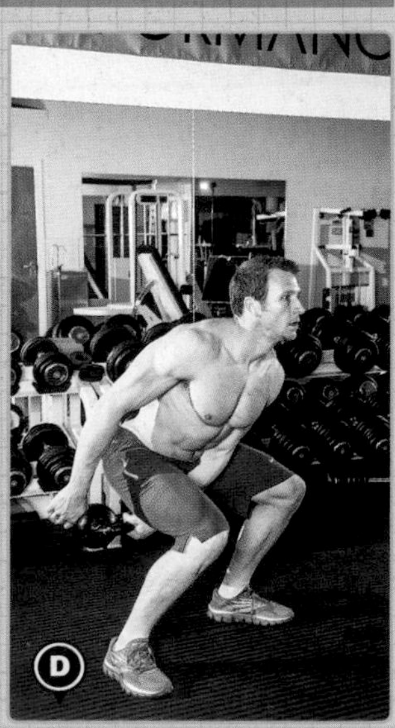

Letting go of the weight from one hand and catching it with your other improves co-ordination.

KETTLEBELL CLEAN

Targets ***Total body***

This classic kettlebell move works every muscle in your body to build explosive power and a strong core

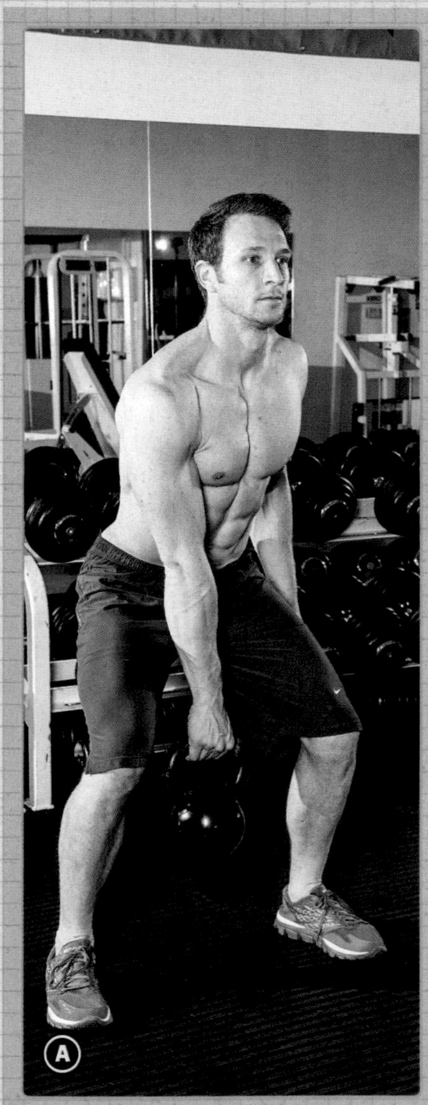

A

Start the move as with the kettlebell swing (see the previous page). Swing the kettlebell upwards with a pop from your hips.

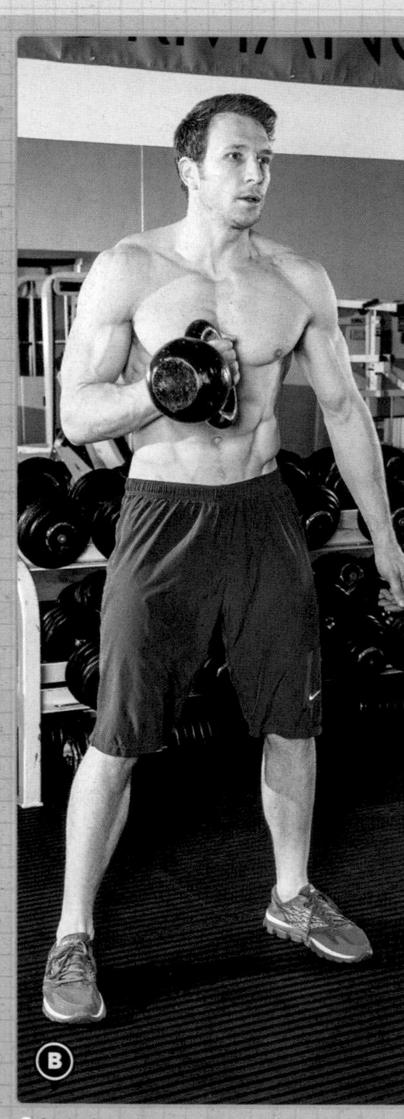

B

As the kettlebell moves upwards, bend your elbow and let the handle slide from your fingers down into your palm to rack the kettlebell on the front of your shoulder, keeping your elbow tucked into your body.

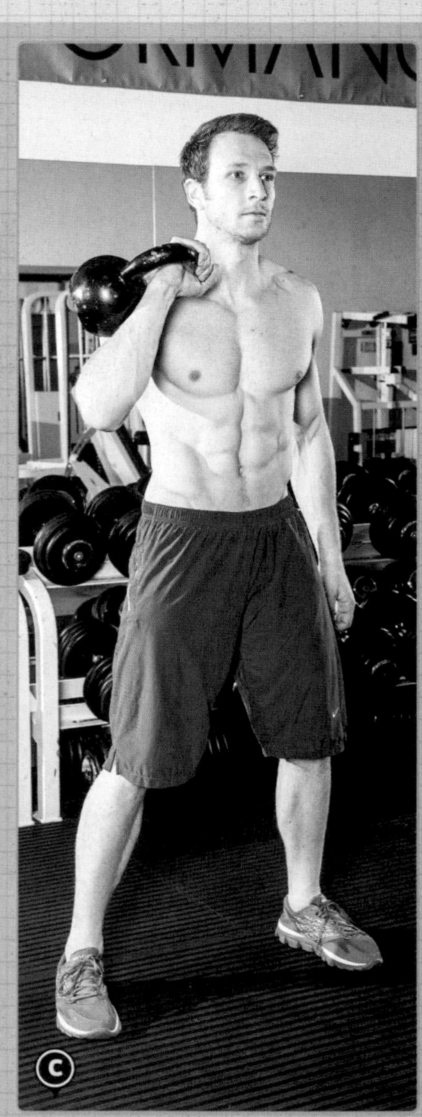

C

Reverse the movement to return to the start position.

Kettlebell clean and press

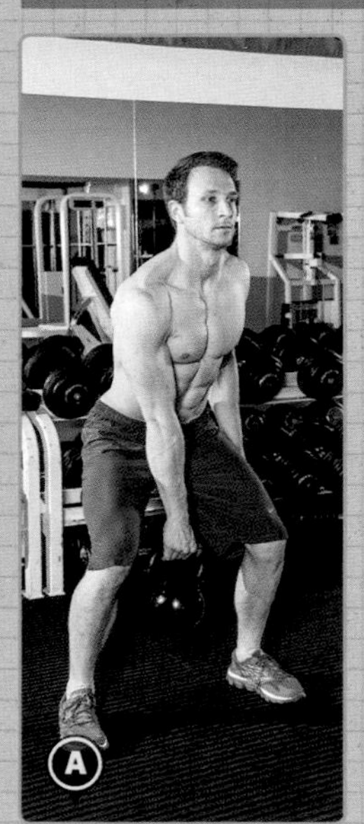

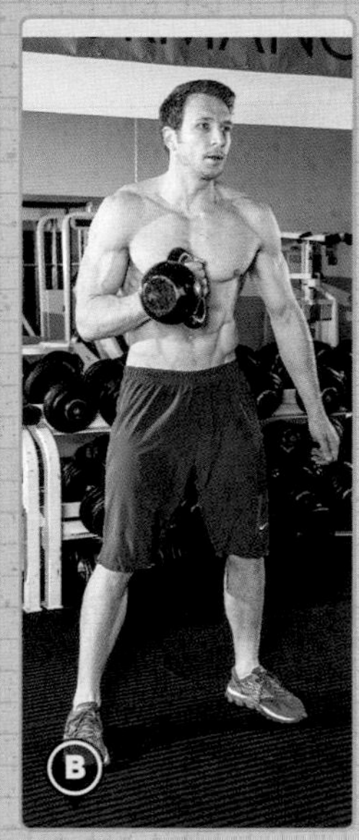

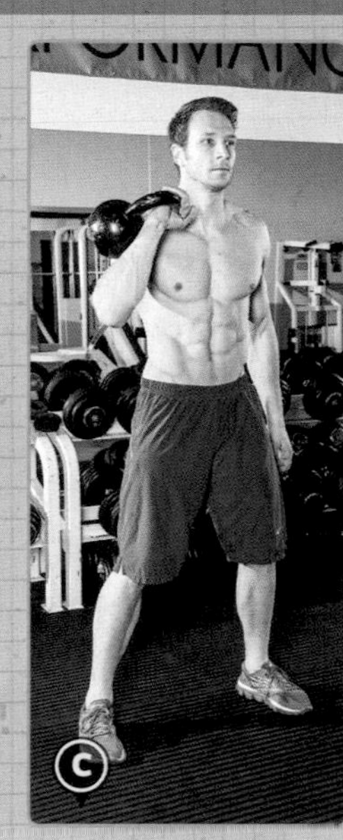

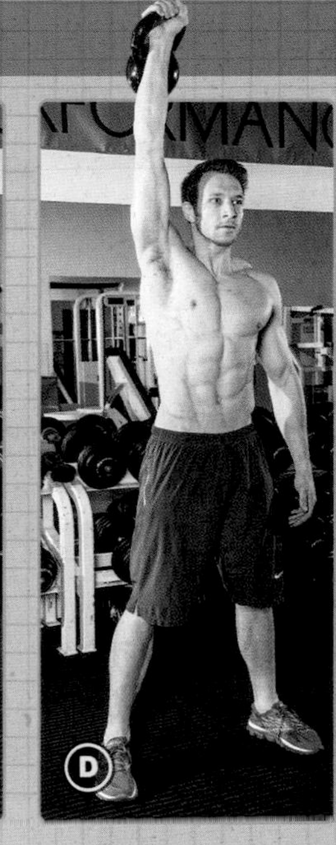

- As the kettlebell moves upwards, bend your elbow and let the handle slide from your fingers down into your palm to rack the kettlebell on the front of your shoulder.
- From this position, straighten your arm to extend the weight directly above your head.
- Reverse the move back to the start.

Kettlebell snatch

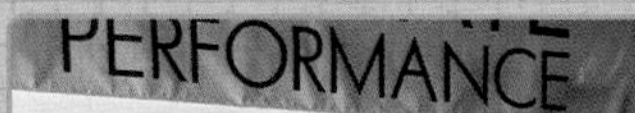

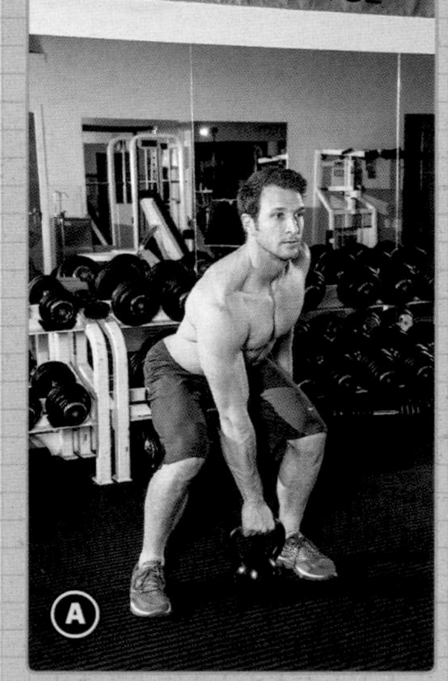

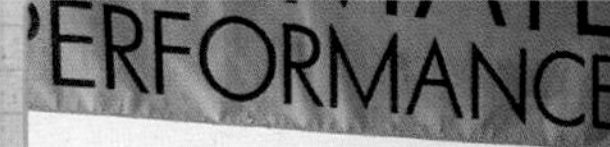

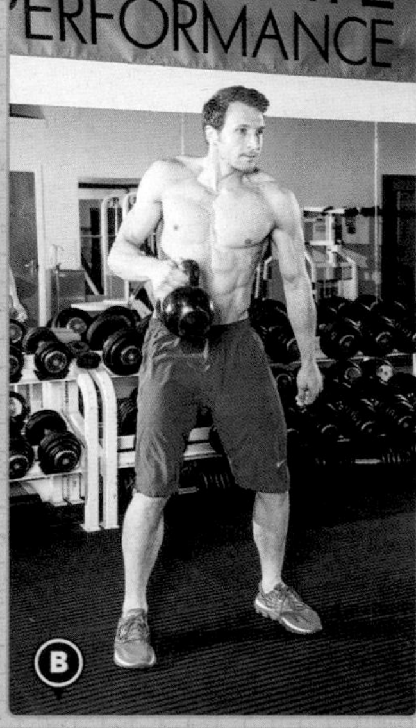

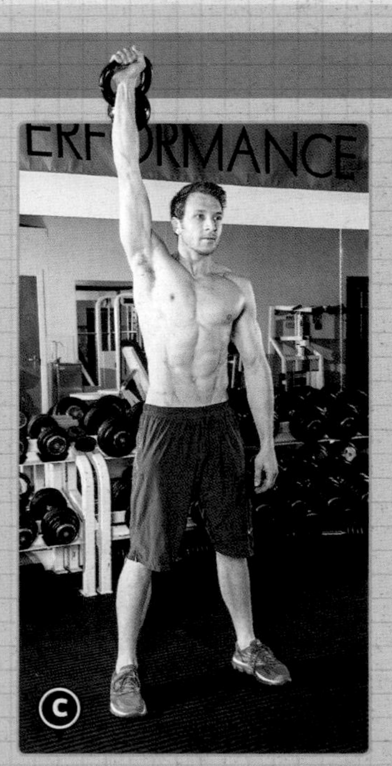

- Swing the kettlebell to start the move, then as it reaches eye level pull your elbow back and 'punch' your hand upwards to catch it at the top of the move – your arm only straightens at the very top. If you do it right, the bell shouldn't bang into your forearm.
- From the top of the move, flip the kettlebell over and progress smoothly into the next swing.

KETTLEBELL SLINGSHOT

Targets *Total body*

This simple but effective moves works your abs and small hip muscles while also improving co-ordination

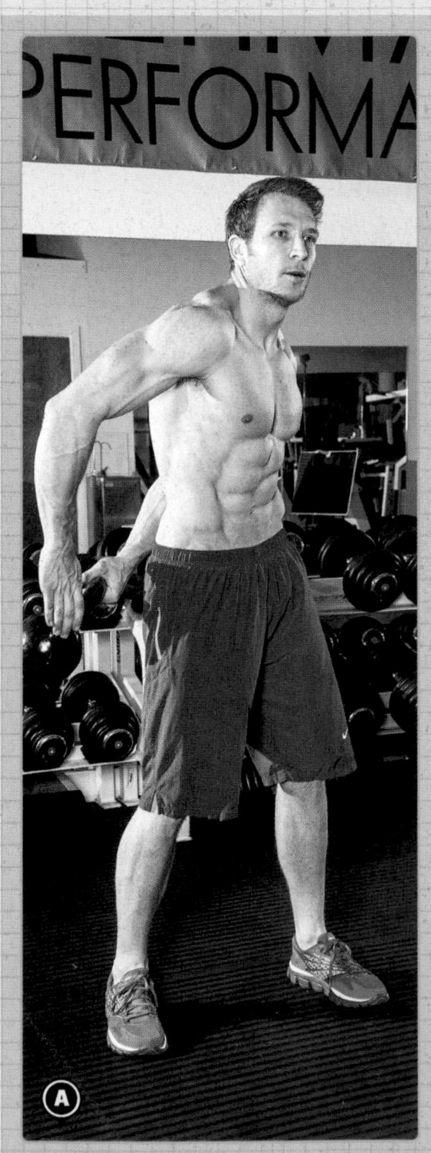

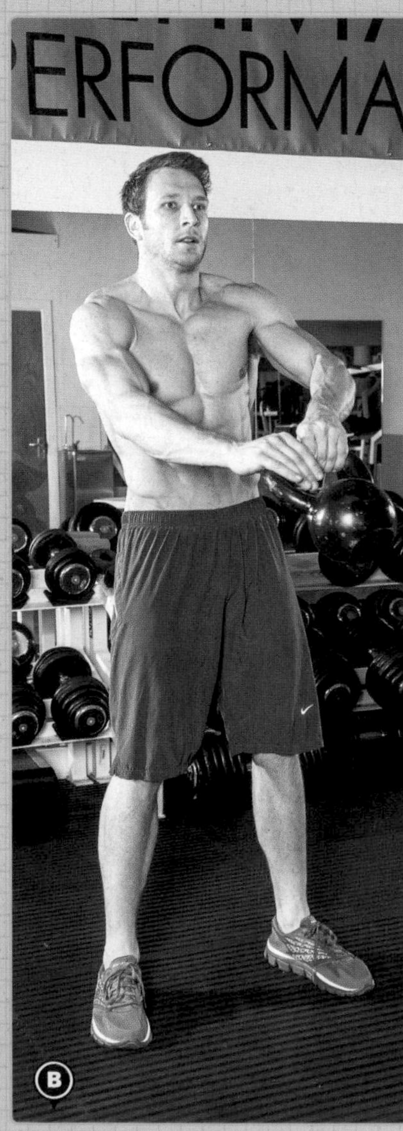

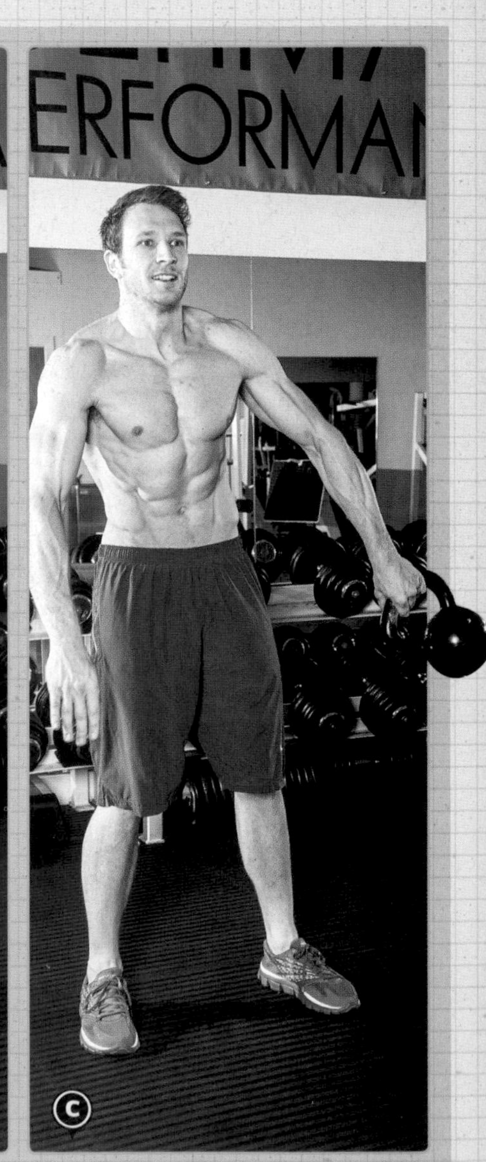

Start to swing the kettlebell around your body, passing it from hand to hand as you go.

Try to keep the movement fluid, while keeping your core braced and back straight.

Kettlebell figure of eight

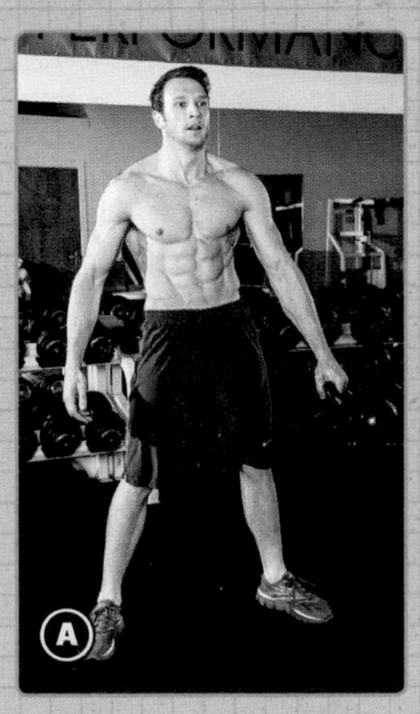

Swing the kettlebell around your body, as with the kettlebell slingshot (left).

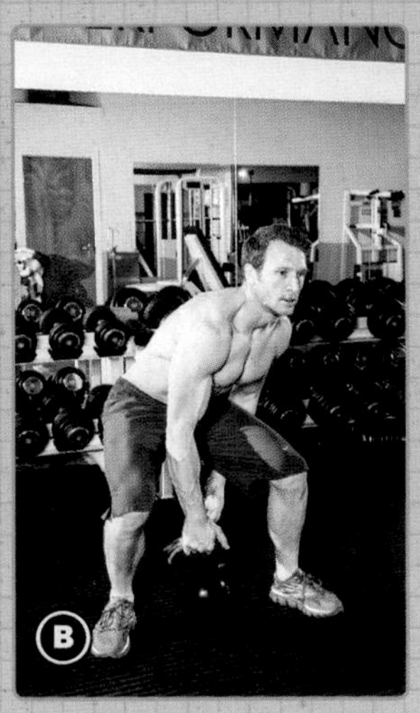

Dip down and pass the kettlebell through your legs in a figure-of-eight motion.

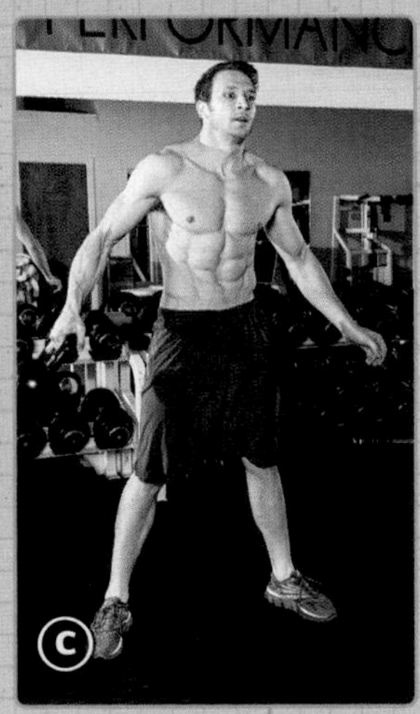

Try to keep the movement fluid, while keeping your core braced and back straight.

Kettlebell halo

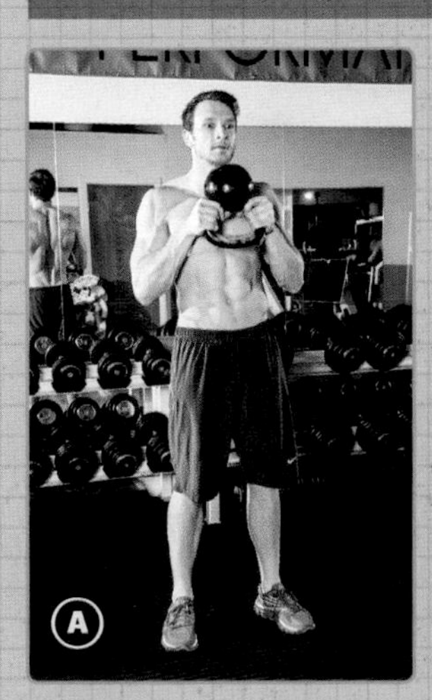

Stand with your feet shoulder-width apart and hold a kettlebell upside down with both hands in front of your face.

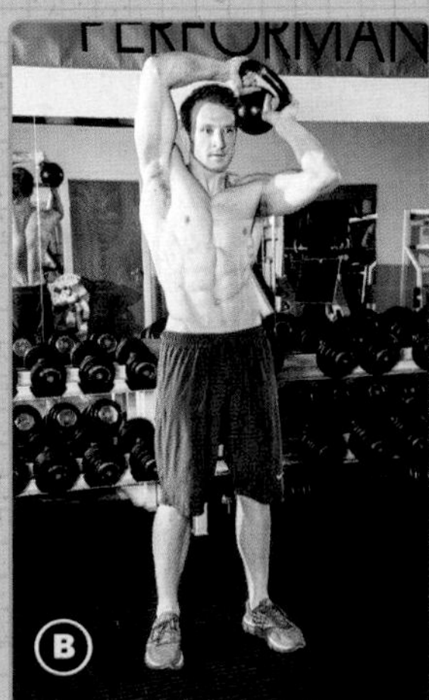

Rotate the kettlebell around your head, keeping your core braced.

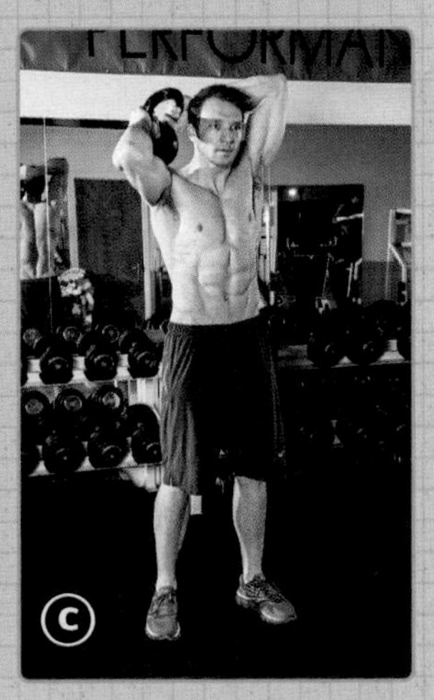

Rotate the kettlebell in both directions equally to work your muscles from every angle.

Kettlebell windmill

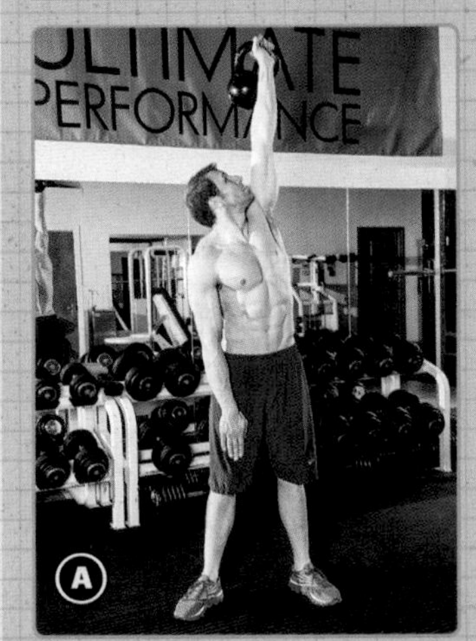

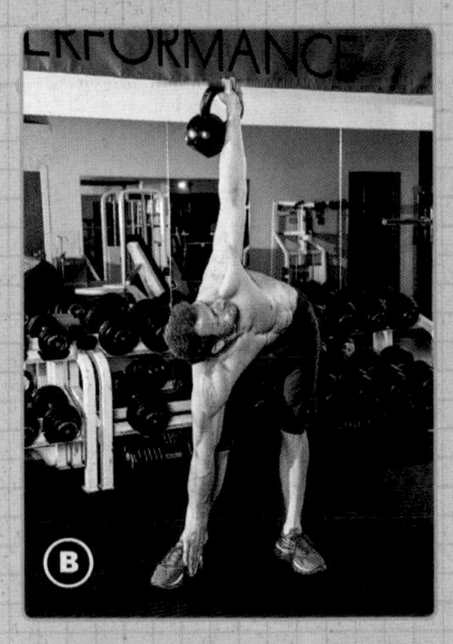

Press the kettlebell above your head into the start position. Keeping the leg under the bell straight and the other one slightly bent, lean your torso forwards and to one side so the other hand travels down your leg. Keep your arms straight throughout.

Turn to face the kettlebell so it's directly overhead at the bottom of the move. Reverse the movement to return to the start.

TURKISH GET-UP

Targets ***Total body***

The classic move popularised by Turkish Olympic lifters builds strength, stability and co-ordination

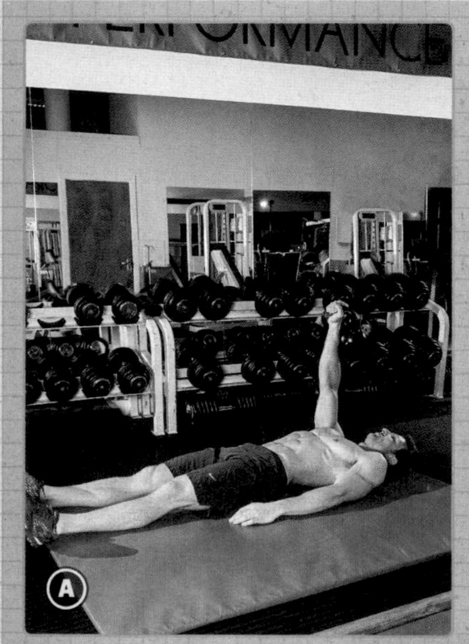

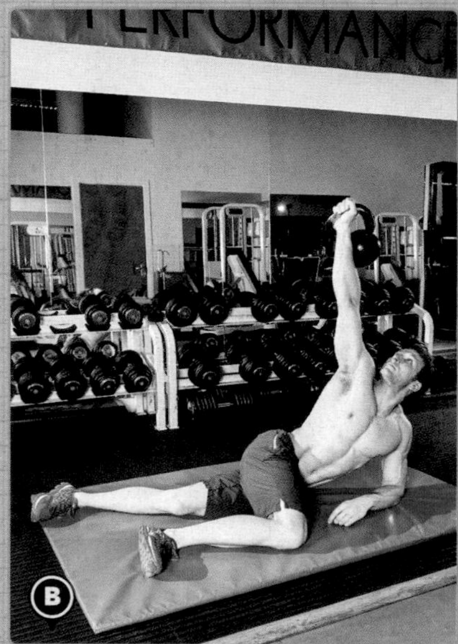

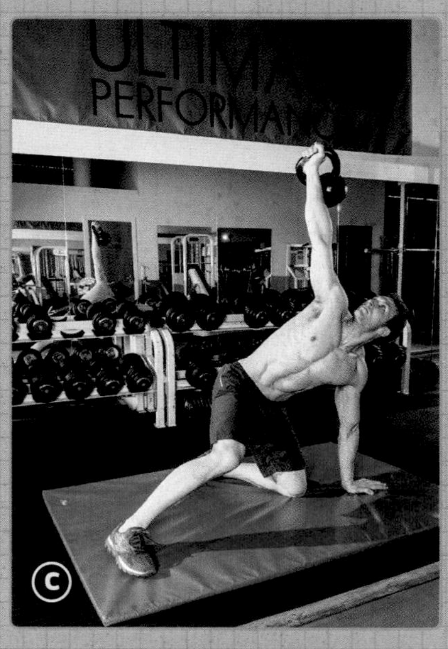

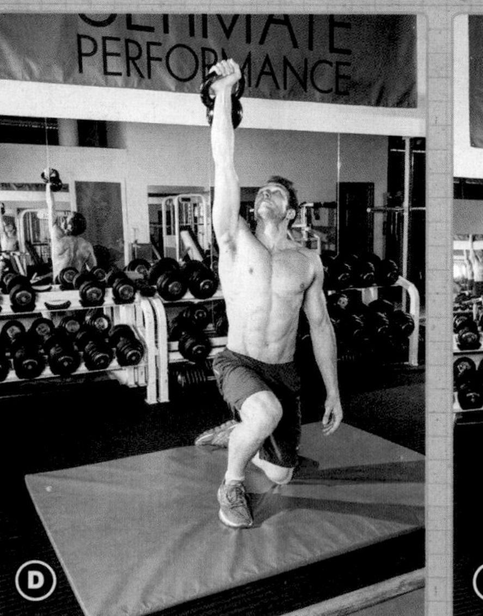

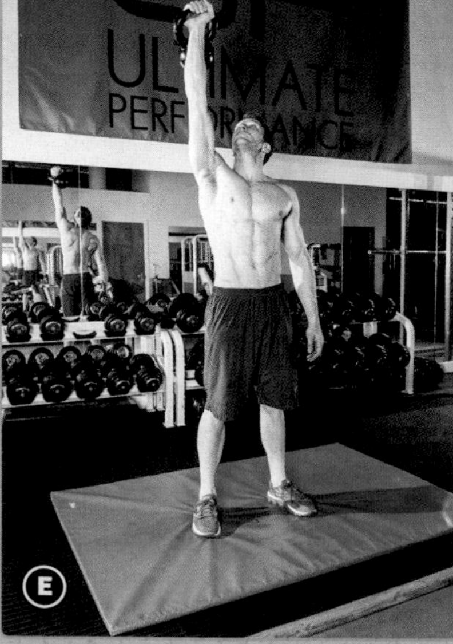

- Lie flat on the floor with one hand by your side and the other directly above you holding a kettlebell.
- Keeping the kettlebell elevated, swing one leg over the opposite leg and rise up on to the elbow of your supporting arm.
- Extend your supporting arm fully and shift your weight forwards to stand up, finishing with the weight over your head before reversing the move back to the start position.

Two-hand anyhow

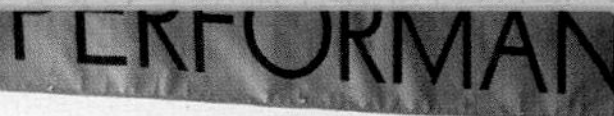

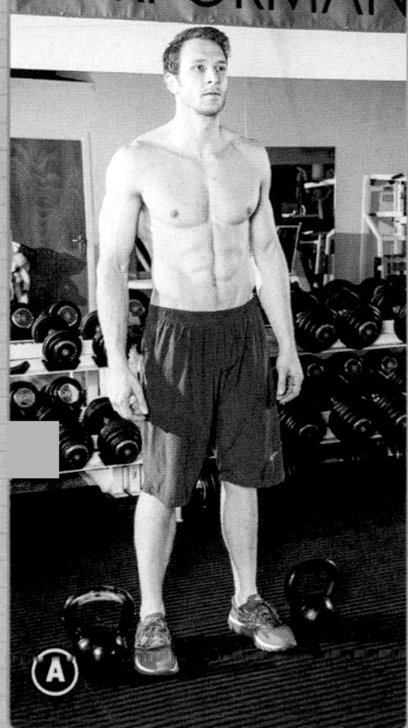

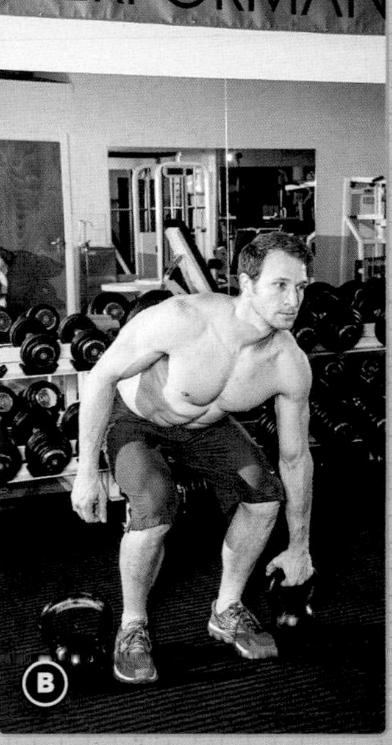

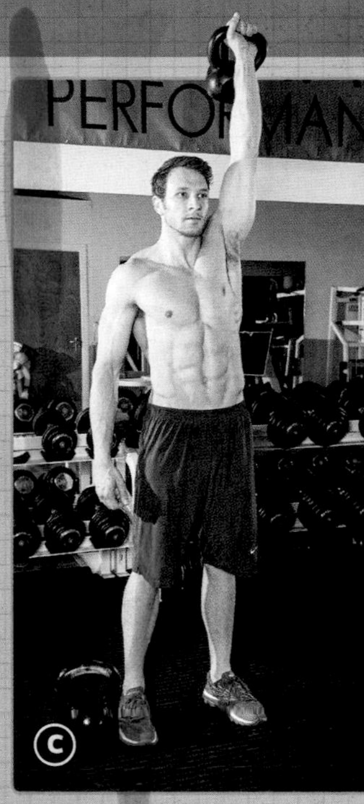

- Stand in front of two kettlebells of equal weights.
- Clean and press the first one directly overhead.
- Perform a windmill to pick up the other kettlebell with your free hand.
- Go into a squat then stand up, curling that kettlebell into the rack position.
- Straighten your arm overhead so both arms are holding kettlebells directly above your head.
- Lower one kettlebell back into the rack position and windmill it to the floor.
- Repeat with the other kettlebell.

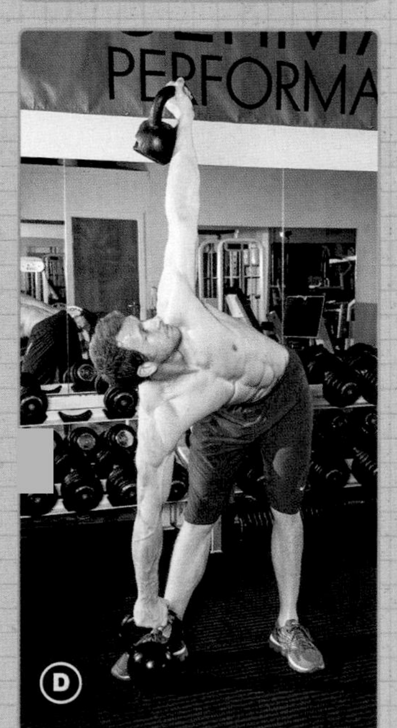

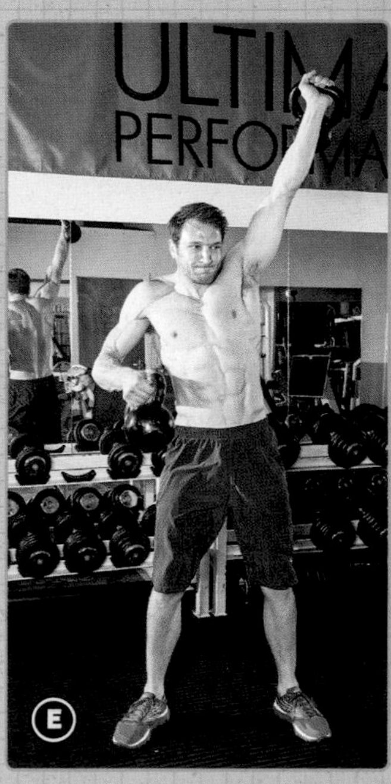

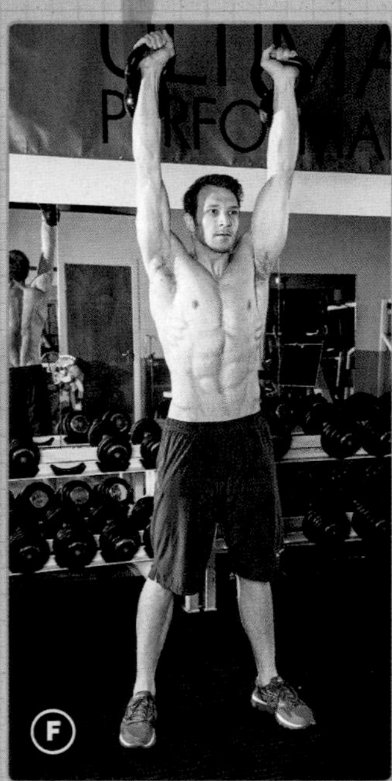

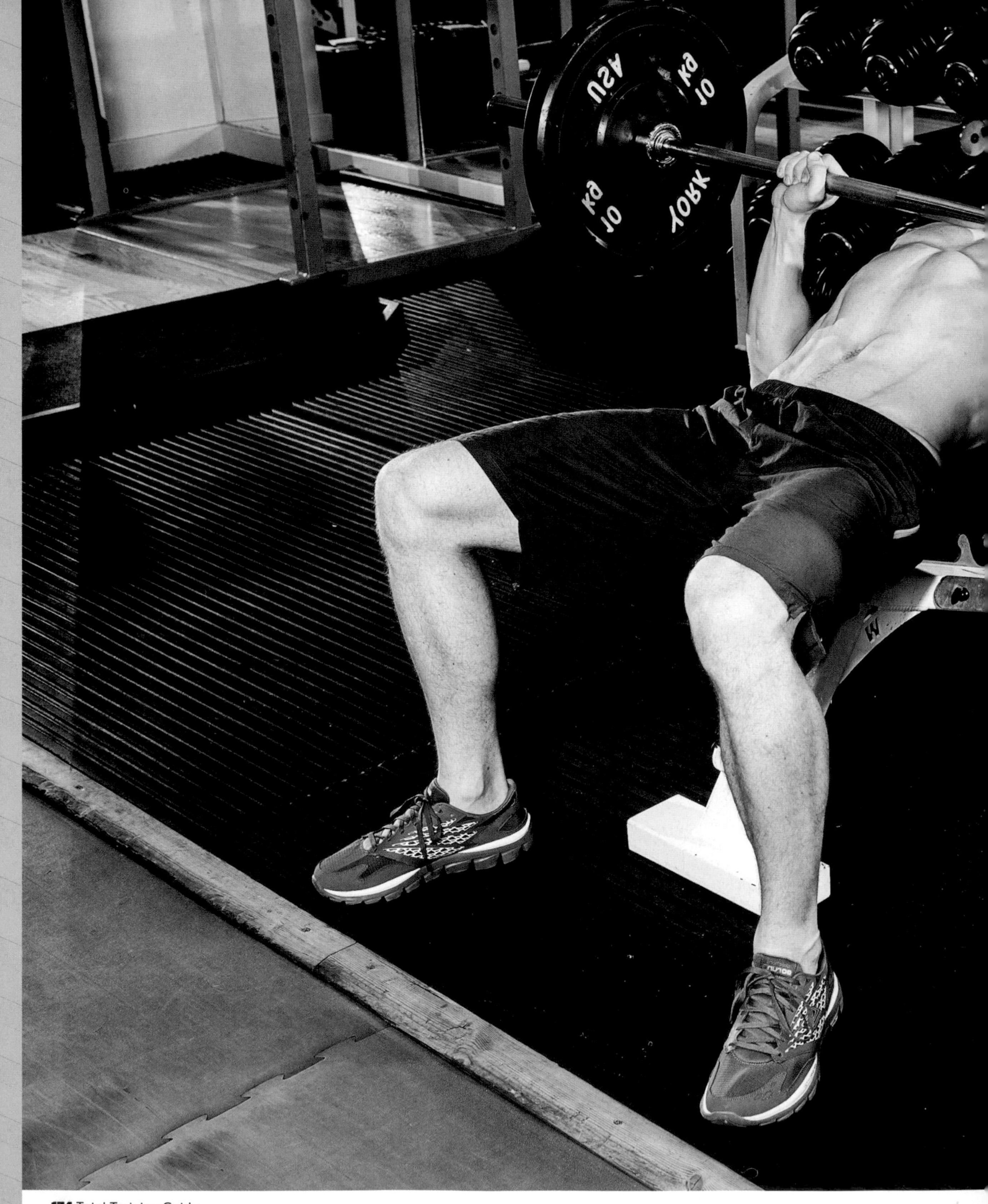
USA
YORK

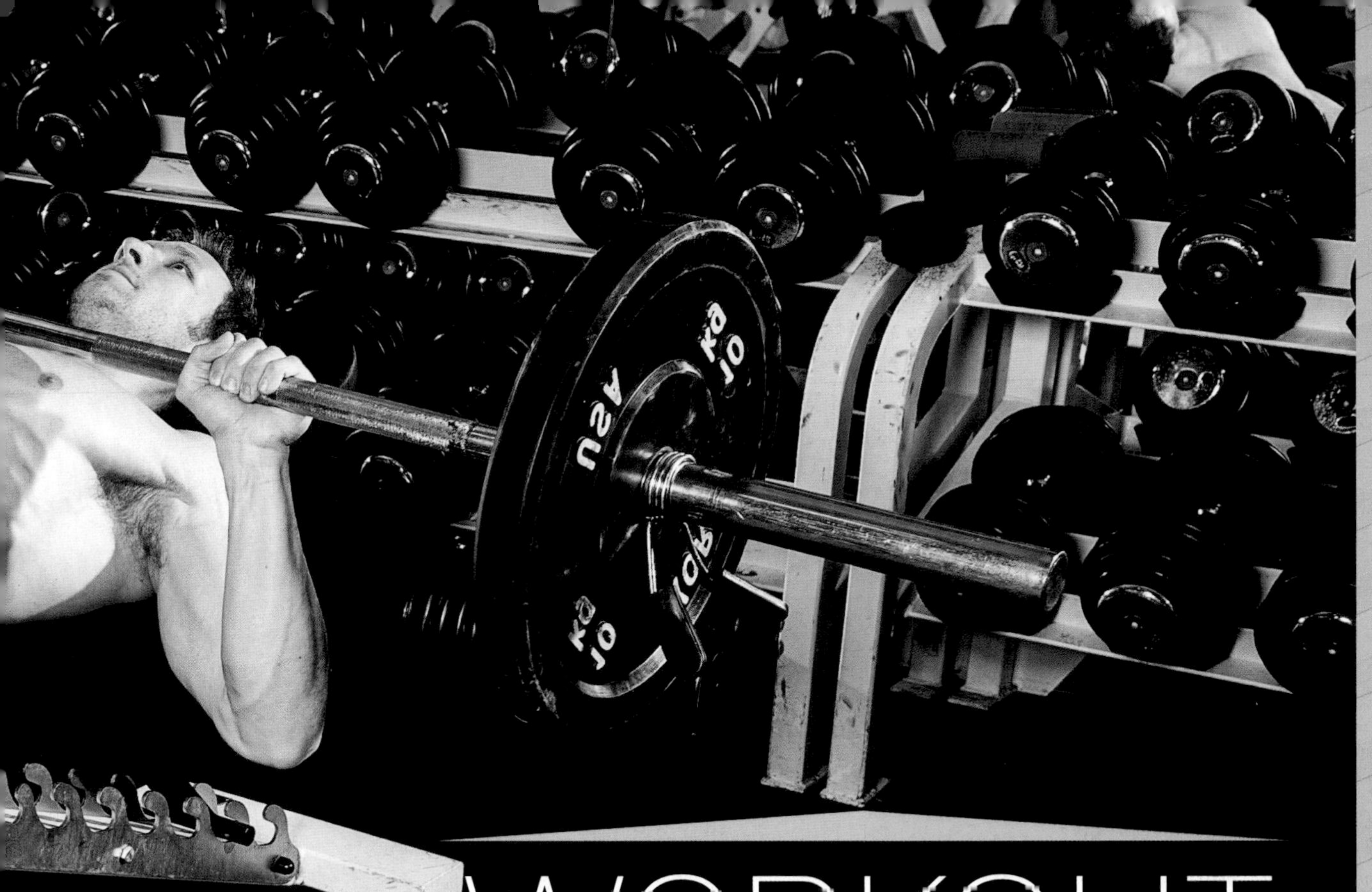

WORKOUT THEORY

Putting workouts together p176

Sets and reps p178

Warming up p180

Training frequency p182

Periodisation p184

Straight sets and supersets p186

Session strategies p188

Pyramids and drop sets p190

Putting workouts together

You know the moves – now it's time to learn how to choose the right ones for the most effective workout

You could learn every exercise in this book but it won't help you get bigger, stronger or leaner. To change your physique you need to understand how these moves should be put together to create an effective training session, and how these sessions come together to form a training programme that will get you to where you want to be.

This chapter looks at the most common, popular and effective workout programmes so you can build one that suits your needs. But before that you need to know the key elements that make up every single workout, regardless of your goal.

The basics

A workout is comprised of six variables.

Exercise selection The lifts you choose to perform in any given workout.

Reps The number of times you perform that move without stopping for rest.

Sets The number of times you perform a certain number of reps.

Weight The amount of resistance you lift for each set.

Tempo The speed at which you perform each rep.

Rest The amount of time you rest between sets and exercises.

The most obvious variable to change between workouts is exercise selection. If you only ever perform the same exercises in the same order at every session, your muscles will quickly adapt and no longer have an incentive to get bigger or stronger. That's why it's also important to increase the weight you lift so your muscles have to lift more than they did before, which provides the stimulus for increased muscle strength and size.

Exercise selection and weight are the two most important variables to change regularly for continued muscle growth, but tampering and tweaking with the other key variables can also have a big impact on your results.

> **"Tweaking the key variables can have a big impact on your results"**

The basics

This chapter explains everything you need to know about putting together a workout, from the very basics (how to select the correct sets and reps range for your training goal) to the more advanced workout strategies (how periodisation can help you to add 20% to any lift in as little as nine weeks). It also covers everything in between, such as how often you should train, how fast you should lift and how long you should rest between exercises.

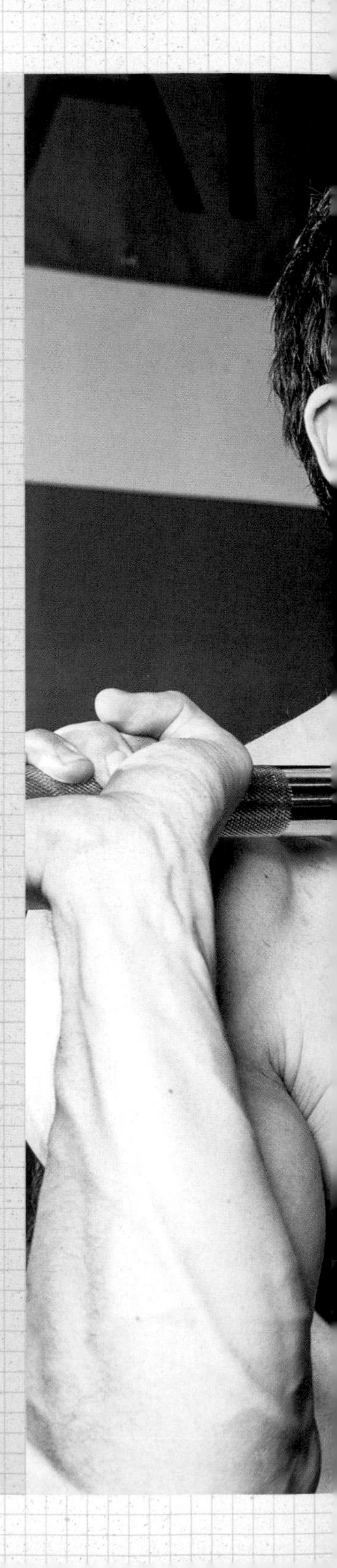

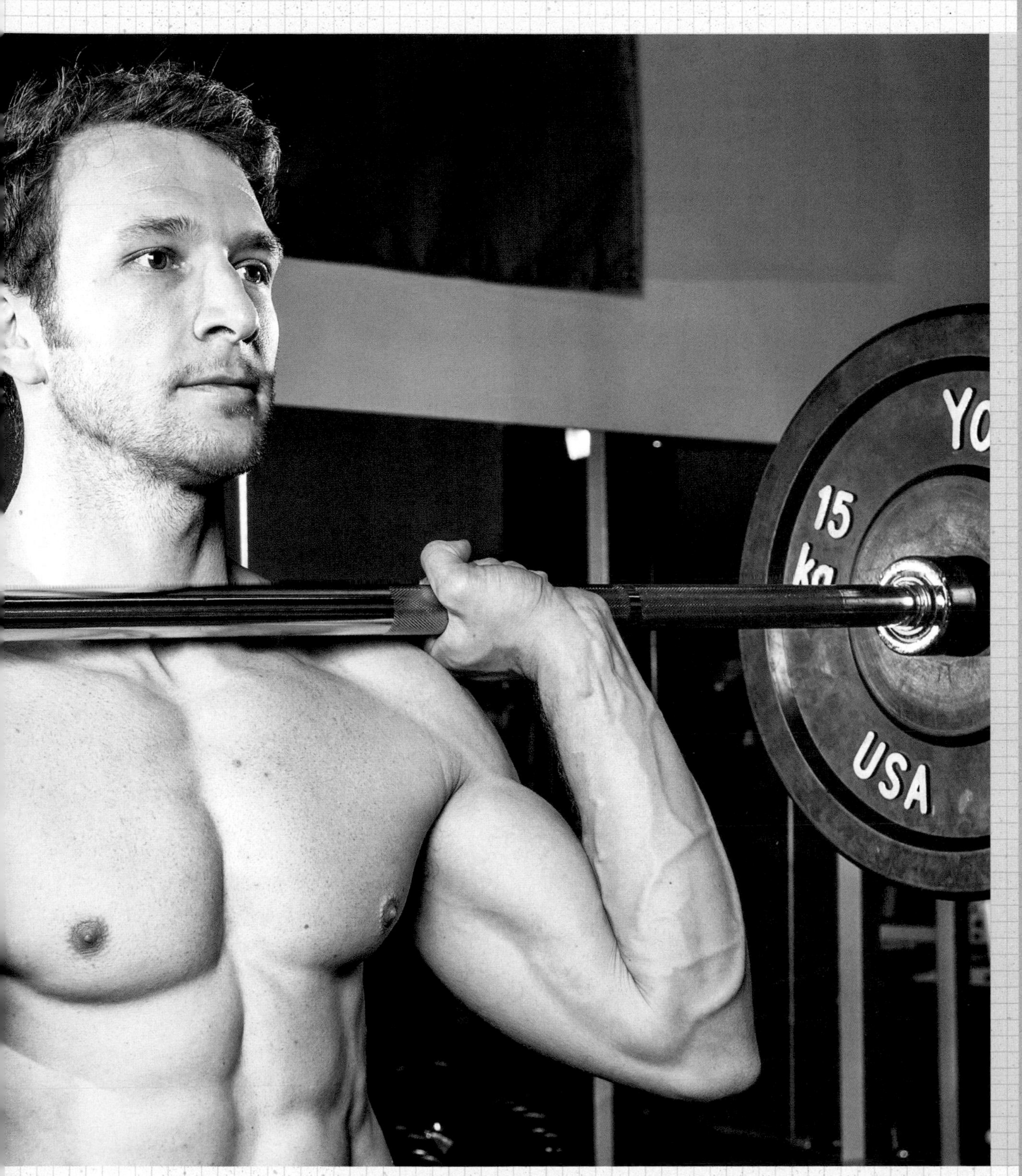
15
USA

The joy of sets

If you don't know how many sets and reps you should be performing you'll never get bigger, stronger or leaner. Here are the basics

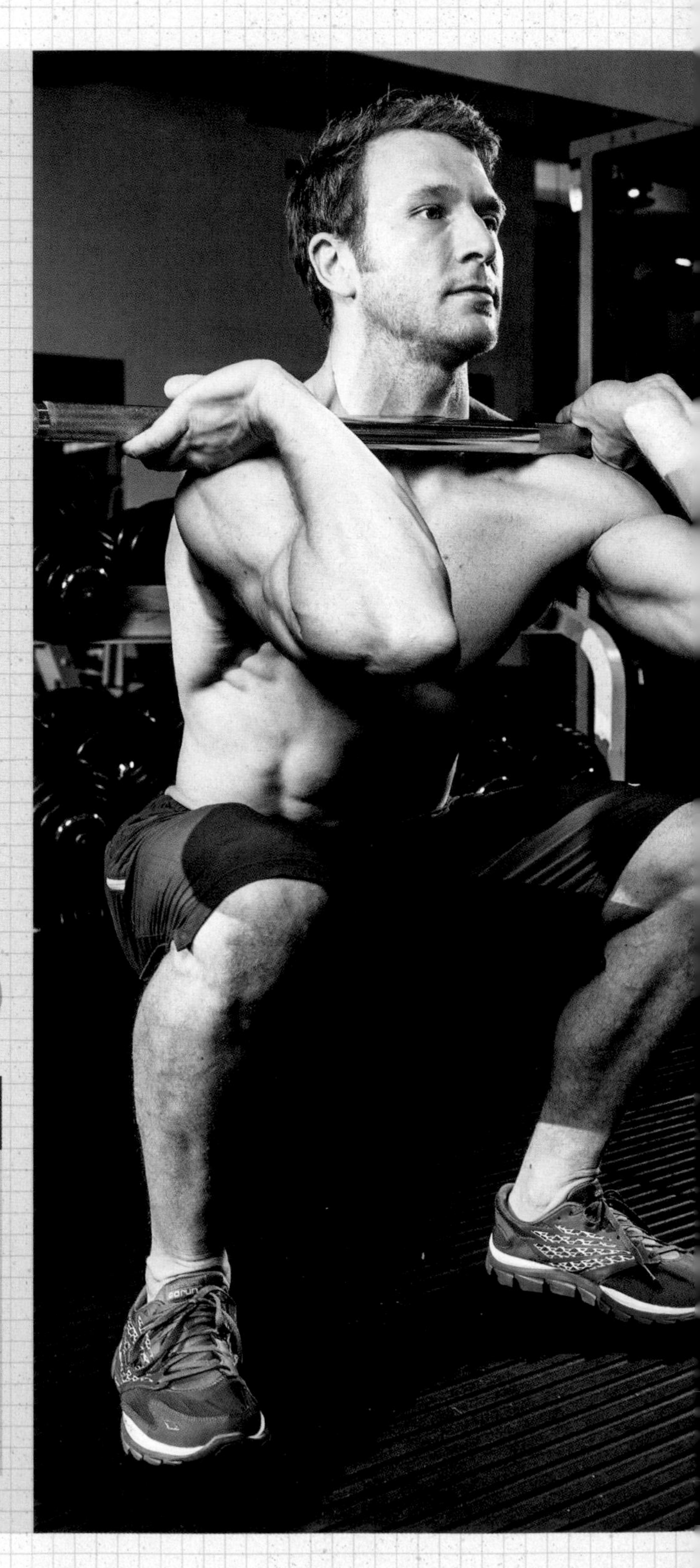

Sets and reps are the bread and butter of your workout. In fact you can't weight train without them. As soon as you lift a weight, even if it's only once, you've completed a rep and a set. But that's not necessarily the best way to build muscle.

Instead you need to lift a weight a certain number of times, rest for a given amount of time, then repeat this process a certain number of times. How many reps you perform per set, and how many sets you perform per exercise, depends entirely on your fitness goals. Here's everything you need to know.

> **The most effective way to build muscle mass is for each set to last between 40 and 70 seconds**

What are reps and sets?

Reps
An abbreviation of repetition, one rep is the completion of a given exercise from start to finish.

Sets
A set is a given number of reps performed consecutively without rest. The number of reps per set can vary from one to more than 20, depending on your training goals. The number of sets performed of each exercise can also vary, but three or four is most effective for building muscle mass.

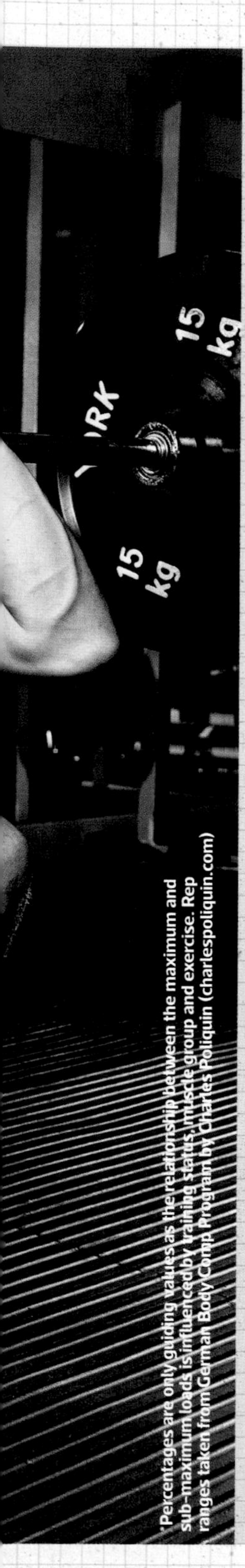

How to pick the right rep range

Performing the appropriate number of reps per set is critical to achieving your goals

1 to 5 reps

Training aim Increase muscle strength and power.
Target weight 85-100% of one-rep max.*
Why? Low-rep sets of heavy weights build strength and power because they recruit, work and fatigue your fast-twitch muscle fibres. It's these fibres that are responsible for your muscles' explosiveness and this approach makes them grow back bigger. This low rep range also improves the communication pathways between your brain and the muscle in question, enabling it to react and contract more quickly and with greater force.

6 to 8 reps

Training aim Optimal compromise between an increase in muscle strength and size.
Target weight 78-83% of one-rep max.*
Why? Completing sets in this rep range will still work your fast-twitch muscle fibres and improve the brain-muscle connection, but performing the extra reps will also fatigue your muscles more thoroughly, resulting in improvements in strength and size.

9 to 12 reps

Training aim Increased muscle mass and improved strength.
Target weight 70-77% of one-rep max.*
Why? The most effective way to build muscle mass is for each exercise set to last between 40 and 70 seconds. Sets of nine to 12 reps are perfect for this because the weight is heavy enough to fatigue the muscles thoroughly but still manageable for you to maintain correct form for the desired length of time.

13+ reps

Training aim Increase in muscle strength endurance with some mass gains.
Target weight 60-69% of one-rep max.*
Why? Using lighter weights for a higher-rep sets recruits, works and fatigues your slow-twitch fibres, instead of your fast-twitch fibres. This rep range also improves the ability of these slow-twitch fibres to deal with lactic acid and the other waste products that accumulate during exercise. You'll see some muscle mass gains, however, especially if you're new to weight training.

*Percentages are only guiding values as the relationship between the maximum and sub-maximum loads is influenced by training status, muscle group and exercise. Rep ranges taken from German Body Comp Program by Charles Poliquin (charlespoliquin.com)

Different types of reps

Because not all reps are created equal

In addition to normal reps, try these variations to keep your muscles guessing – and growing.

Negative reps

Your muscles are stronger in the eccentric, or lowering, phase of each lift than they are in the concentric, or raising, stage. Negative reps take advantage of this strength by using a much heavier weight and starting at the 'top' position of a move and then lowering that weight as slowly as possible, ideally taking more than four seconds to do so.

A good example would be jumping to the top of the pull-up position then slowly lowering yourself back to the start, or having a spotter help you to lift a barbell to the top of a biceps curl before you lower it slowly under your own strength.

Forced reps

Once you reach the stage where your muscles fail and can no longer perform even a single extra rep, a training partner or spotter can step in to help you force out a few extra reps to break down even more muscle tissue.

They do this by helping you get past the 'sticking point' of a given exercise – for example the first half of a biceps curl – before you take over to complete the rep's full range of motion on your own.

Partial reps

These reps only involve movement through a certain part of an exercise's normal full range of motion. In most cases, this is the easiest part of each rep, allowing heavier weights to be used.

Warming up

Get all the elements of your warm-up right and be stronger when you start lifting

Dashing straight from the changing room into your first set without warming up isn't only dangerous, it's also stupid. A proper warm-up not only prepares your muscles for what lies ahead – helping to prevent an unnecessary injury – it also fires up your central nervous system, which means your muscles will contract quicker – making you stronger – when the real workout begins.

But if you thought the best way to warm-up was five or ten minutes on the treadmill, it's time to think again. How can a gentle jog prime your muscles for a hard weights session, especially if you're training your upper body? Here's what you need to do.

Steady progression

The most effective way to warm up your muscles is to perform progressively heavier versions of the moves you'll do in your workout. Start with a few reps at an easy weight then gradually increase the weight – keeping the reps low to minimise fatigue – until you reach your work-set weight. Here's the formula you should stick to ensure you select the right weights for each warm-up set.

Say the first move of your workout is the squat and your target work-set weight is 100kg for 10 reps.

Warm-up set one
8 reps at 30% (33kg), minimal rest

Warm-up set two
5 reps at 50% (50kg), 30-60sec rest

Warm-up set three
3 reps at 70% (70kg), 45-75sec rest

Warm-up set four
2 reps at 85% (85kg), 60-75sec rest

Warm-up set five
1 rep at 95% (95kg), 60-75sec rest

Start first work set

You only need to do this for the first two moves of the workout. For all other moves for the same or similar body parts, select a weight about two-thirds of your work-set weight and perform four to six reps to get your muscles working. However, if you're moving to a new muscle group, do this warm-up sequence again to be protected against injury. If chin-ups, pull-ups or dips are among your first two moves, use a resistance machine to warm up instead.

Activation advantage

Do explosive movements before your set to fire up your muscles even further

- Explosive movements before your initial work set can further activate your central nervous system to elicit greater reaction and force from your muscles. Before pushing exercises, for example, hurl a medicine ball at the ground as hard as possible, do a couple of clap press-ups or unleash a couple of left and right hooks on punch bag. For lower-body exercises, a couple of hard kicks to a heavy bag will do the trick, or a few jump squats.
- These sets really tax the muscles, so leave a good few days between sessions to allow for sufficient recovery.

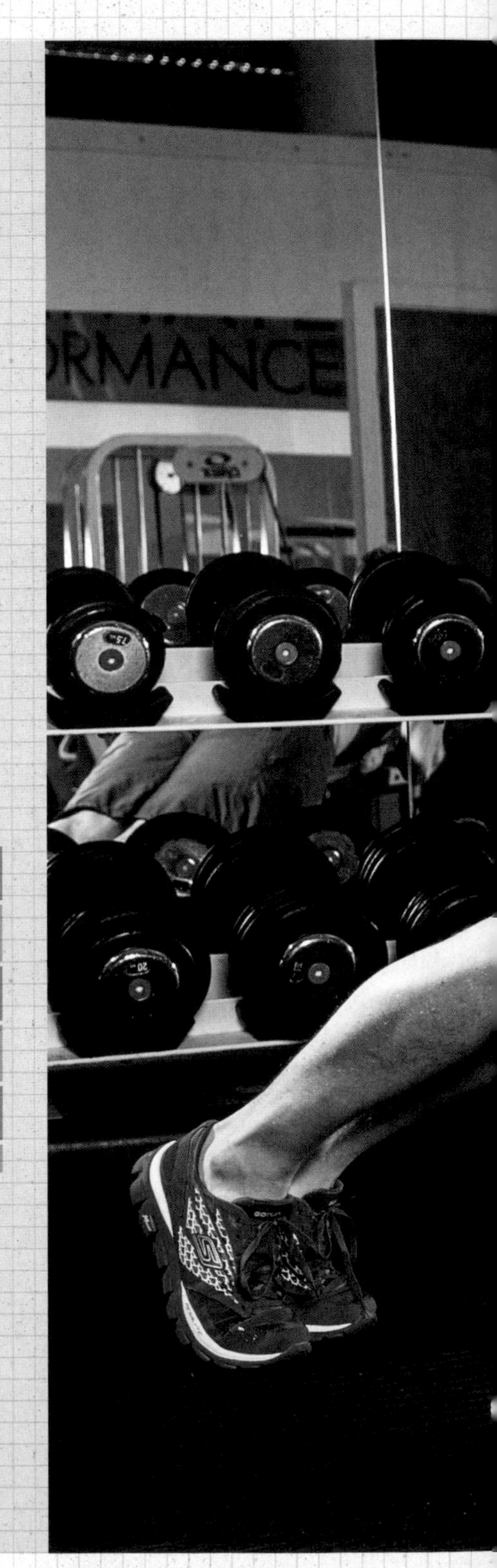

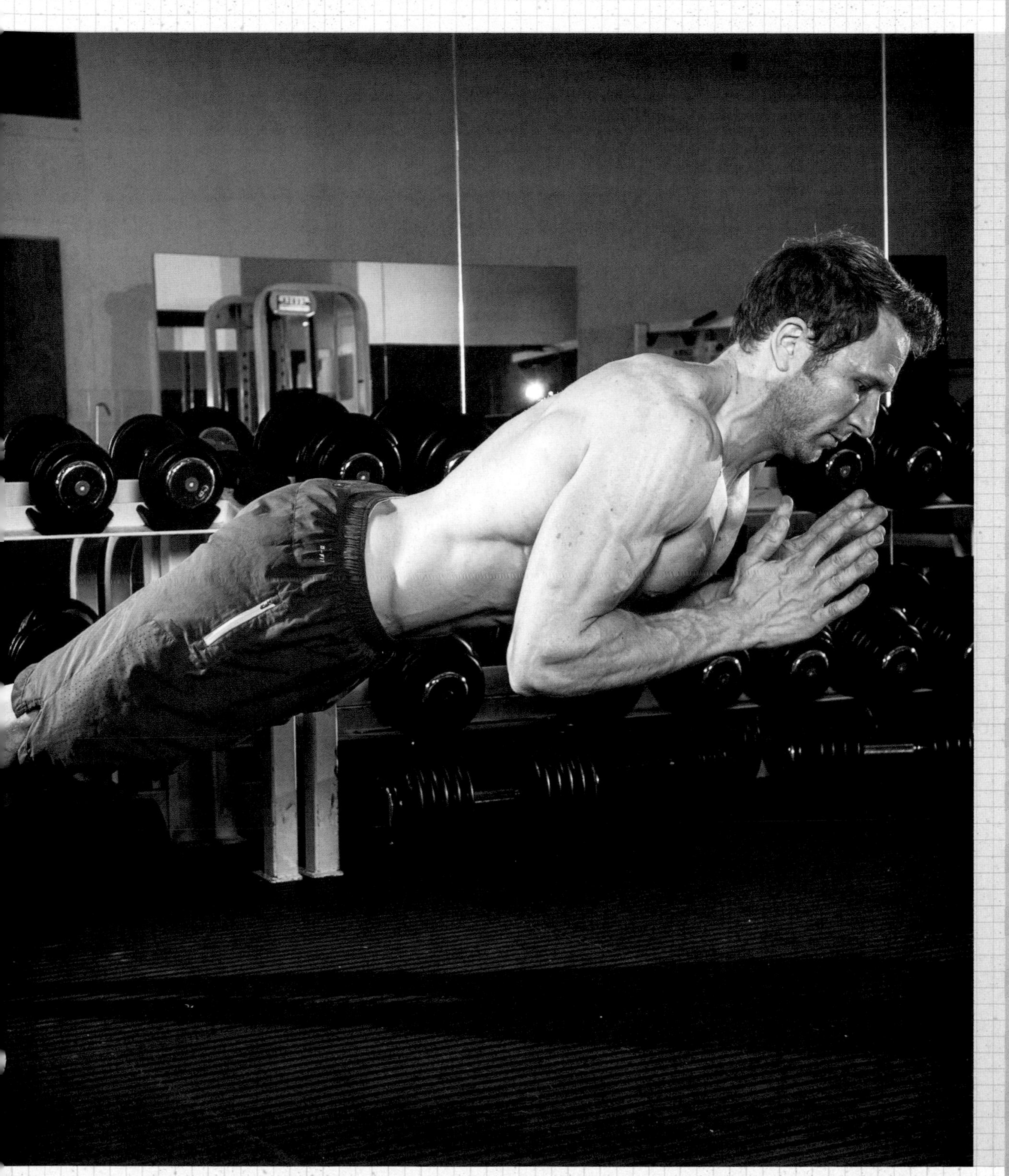

Training frequency

What's the ideal number of weekly training sessions for the best results? And how much rest do you really need between them?

What many people don't realise is that your muscles don't grow while you're in the gym. Of course, they appear bigger when you lifting, but that's only because they are filled with blood that creates that 'pumped' look.

So although weight training is required for making muscles bigger and stronger, it's in between sessions when the damaged muscle fibres are repaired that your muscles grow. This means that planning your rest is as important as planning your training.

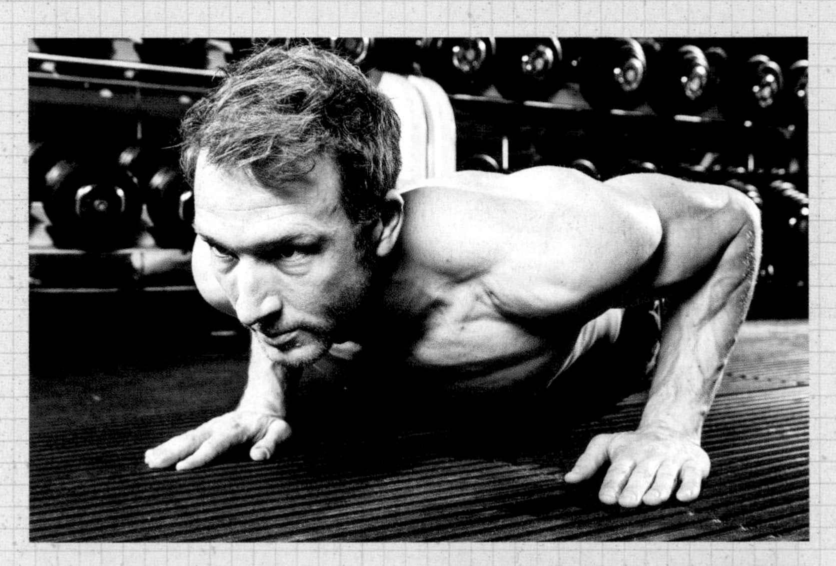

Rest assured

Taking too long between sessions can reduce stimulus momentum, whereas too little recovery time can limit gains while also increasing the risk of fatigue, overtraining, injury and mental boredom.

You'll know when you have had sufficient rest because you'll feel fresh and strong. That's because your body has 'super-compensated' from the training so you are stronger. At this point you can push yourself harder than you did before, and the positive adaptive process repeats itself so you keep getting bigger and stronger.

Own goals

So what's the perfect amount of time needed to recover from a session so that you are in prime condition when you next hit the gym? Again, everything depends on your goals.

If you are training for power then you'll need to leave up to three days between sessions, because power training involves low-rep, high-weight, multi-joint moves, which are very taxing on both the muscles and your central nervous system.

If you're increasing strength, aim to train each muscle group twice a week, which means you should leave between 24 and 48 hours between sessions that target the same muscle group. If you are following a split programme, rather than doing total-body sessions, it's fine to do upper body one day and legs the next, but you still need to factor in some good-quality rest each week. The same rules apply for building muscle size.

Strong sense

For muscular endurance, which uses lighter weights for a high number of reps, you don't need as much rest because this type of training doesn't do so much fibre damage to the muscle as the others, and so can be performed more frequently. That said, still leave at least 24 hours between sessions, and take one or two rest days a week.

At a glance: Training frequency

- Rest is as important as training in your muscle-building goals because it's during the time between sessions that your muscles are repaired and grow.
- Too little rest between workouts means your muscles won't have fully recovered, so you may struggle to lift the same weights for the same sets and reps as before.
- Too much rest between workouts means you are won't be pushing your muscles at the required intensity or giving them sufficient stimulus to grow.

Rest

Getting your rest periods between sets right will help you achieve your fitness aims sooner

Rest is a training variable just as important as sets, reps, weight and tempo in ensuring you hit your fitness target.

When you lift weights, you do so to push your muscles out of their comfort zone because this stress makes them stronger. But there is only so much work they can perform before their energy stores become depleted, hampering their ability to perform additional reps with good form. By resting for a predetermined period you give your body time to resupply the muscle cells with fuel so they can do more lifting.

Time out

How long you rest between sets depends on your objectives. When training for power, you need to lift moderate to high weights at speed, which taxes your central nervous system. This neuromuscular fatigue clogs up the pathways between your brain and muscles, so without sufficient rest you are unable to send the signal that fires up the muscles as quickly as you need to get the bar moving on the next set. Rest of at least three minutes is needed between sets, if not four or five.

When training for gains in strength you need to rest for about the same time as when lifting for power because the volume and intensity is such that it causes both muscular and neuromuscular fatigue.

Hypertrophy, or size increase, is all about working the muscles so hard they start to break down, which stimulates your body to repair them so they get bigger. Because you need to work your muscles for between 40 and 70 seconds per set to stimulate growth, this increased time under tension creates a build-up of lactic acid in the muscles, which is painful. So rest for between 60 and 90 seconds between each set, which should be enough time for most of the lactic acid to be removed so you can hit the muscles hard again.

If you want your muscles to be able to handle a load for a longer period of time, you should train with a light weight for high reps and with little time to recover. This trains your muscles to deal with lactic acid build-up more efficiently so you can keep going for longer so keep rest periods as brief as possible, ideally under 60 seconds.

At a glance: Rest

- Rest between sets and exercises allows your muscles to replenish their energy stores.
- Not resting for long enough means your muscles won't be as capable of performing the set with good form.
- Resting for too long can result in you not testing your muscles enough to force them to grow back bigger and stronger.

Tempo

The most often neglected training variable is one you can't afford to ignore if you want to add serious muscle

Tempo is the speed at which you lift and lower the weight during each rep. The longer you take over each rep, the harder your muscles must work to manage and control the load. The duration of time your muscles are working is commonly known as 'time under tension' (TUT).

Research shows that your muscles need to be under tension for between 40 and 70 seconds per set to elicit a muscle-building response. If you currently perform quick reps and complete sets in less than 40 seconds then start by with a 'two seconds up, two seconds down' approach for sets of ten reps, which should be enough of a change to result in a significant increase in muscle mass. You can then stick to this tempo and up the weight, or slow the tempo even more.

At first, reduce the amount of weight you lift to ensure you hit the correct tempo on every rep of your set. Although it is important to lift heavy to build muscle, it's better to go a little lighter but increase the time under tension. This will have a far more beneficial effect than going a bit heavier in the short term.

If you're unsure of how fast or slowly you should be lifting, ask yourself what you are training for. If you want to train for speed, lift quickly; for maximal strength then lift heavy; for maximal size lift less heavy but slower; and for improved endurance capacity then lift lighter for longer. Those are the rules to stick to.

At a glance: Tempo

- Tempo is the speed at which you lift and lower a weight.
- The slower the tempo, the longer your muscles are exposed to the stress of managing the weight. This is called 'time under tension'.
- The more damage you do to your muscles during training, the bigger and stronger they will grow.
- Performing each rep very quickly can help build explosive power, but only if you maintain perfect form throughout otherwise you risk injury.

Periodisation

Increasing the weight you lift each session will ensure you keep progressing

Never mind the advances in science and cutting-edge fitness thinking – sometimes you'll find the best advice has been around for some time. Thousands of years, in fact.

Varying the intensity of training over a series of cycles to avoid a plateau – or 'periodisation' – became popular in the 20th century, but it was the Ancient Greeks who first realised the benefits. Legend says the strongman Milo of Croton used a calf as his training tool of choice. As the young cow grew, the weight he had to lift increased.

Repetitive strain

Periodisation may be well established but that doesn't mean it's common knowledge in every weights room. One of the most common mistakes made in the pursuit of new muscle is doing the same thing week in, week out.

If you keep doing the same thing, eventually you'll stop improving. But if you increase the load you're lifting you'll gain muscular size and strength.

This phenomenon, known as general adaptation syndrome, is something periodisation seeks to exploit. And the key is to incrementally increase the amount of weight you lift for a given lift – while performing the same number of sets and reps at the same tempo – each time you do that move. A good starting point is to add 2.5% each session on upper-body moves, and 5% for lower-body lifts.

Weighting game

So, if you use realistic load increases and well-timed rest weeks you can keep getting bigger and stronger, right? Not quite. It was just as well for old Milo that eventually his cow stopped growing. That's because progression isn't linear and you can't keep adding 2.5% or 5% to your lifts every week indefinitely. There's only so much your body can do. You'll experience a steep improvement curve to start off with and that will slow to incremental changes. It's important to realise that the longer you train the harder it is to make progress.

"If you keep doing the same thing, eventually you'll stop improving. But if you increase the load you lift, you'll gain size and strength"

It may become increasingly challenging to get bigger and stronger once you've been training for years, even if you do use periodisation. But without using periodisation, it's virtually impossible.

Log your progress

A key part of periodisation is keeping a training log to track your progress. If you don't record what you do, you have no way of knowing whether you're increasing the stress you're placing on your body or whether you're improving. Another important aspect of periodisation is taking rest or recovery weeks. You can use the same workouts for four to six weeks, improving week on week, but after that you may find you're not able to push on so it's a great idea to take a week off or a week of active recovery by doing half the volume you would usually do.

At a glance: Periodisation

- Structure your periodisation programme according to your goal. If you want strength and hypertrophy, keep your sets and reps the same but increase the weight.
- Don't increase the load you lift each week by more than 2.5% for upper-body moves and 5% for lower-body exercises.
- Include a rest week at the end of each cycle of weekly load increases. Cycles can last between two and 12 weeks, but four to six is likely to give you the best results.
- You can vary the load you lift within a short amount of time. Known as a microcycle, this will increase your chances

Serious gains

Use periodisation to add 20% to any exercise in nine weeks

This chart shows the progression you could make using periodisation over nine weeks. This is based on someone who starts by bench pressing 60kg – but it's the structure of the progression, rather than the type of exercise, that's key. If you lift more or less than 60kg, adjust the starting weight but follow the same level of progression, making sure you don't add more than about 2.5% each week.

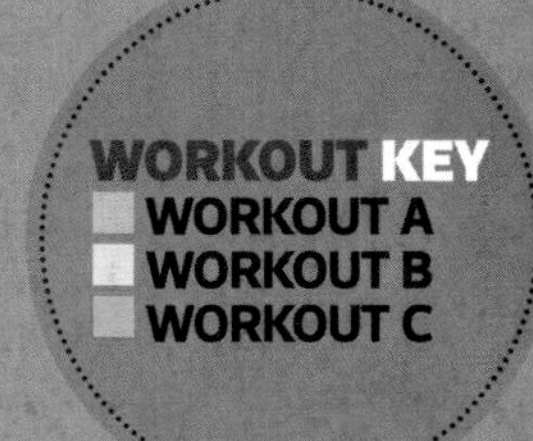

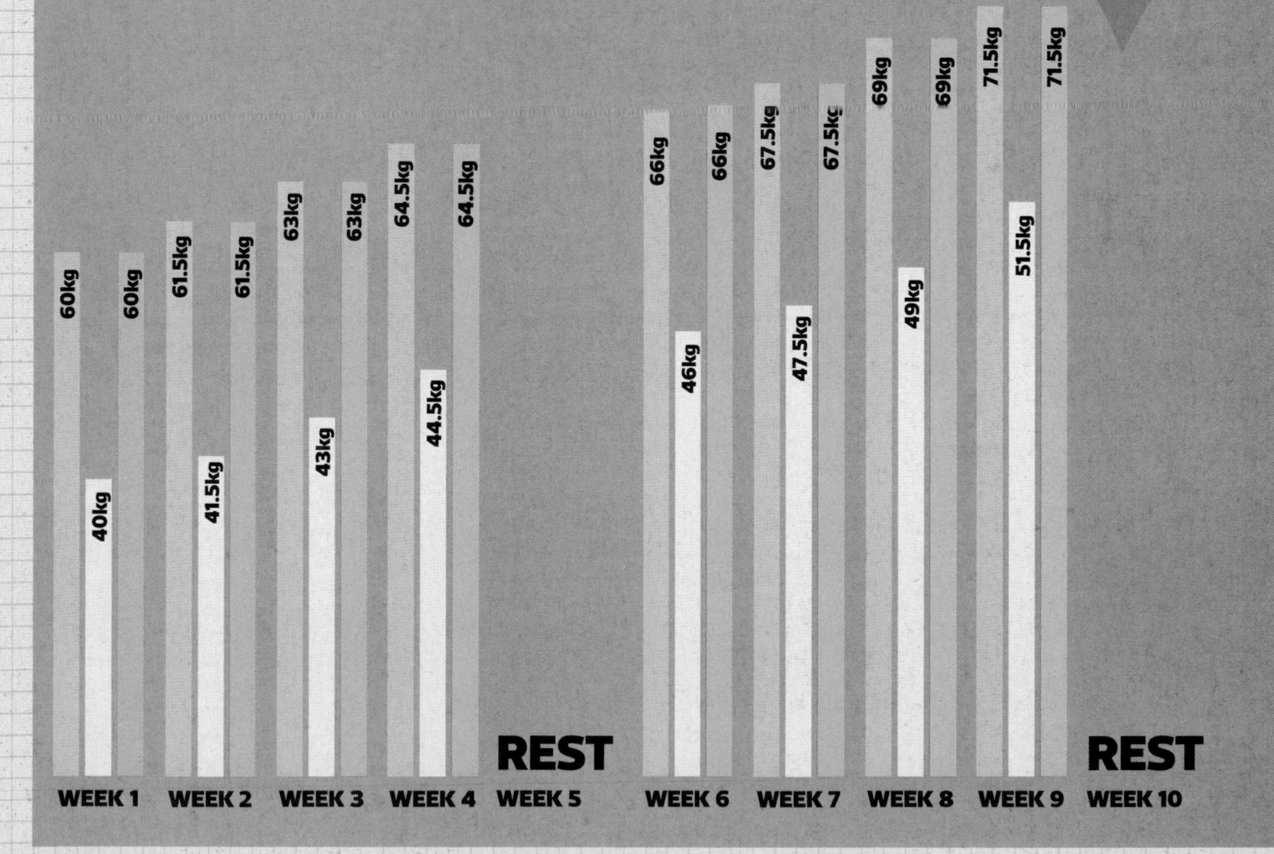

Straight sets and supersets

Add muscle size and strength with these set strategies

These simple but highly effective exercise strategies should form the basis of your workouts when you start to put your training routine together. Here's everything you need to know about how straight sets and supersets work.

Straight sets

Straight sets require you to perform one exercise for a certain number of repetitions, usually eight to 12 for muscle-building programmes, followed by a short rest, then another set the same. This is the most basic approach to weightlifting but it can be the most effective, especially if you are new to training with weights.

Straight sets

What are they?
Performing a certain number of reps of the same exercise before resting and repeating.

Such as?
Three sets of ten reps of the bench press is a typical straight-sets workout.

Why should I do them?
The aim is to work the target muscle group to failure. In this case you would select a weight you can lift ten times for the first two sets, so that by the end of the third set of repetitions your muscles are so fatigued you can't do a single extra rep. Straight sets are also great for preparing a muscle group, and its stabilising muscles, for more advanced workouts.

Supersets

Supersets involve doing two different exercises back to back and they're a great way to shake up your existing training regime: they shock your muscles into growing because of the increased workload and they allow you to work out harder in less time, improving your muscles' ability to work harder without as much rest.

There are many different superset workouts you can do. Here are some of the most popular and effective set strategies to add serious muscle in less time.

Antagonistic supersets

What are they?
A superset of two exercises that works opposing muscles groups, affording each group additional recovery time between sets.

Such as?
A set of dumbbell bench presses (chest and triceps) followed immediately by a set of one-arm rows (back and biceps), followed by a short rest. Repeat three times.

Why should I do them?
Focusing on different muscle groups provides a more balanced workout in less time and allows you to lift heavier weights during each set, promoting greater muscle gains.

Peripheral heart action (PHA) supersets

What are they?
A superset of two exercises, one of which works a muscle group in the upper body and the other one in the lower body, done without any rest in between.

Such as?
A set of bench presses (upper body) then lunges (lower body).

Why should I do them?
Alternating between working muscles in opposite ends of your body forces your heart to work really hard to pump blood into the target muscles. This makes the workout more intensive to build muscle and burn fat at the same time.

> **"Supersets improve your muscles' ability to work harder with less rest"**

Pre-exhaustion supersets

What are they?
Two exercises performed back to back that target the same muscle group. The first move is an isolation exercise, the second is a compound lift.

Such as?
Leg extensions followed by squats.

Why should I do them?
Fatiguing the muscle with an isolation exercise before exhausting it with a compound move is a highly effective way to break down the most amount of muscle tissue. However, performing a heavy compound lift when tired makes this set strategy more dangerous than most, so always use a spotter.

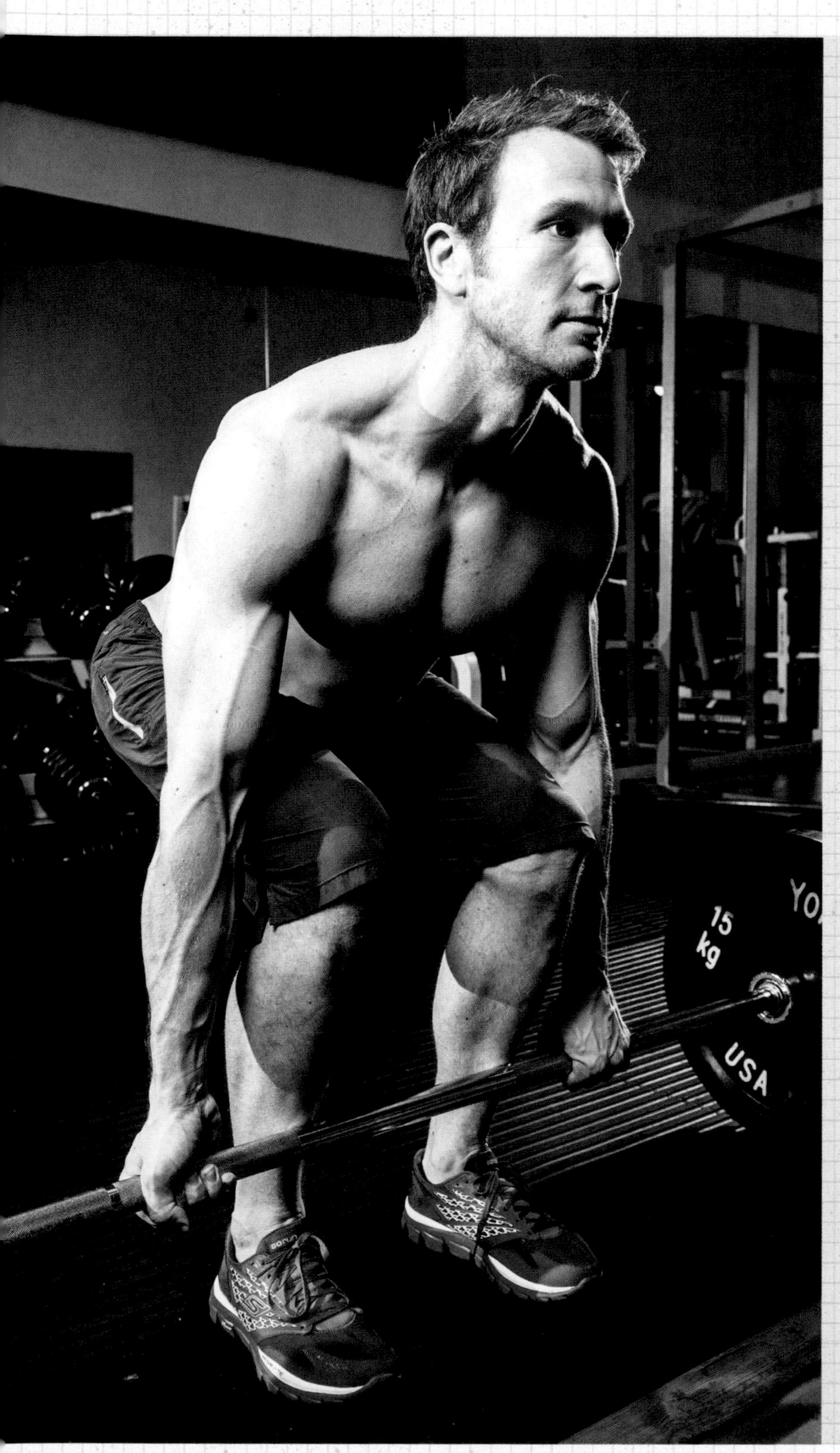

Post-exhaustion supersets

What are they?
Reversing the pre-exhaustion tactic, in this version you perform two exercises back to back that target the same muscle group. The first move is an compound lift, the second is an isolation exercise.
Such as?
Chin-ups followed by EZ-bar biceps curls.
Why should I do them?
Performing the compound move first when you are fresh means you can fatigue your muscles, plus the supporting ones, before really blitzing the target muscle with an isolation move. This is a safer strategy than pre-exhaustion and is as effective for building muscle.

Staggered supersets

What are they?
These are like straight sets, but you use the rest periods between them to work on a hard-to-grow muscle group that requires additional training, such as your calves or biceps.
Such as?
After completing a set of chin-ups, deadlifts or squats, use your rest period to do a set of dumbbell biceps curls, calf raises or triceps press-downs, then return to your main exercises without resting.
Why should I do them?
Smaller muscle groups require greater stimulation for growth, and using staggered sets means you can work them even on days when not training them exclusively.

Session strategies

Here are the three most common approaches to designing a training session to suit your needs

Split body training

Working different body parts on different days can reap big rewards

Split training, or body part training, involves working specific muscle groups in one session, then focusing on another group of muscles in the next workout.

This approach allows you to exhaust certain muscles fully one day, then giving them several days to recover before training them again, during which time you can train other muscle groups.

A typical split routine may look like this:

Day one	Chest and back
Day two	Legs
Day three	Rest day
Day four	Arms and shoulders
Day five	Rest day

Then you start again at day one. Each muscle group is typically worked twice per week, with around 48 to 72 hours between these sessions to allow sufficient time for recovery.

Split training is an advanced approach because it allows you to lift heavy weights on a frequent basis, making it one of the best approaches for adding muscle mass quickly and efficiently.

However, this strategy relies on having a structured training programme so you can successfully increase the weights you are lifting to ensure muscle growth. And while missing the odd session isn't a problem, failure to stick to the body-part routine can result in you resting for too long between training the same muscle groups, which will stall your progress. Lifting heavy can also result in more muscle soreness, so adequate recovery time is essential for success.

At a glance: Split body training

Advantages

- Great way to add serious muscle mass
- Effective approach requiring as few as three workouts each week
- Allows you to focus on hard-to-grow muscle groups

Disadvantages

- Requires a structured, progressive training programme to be effective
- The use of heavy weights may require a spotter
- Doesn't have much transfer value to sports because it doesn't require the body to work as a unit

Total-body training

Working your whole body every session will add muscle and torch fat

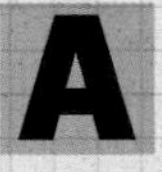

A total body routine involves training every major muscle group each time you hit the gym.

So you'd perform one body-part specific move for a certain number of sets and reps before moving on to another body part.

A typical workout might look like this:

1. **Bench press** (chest and triceps)
2. **Bent-over row** (upper back and biceps)
3. **Squat** (legs)
4. **Good morning** (lower back)
5. **Shoulder press** (shoulders and triceps)
6. **Plank** (abs and core)

Alternatively, you could superset antagonistic muscle groups for an even faster and more taxing workout.

Using compound lifts promotes muscle gain and burn fat through an increase in the release of testosterone and other growth hormones. Apart from that, this approach is also great for working your heart and lungs as you move quickly between exercises that target different muscles and for keeping your body guessing as to what it can expect next.

However, it is vital that no muscle groups are neglected during this approach, especially those moves that you don't like. Failing to work the whole body to the same extent can increase your odds of injury and developing muscular imbalances.

At a glance: Total-body training

Advantages

- Intensive approach that builds muscle and burns fat
- A session based around compound lifts boosts the release of testosterone and growth hormones
- Sessions can be performed quickly to minimise time spent training
- Can provide a good aerobic workout

Disadvantages

- Working the whole body in one session makes it difficult to really fatigue every muscle group
- Does not always target minor muscle groups effectively
- Every session can start to feel the same, leading to boredom and a lack of motivation

Circuit training

If you're struggling to find the time to squeeze your sessions into an already busy schedule, then circuit training could be the answer

If you have a membership to a big gym chain then you've probably seen circuit training classes advertised in the foyer.

This type of session is popular because it allows people to work their whole body in a short space of time.

That's because circuit training is a variety of different moves or stations – anywhere between six and 12 exercises – performed back to back without rest. After all the stations have been completed you rest for up to three minutes before repeating the circuit again, typically doing three or four full circuits in one session.

The quick pace and constant switching between exercises and equipment shocks your body and tackles all your major muscle groups, meaning you can get an effective full-body workout in as little as 45 minutes.

The intensive nature of this session means that you won't be lifting heavy weights – some stations may only be bodyweight moves – so circuits are better suited for building muscular endurance, burning fat and a decent aerobic workout than adding serious muscle mass.

Many gym chains run circuit classes in studios, but you can create your own circuit wherever you train using resistance machines, free weights and bodyweight moves, or a combination of all three.

At a glance: Circuit training

Advantages

- Works the whole body in a short amount of time
- Provides a good aerobic workout, builds muscular endurance and burns fat
- Can be done anywhere, anytime, using bodyweight exercises
- Has a great transfer value to sports performance

Disadvantages

- Not ideal for building muscle mass because of the light weights involved
- Can require a lot of equipment and working in with other people if performed in a gym
- You need to be highly motivated to work consistently without stopping for rest

Pyramid sets and drop sets

Pyramid sets

Increase the weight, but lower the reps, and watch your muscles grow

Pyramid sets

What are they?

A series of sets of the same exercises in which you increase the weight after each set but reduce the number of reps.

Such as?

To take the deadlift as an example: 15 reps of 60kg, ten reps of 70kg, eight reps of 80kg, four to six reps of 90kg. You can then work back down again.

Why should I do them?

For larger muscle groups, doing pyramid sets is a great way to add mass and strength because your muscles must work harder as the sets progress. This keeps them guessing and puts them out of the comfort zone, resulting in bigger gains.

PYRAMID TIP

Proper form is critical in pyramid sets to avoid injury, especially as the weight increases. Make sure you are comfortable with each phase of a move and with the entirety of the move before attempting heavy lifts.

Drop sets

Working past failure by dropping the weight will fatigue your muscles fast

Drop sets

What are they?

A series of sets of the same exercise in which you start with a heavy weight and lift until fatigued, then reduce the weight and do a new set to fatigue, pausing to rest between sets.

Such as?

Starting a biceps curl workout with 25kg dumbbells, working to failure, then immediately grabbing the 20kg weights and continuing, repeating this sequence until you can't do a single rep, even with a really light dumbbell.

Why should I do them?

To work the target muscle to complete fatigue and damage as many muscle fibres as possible so that they grow back faster. Keep the weight drops small between sets and your final set should be with a weight about 20% of the start weight. These sets really tax the muscles, so leave a good few days between sessions to allow for sufficient recovery.

> **"Doing pyramid sets keeps your muscles guessing, resulting in bigger gains"**

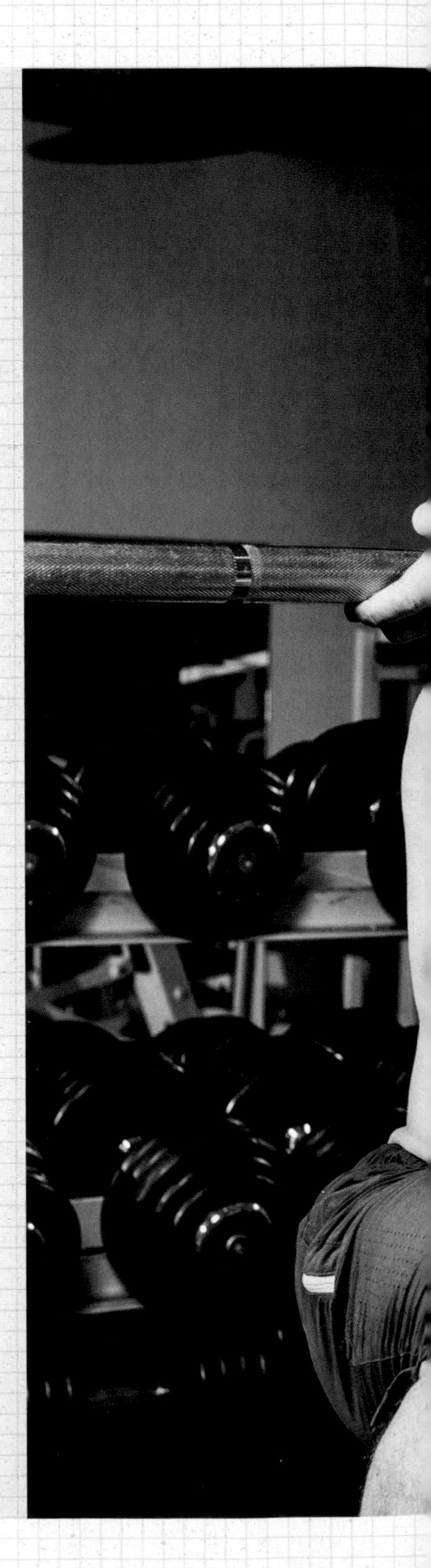

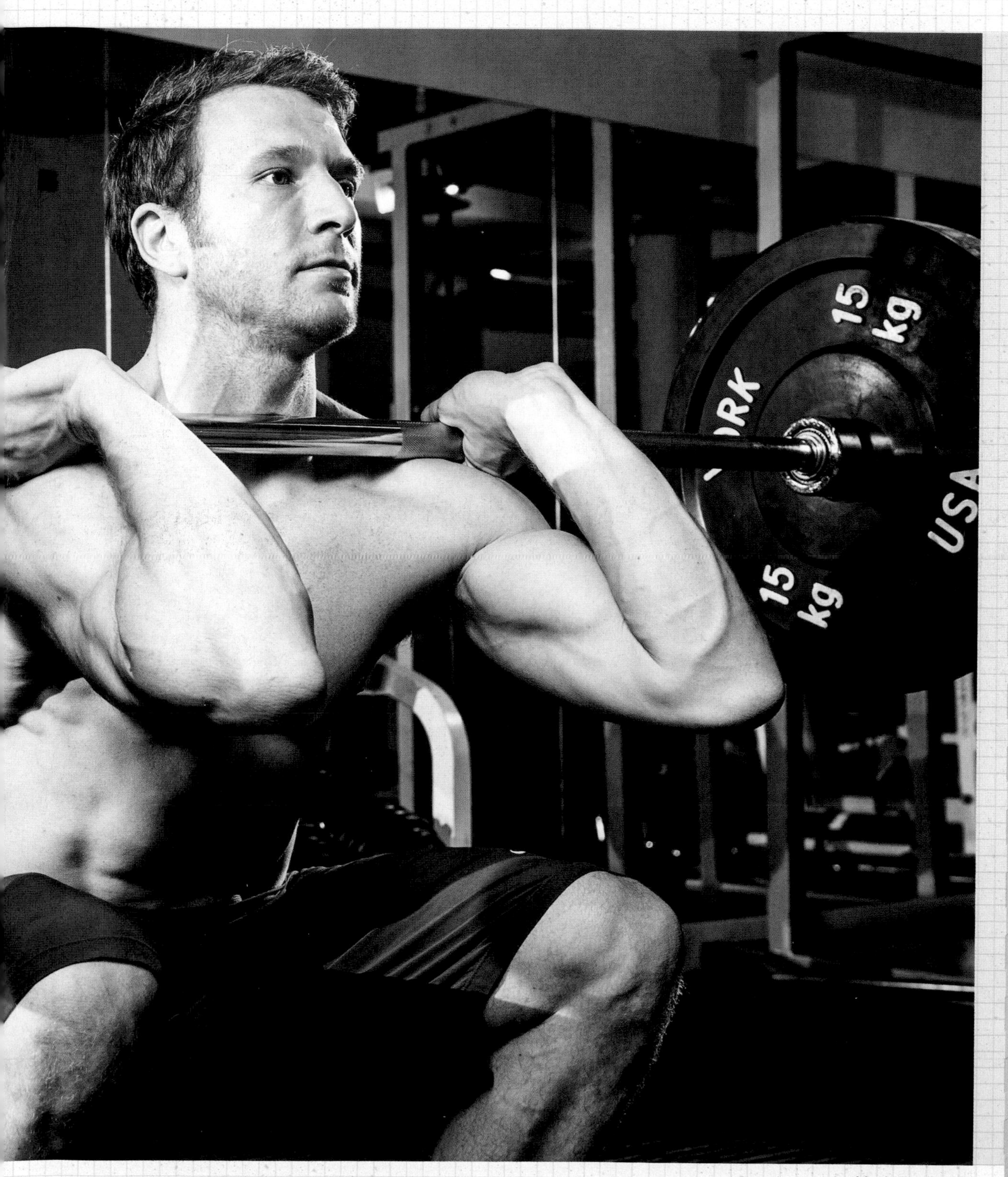
15
kg
USA
15
kg

Index

KEY
Abs
Arms
Back
Chest
Shoulders
Legs
Total body

A

Alternating box jumps ... 125
Alternating dumbbell shoulder press... 142
Alternating raise ... 145
Alternating wide dumbbell shoulder press ... 142
American kettlebell swing ... 167
Aquaman ... 93
Arnold press ... 141
Assisted triceps dip ... 65

B

Ballistic bench press ... 99
Barbell biceps curl ... 54
Barbell lunge ... 118
Barbell rollout ... 48
Barbell shrug ... 88
Bastard burpee ... 161
Bench leg raise ... 42
Bench press ... 98
Bent-over flye ... 81
Bent-over row ... 80
Bicycle ... 33
Bodyweight lunge ... 113
Bodyweight squat ... 112
Box jumps ... 125
Bulgarian split squat ... 122
Burpee ... 160

C

Cable crossover ... 105
Cable crunch ... 27
Cable EZ-bar triceps press-down ... 73
Cable flye ... 105
Cable kickback ... 75
Cable lateral raise ... 145
Cable pull-over ... 109
Cable rope curl ... 61
Cable triceps press-down ... 72
Chin-up ... 62
Clap press-up ... 107
Clean ... 158
Clean and jerk ... 159
Close-grip bench press ... 66
Close-grip lat pull-down ... 83
Concentration curl ... 57
Crossover crunch ... 32
Crunch ... 26

D

Deadlift ... 156
Decline alternating dumbbell press.. 103
Decline back extension ... 95
Decline bench press ... 102
Decline close-grip bench press ... 67
Decline dumbbell press ... 103
Decline plank ... 39
Decline plank with alternate foot touch ... 39
Decline press-up ... 101
Deficit deadlift ... 157
Diamond press-up ... 67
Dorsal raise with shoulder rotation ... 93
Dumbbell bench press ... 99
Dumbbell bent-over row ... 81
Dumbbell biceps curl ... 55
Dumbbell crunch ... 27
Dumbbell Cuban press ... 151
Dumbbell floor press ... 107
Dumbbell flye ... 104
Dumbbell kickback with lift ... 75
Dumbbell lunge ... 119
Dumbbell lunge to press ... 165
Dumbbell overhead triceps extension ... 71
Dumbbell pull-over ... 108
Dumbbell pull-over press ... 109
Dumbbell shoulder press ... 140
Dumbbell shrug ... 89
Dumbbell side bend ... 31
Dumbbell side step-up ... 125
Dumbbell squat ... 115
Dumbbell squat to curl to press ... 165
Dumbbell step-up ... 124
Dumbbell triceps kickback ... 74
Dumbbell upright row ... 149

E

Elevated front foot split squat ... 119
External cable rotation ... 153
External dumbbell rotation ... 153
EZ-bar biceps curl ... 55
EZ-bar preacher curl ... 58
EZ-bar upright row ... 149

F

Face pull ... 87
Front raise ... 145
Front squat ... 116

G

Garhammer raise ... 37
Glute bridge ... 133
Good morning ... 90
Gym ball back extension ... 95
Gym ball dumbbell Bulgarian split squat ... 123
Gym ball Bulgarian split squat with twist ... 123
Gym ball crunch ... 27
Gym ball dumbbell pull-over ... 109
Gym ball glute bridge ... 133
Gym ball hamstring curl ... 133
Gym ball jackknife ... 45
Gym ball oblique crunch ... 31
Gym ball one-arm overhead triceps extension ... 71
Gym ball passing jackknife ... 45
Gym ball rollout ... 49
Gym ball Russian twist ... 47
Gym ball side plank ... 41
Gym ball twist crunch ... 33

H

Hammer curl ... 60
Hang clean ... 159
Hanging knee raise ... 34
Hanging leg raise ... 35
High cable reverse flye ... 147
High pull ... 148
High-cable woodchop ... 51
Hip raise ... 43

I

Incline alternating dumbbell press ... 101
Incline back extension ... 94
Incline bench press ... 100
Incline dumbbell press ... 101
Incline Cuban press ... 151
Incline dumbbell flye ... 105
Incline plank ... 39
Incline press-up ... 103
Incline reverse bench shrug ... 149
Incline reverse lateral raise ... 146
Internal cable rotation ... 152
Internal dumbbell rotation ... 153
Inverted row ... 87
Inverted shoulder press ... 139
Isometric leg raise ... 37

J

Jackknife ... 44
Jump lunge ... 113
Jump squat ... 113

K

Kettlebell clean ... 168
Kettlebell clean and press ... 169
Kettlebell figure of eight ... 171
Kettlebell goblet squat ... 128
Kettlebell halo ... 171
Kettlebell hand switch ... 167
Kettlebell pistol squat ... 129
Kettlebell rack squat ... 129
Kettlebell slingshot ... 170
Kettlebell snatch ... 169
Kettlebell windmill ... 171

L

Lat pull-down ... 82
Lateral lunge ... 120
Lateral lunge and touch ... 121
Lateral raise ... 144
Leg extension ... 131
Leg press ... 130
Low-cable woodchop ... 51
Low-to-high cable raise ... 147
Lower-body Russian twist ... 47
Lying EZ-bar triceps extension ... 68
Lying hamstring curl ... 132
Lying reverse lateral raise ... 147
Lying triceps extension and pull-over ... 69

M

Medicine ball sledgehammer ... 91
Medicine ball close-grip press-up ... 67
Medicine ball knee raise ... 35
Medicine ball leg raise ... 43
Medicine ball leg raise and hold ... 43
Medicine ball reverse crunch ... 29
Modified V-sit ... 45
Mountain climber ... 49

N

Narrow-stance leg press ... 131
Negative chin-up ... 63
Negative pull-up ... 79
Negative triceps dip ... 65
Neutral chin-up ... 63
Neutral shoulder press ... 141

O

Oblique crunch ... 30
Offset press-up ... 107
One-arm cable cross crunch ... 33
One-arm cable row ... 85
One-arm dumbbell clean ... 162
One-arm dumbbell clean and press ... 163
One-arm dumbbell row ... 84
One-arm dumbbell snatch ... 163
One-arm dumbbell swing ... 163
One-arm lat pull-down ... 83
One-arm medicine ball slam ... 31
One-arm preacher curl ... 59
One-arm reverse flye ... 85
One-arm triceps extension ... 70
One-arm triceps press-down ... 73
One-hand kettlebell swing ... 167
One-leg good morning ... 91
One-leg kettlebell deadlift ... 129
One-leg squat ... 115
Overhead squat ... 117

P

Pistol squat ... 115
Plank ... 38
Press-up ... 99
Pull-up ... 78
Pull-up burpee ... 161
Push press ... 164

R

Rack pull ... 157
Reverse crunch ... 28
Reverse lunge ... 121
Reverse-grip bent-over row ... 81
Reverse-grip biceps curl ... 55
Reverse-grip lying triceps extension ... 69
Reverse-grip preacher curl ... 59
Romanian deadlift ... 126

S

Seated behind-the-neck press ... 139
Seated cable row ... 86
Seated calf raise ... 135
Seated dumbbell curl ... 56
Seated dumbbell shoulder press ... 141
Seated EZ-bar overhead triceps extension ... 71
Seated hammer curl ... 57
Seated incline dumbbell curl ... 57
Seated reverse crunch ... 29
Seated Russian twist ... 46
Seated shoulder press ... 139
Shoulder press ... 138
Side plank ... 40
Side plank with lateral raise ... 41
Side-plank star ... 41
Single-arm dumbbell press ... 143
Snatch ... 159
Snatch pull ... 89
Snatch-grip deadlift ... 157
Snatch-grip shrug ... 89
Spider curl ... 59
Split dumbbell Romanian deadlift ... 127
Split good morning ... 91
Split squat ... 119
Split squat to one-arm row ... 85
Squat ... 114
Standing barbell rollout ... 49
Standing cable overhead triceps extension ... 73
Standing cable Russian twist ... 47
Standing calf raise ... 134
Standing dumbbell calf raise ... 135
Standing EZ-bar triceps extension ... 69
Stiff-leg Romanian deadlift ... 127
Sumo squat ... 117
Superman raise ... 93
Supine gym ball calf raise ... 135

T

T press-up ... 106
Toes to bar ... 36
Transverse lunge ... 121
Triceps dip ... 64
Tuck and crunch ... 29
Tuck-jump burpee ... 161
Turkish get-up ... 172
Twisting knee raise ... 35
Two-arm kickback ... 75
Two-hand anyhow ... 173
Two-hand kettlebell swing ... 166
Two-point box ... 92

U

Underhand lat pull-down ... 83

W

Weighted back extension ... 95
Weighted chin-up ... 63
Weighted pull-up ... 79
Weighted triceps dip ... 65
Wide-grip cable row ... 87
Wide-grip pull-up ... 79
Wide-stance leg press ... 131
Windscreen wiper ... 37
Woodchop ... 50
Woodchop lunge ... 51

Z

Zottman curl ... 61